HEALTH SERVICE GOVERNANCE HANDBOOK

Claire Lea

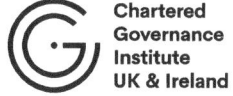

First published 2015

Published by
CGI Publishing Limited
Saffron House, 6–10 Kirby Street
London EC1N 8TS

© CGI Publishing Limited, 2019

All rights reserved. No part of this publication may be reproduced, stored in a retrieval system, or transmitted, in any form, or by any means, electronic, mechanical, photocopying, recording or otherwise, without prior permission, in writing, from the publisher.

The right of Claire Lea to be identified as author of this Work has been asserted by her in accordance with sections 77 and 78 of the Copyright, Designs and Patents Act 1988.

Typeset by Paul Barrett Book Production, Cambridge
Edited by Sheida Heidari
Cover designed by Anthony Kearney

British Cataloguing in Publication Data
A catalogue record for this book is available from the British Library.

ISBN 978-1-86072-771-9

As with all legislation, the provisions of the Companies Acts and related legislation are open to interpretation and must be assessed in the context of the particular circumstances at hand, the articles of association of the company in question, and any relevant shareholders' agreement or other pertinent ancillary agreements. While every effort has been made to ensure the accuracy of the content of this book, neither the author nor the publisher can accept any responsibility for any loss arising to anyone relying on the information contained herein.

Contents

Dedication	ix
Preface	x
Endorsements	xii
About the author	xiii
Acronyms and abbreviations	xiv

1 DEFINITIONS AND ISSUES IN GOVERNANCE — 1

Introduction	1
Defining governance	1
Principles of good corporate governance	6
Key issues in governance	9
A brief history of corporate governance	13
Governance in the public and voluntary sectors	19
Arguments for and against governance regimes	26
Summary	27

2 THEORETICAL FRAMEWORKS — 29

Introduction	29
Agency theory	29
Stakeholder theory	33
Stewardship theory	37
Transaction cost theory	39
Generative governance theory	42
Summary	43

3 DEFINITIONS AND ISSUES IN HEALTH SERVICE GOVERNANCE — 45

Introduction	45
Defining health service governance	45
Why does health service governance matter?	46
Common themes in poor governance	49
The NHS Constitution	49
The Five Year Forward View and the 2018 funding settlement	53
Summary	58

4 THE STRUCTURE OF THE NHS — 60

Introduction	60
The NHS	60
The Statement of Accountability	61

Providing care	64
Commissioning care	66
Improving public health	71
Empowering people and local communities	73
Supporting the healthcare system	77
Education and training	80
Safeguarding patients' interests	81
Summary	84

5 HEALTH SERVICE GOVERNANCE AND THE LAW — 86

Introduction	86
Governance and the law	86
Company law and other legislation	109
Summary	110

6 VOLUNTARY CODES OF BEST PRACTICE — 112

Introduction	112
Compulsory regulation and voluntary best practice	112
Codes for health service governance	116
Other corporate codes	126
Summary	129

7 THE BOARD'S STRUCTURE AND ITS COMMITTEES — 130

Introduction	130
Company purpose	130
Board structures	134
Matters reserved for the board	138
Size and composition of the board	139
Board committees	142
Governance checklist	149
Summary	150

8 DIRECTORS' DUTIES AND LIABILITIES — 151

Introduction	151
Who can be a director?	151
NHS directors	152
The powers of directors	154
The duties of directors to their organisation	154
The common law duties of directors	155
The statutory duties of directors	157
Other statutory duties	162
Liability of directors	164
NHS Code of Conduct and Accountability	167
Conflicts of Interest	168
Governance checklist	176
Summary	177

9 MAINTAINING AN EFFECTIVE BOARD — 178

Introduction — 178
The board and culture — 179
Culture and constructive challenge — 181
Constructive challenge and effective decision making — 185
Effective decision making and stakeholder engagement — 187
Other factors affecting board effectiveness — 187
Appointments to the board — 189
Nomination committee — 195
Succession planning and refreshing board membership — 197
Induction and training of directors — 199
Performance evaluation of the board, its committees and individual directors — 201
Governance checklist — 206
Summary — 206

10 THE CHAIR OF THE BOARD — 208

Introduction — 208
The role of the chair — 208
Separating the role of chair and chief executive officer — 216
The chair and the company secretary — 218
The chair and the senior independent director — 219
The chair and the stakeholders — 221
Governance checklist — 222
Summary — 222

11 EXECUTIVE DIRECTORS — 224

Introduction — 224
The role of executive directors — 224
The appointment of executive directors — 225
The role of the CEO — 227
The role of the director of finance or chief finance officer — 230
Other executive director roles — 231
The remuneration of executive directors — 232
Why is remuneration a governance issue? — 238
Principles of executive director remuneration — 239
The remuneration committee — 242
Severance payments — 244
Disclosure of directors' remuneration details — 247
Governance checklist — 248
Summary — 249

12 NON-EXECUTIVE DIRECTORS — 250

Introduction — 250
The appointment, induction and evaluation of non-executive directors — 251
Independence of non-executive directors — 256

The effectiveness of non-executive directors	259
Barriers to effectiveness	261
Non-executive director remuneration	263
Resignation	265
Governance checklist	265
Summary	266

13 THE COMPANY SECRETARY — 267

Introduction	267
The skills and knowledge required to be a company secretary	268
The company secretary as an officer of the company	269
The responsibilities of the company secretary	271
Additional duties of the company secretary	275
The conscience of the company	275
The company secretary and the in-house lawyer	277
The development of company secretaries in the NHS	278
Fit for the future	285
Governance checklist	286
Summary	286

14 NHS FOUNDATION TRUSTS — 288

Introduction	288
The history of foundation trust status	289
The legal and regulatory framework for FTs	290
Foundation trust membership	293
Foundation trust council structure and its committees	295
Duties, rights and powers of the council of governors	300
Foundation trust board structure and its committees	305
Maintaining an effective foundation trust board	309
The foundation trust governance challenge	311
Governance checklist	313
Summary	314

15 CLINICAL COMMISSIONING GROUPS — 315

Introduction	315
The history of CCGs	316
The legal and regulatory framework for CCGs	318
CCG membership	321
CCG governing body and its committees	324
Duties, rights and powers of the CCG and its governing body	331
Maintaining an effective governing body	331
The CCG governance challenge	336
Governance checklist	342
Summary	342

16 NEW MODELS OF CARE 344

Introduction 344
Five Year Forward View 345
Integrated Care 346
Models of care 347
Corporate forms 349
Contractual forms 353
Regulation of new models of care 355
Governance implications 356
A way forward 359
Governance checklist 363
Summary 363

17 RISK MANAGEMENT 365

Introduction 365
The regulatory framework for risk management and internal control 366
The nature of risk 368
Types of risks 371
Responsibilities for risk management and internal control 374
Risk management systems and procedures 376
Internal control systems and procedures 379
Reviewing the effectiveness of risk management and internal control 383
Emergency preparedness and business continuity 383
High reliability organisations 386
Governance Checklist 388
Summary 389

18 ASSURANCE 391

Introduction 391
Regulatory reporting 392
Failure regimes/special measures 397
Quality governance 402
Financial reporting 406
The corporate governance statement 412
The annual governance statement 413
The board assurance framework 414
Governance checklist 417
Summary 417

19 AUDIT 419

Introduction 419
The role of internal audit 419
The role of external audit 422
Independence of external audit 426

The audit committee	431
Raising concerns procedure	439
Governance checklist	442
Summary	443
Glossary	444
Index	455

Dedication

For Tim, Jack and Daniel

"Will you come with me to the mountains? It will hurt at first, until your feet are hardened. Reality is harsh to the feet of shadows. But will you come?"

The Great Divorce, CS Lewis

Preface

This is the third edition of the *Health Service Governance Handbook*, which has been compiled to update the HSG Handbook originally written in 2015. It will come as no surprise to NHS governance practitioners that yet again there is plenty of new material and debate in the governance arena within the NHS. However, on this occasion there is also a considerable amount of new material from the corporate sector with the introduction of the new UK Corporate Governance Code and the FRC Guidance on Board Effectiveness.

The aim of the Handbook is to provide a comprehensive guide for governance practitioners within the NHS with governance checklists to support in the delivery of best practice

These are interesting times within health service governance with work arounds being frequently considered in order to counter the inflexibility of the Health and Social Care Act 2012 when the drive from the government and NHS England is to innovate and collaborate in a way which the Act never envisaged. Despite this, the basic tenets of best practice in governance remain the same– namely, ensuring that the appropriate checks and balances continue to be rigorous and adaptive, so those who have been entrusted with high levels of decision-making powers do so in the best interests of patients and the general public.

The wider corporate debates that result from scandals created by poor governance both at home and abroad along with the uncertainty created by the decision to exit the European Union have led to a greater focus on the board's role in leading on culture, values and behaviour. This only seeks to reinforce the fact that governance is never just about processes but is also about people.

I can only hope that NHS boards and governing bodies capture this zeitgeist and as leaders of healthcare organisations lead by example, so that not only does the public benefit from improved health outcomes but also staff are developed and encouraged in their caring vocation.

And whilst I will never receive an OSCAR, I can't complete this preface without thanking the many people who enable this work to be completed.

The ICSA is the chartered membership and qualifying body for people working in governance, risk and compliance, including company secretaries. With over 120 years' experience of the skills, knowledge and experience required for governance professionals, the ICSA is the home of good governance! Thank you for continuing to foster the development of governance within the NHS.

NHS Providers, who have continued to work with me to ensure that this handbook is as accurate as it can be at the time of publication.

My colleagues, both NHS and otherwise, who keep me on my toes and whose tenacity and resilience in what is often a misunderstood and under-appreciated role always inspires me to keep going in the updating of the Handbook.

My family and friends, who have walked the dog when I didn't have time and supplied an endless supply of coffee and encouragement – thank you!

Claire Lea
Director, Charis Consultants Limited
April 2019

Endorsements

Dr John Bullivant FCQI, Chair

Good Governance Institute

NHS Providers

About the author

Claire has over 15 years of NHS experience, during which she has worked across a wide number of NHS providers including mental health, acute and community services. She is a qualified Chartered Secretary with the Institute of Chartered Secretaries and Administrators (ICSA) and has a degree in Law (LLB-Lancaster). Her experience includes being the company secretary at Heart of England NHS Foundation Trust, which she joined after having advised on the merger with Good Hope Hospital NHS Trust and serving as a non-executive director at George Eliot Hospital NHS Trust, in the role of Chair of Audit, Chair of Quality and the non-executive lead for freedom to speak up. Prior to that, she was a company secretary in the pensions and merchant banking sector.

As a freelance governance specialist, Claire now works with a wide number of trusts, particularly those under intense governance scrutiny by the regulators. Claire is currently the Examiner for the Health Service Governance module for the Institute of Chartered Secretaries. She is an Associate of NHS Providers developing and delivering Governwell, the national training programme for FT governors. She delivers bespoke training events for governors and boards of aspirant and foundation trusts.

She is particularly interested in how the behaviour and culture of boards and their organisations influence the effectiveness of their governance arrangements.

Acronyms and abbreviations

5YFV	Five-year Forward View
A&E	Accident & Emergency
ACC	Acute Care Collaboration
ACN	Accountable Clinical Network
ACO	accountable care organisation
ACP	accountable care partnership
ACS	Accountable Care System
AfC	Agenda for Change
AGM	annual general meeting
AGS	annual governance statement
AHA	area health authority
ALB	arm's-length body
AO	accounting officer/accountable officer
BAF	board assurance framework
CA 2006	Companies Act 2006
CA 2014	Care Act 2014
CCA 2004	Civil Contingencies Act 2004
CCG	clinical commissioning group
CCG ARM	Clinical Commissioning Group Annual Reporting Manual
CCG IAF	CCG Improvement and Assessment Framework
CEO	chief executive officer
CFO	chief financial officer
CFSMS	Counter Fraud and Security Management Service
CHAI	Commission for Healthcare Audit and Inspection
CHI	Commission for Health Improvement
CHRE	Council for Healthcare Regulatory Excellence
CIMA	Chartered Institute of Management Accountants
CIP	cost improvement plan
CIPFA	Chartered Institute of Public Finance and Accountancy
CJV	corporate joint venture
CMA	Competition and Markets Authority
COO	chief operating officer
COSO	Committee of Sponsoring Organizations of the Treadway Commission (US)
CPPIH	Commission for Patient and Public Involvement in Health
CQC	Care Quality Commission
CSR	corporate social responsibility

ACRONYMS AND ABBREVIATIONS

CSU	commissioning support unit
DBS	Disclosure and Barring Scheme
DHSC	Department of Health and Social Care
DoF	director of finance
DoLS	Deprivation of Liberties Safeguards
DPA 1998	Data Protection Act 1998
ED	executive director
EHCH	enhanced health in care homes
ENDPB	executive non-departmental public body
ERRA 2013	Enterprise and Regulatory Reform Act 2013
EU	European Union
FOIA 2000	Freedom of Information Act 2000
FRC	Financial Reporting Council
FRC Audit Guide	FRC Guidance on Audit Committees
FRC Board Guide	FRC Guidance on Board Effectiveness (2018)
FRC Risk Guide	FRC Guidance on Risk Management, Internal Control and Related Financial and Business Reporting
FReM	Financial Reporting Manual
FT	foundation trust
FT ARM	Foundation Trust Annual Reporting Manual
FT Code	NHS Foundation Trust Code of Governance
FTSU	Freedom To Speak Up
GAM	Group Accounting Manual (Department of Health)
GDPR 2016	EU General Data Protection Regulation 2016
GGI	Good Governance Institute
GMC	General Medical Council
GP	general practitioner
HEE	Health Education England
HFEA	Human Fertilisation and Embryology Authority
HFMA	Healthcare Financial Management Association
HoIA	Head of Internal Audit
HOSC	Health Overview and Scrutiny Committee
HPA	Health Protection Agency
HR	human resources
HRA	Health Research Authority
HRA 1998	Human Rights Act 1998
HRO	high reliability organisation
HSCA 2012	Health and Social Care Act 2012
HWB	health and wellbeing board
IAF	Improvement and Assessment Framework
ICO	Information Commissioner's Office

ICS	Integrated Care System
IMCA	Independent Mental Advocate Service (IMCA)
IT	information technology
JHWS	Joint Health and Wellbeing Strategy
JSNA	Joint Strategic Needs Assessment
KLOE	key line of enquiry
KPI	key performance indicator
LGA	Local Government Association
LINk	Local Involvement Network
LLA	liability limitation agreement
LLP	limited liability partnership
MCA 2005	Mental Capacity Act 2005
MCP	Multispeciality Community Provider
MP	Member of Parliament
NAO	National Audit Office
NAPF	National Association of Pension Funds
NDPB	non-departmental public body
NED	non-executive director
NHS	National Health Service
NHS Act 2006	National Health Service Act 2006
NHS TDA	NHS Trust Development Authority
NHSBTA	National Health Service Blood Transfusion Authority
NHSE	NHS England
NHSI	NHS Improvement
NHSLA	NHS Litigation Authority
NICE	National Institute for Health and Clinical Excellence
NMC	Nursing and Midwifery Council
NPSA	National Patient Safety Agency
NYSE	New York Stock Exchange
OECD	Organization for Economic Co-operation and Development
OSC	overview and scrutiny committee
PACS	Primary and Acute Care System
PHE	Public Health England
PHSO	Parliamentary and Health Service Ombudsman
PIDA 1998	Public Interest Disclosure Act 1998
PPI	Patient and Public Involvement
SI	Statutory Instrument
SID	senior independent director
Solace	Society of Local Authority Chief Executives
SoS	Secretary of State for Health and Social Care

SPAMSOAP	Segregation of duties; Physical controls; Authorisation and approval; Management controls; Supervision; Organisation; Arithmetical and accounting controls; Personnel
STF	Sustainability and Transformation Fund
STP	Sustainability and Transformation Partnership
The Good Governance Standard	The Good Governance Standard for Public Services
TSA	Trust Special Administrator
UECN	Urgent and Emergency Care Network
UK	United Kingdom
UK Code	UK Corporate Governance Code (Financial Reporting Council) (2018)
VFM	value for money
VSM	very senior management

1
Definitions and issues in governance

Introduction

Chapter 1 sets out definitions of governance on which the handbook then relies for the rest of the text. It explores the difference between governance and management and begins to set out the core principles significant for reliable and resilient governance. The chapter explains the history of corporate governance within the UK before considering the central codes and guidance for good practice in the National Health Service (NHS).

Defining governance

'Governance' refers to the way in which something is governed and to the function of governing. However, the term is so commonly used that it is often hard to define exactly what it means and its objectives. The governance of a country, for example, refers to the powers and actions of the legislative assembly, the executive government and the judiciary.

Governance is not an easy concept to understand. In the case of governing a country, it would be concerned with who has the power to rule and what the governors of the country should be trying to achieve. The government of a democratic country sets itself the objective of protecting its people and acting in their best interests, whatever these might be. Powers are shared between the legislative, executive and judiciary, but it is a matter of debate regarding how these powers should be shared and exercised. In the UK, for example, there is healthy political debate about the respective powers of Parliament, the Prime Minister and the Cabinet, the UK law courts, and currently the powers of the government bodies and courts of the European Union (EU). In the case of governing an organisation, NHS or otherwise, governance would be concerned with how powers are shared and exercised by the directors, and how the holders of power in the organisation should be held accountable for what they do.

For the purposes of this handbook, specific definitions have been used to offer clarity about what is being mentioned. These definitions may be used interchangeably in practice but adhering to them within the handbook will enable the reader to distinguish between different landscapes in which governance needs to be understood. The defined meanings are as follows.

- **Governance:** the concepts of governance that are generally applicable regardless of landscape.
- **Corporate governance:** the governance applicable to the corporate commercial business world, including public and private companies.
- **Health service governance:** the governance applicable to NHS organisations.
- **Public sector governance:** the governance applicable across the wider public sector including the NHS.

Health service governance operates on two levels:

1. the manner in which the government department (Department of Health and Social Care (DHSC)) is held to account by the electorate for the way in which it manages the provision of healthcare; and
2. the way in which individual parts of the NHS are governed and to what purpose.

Membership and the balance of power

Companies and NHS organisations alike are legal entities or 'legal persons' established according to statutory obligations such as the Companies Act or Health and Social Care Act legislation. As legal persons, they can enter into contracts and make business transactions. They can own assets and owe money to others, and they can sue and be sued in law. However, decisions about what the company or organisation should do are taken by individuals in the company in the organisation's name. There is a gap, therefore, between the legal entity and its owners (members). This gap is 'bridged' by the individuals who act on the entity's behalf. Governance is the foundation of that 'bridge'.

- The citizens of a country, even in a democracy, have relatively few powers. Power is in the hands of the legislative (Parliament) and the executive (the government). Similarly, shareholders have limited powers, and these are restricted mainly to certain voting rights. Power is in the hands of the board of directors, or perhaps just one or two individual directors on the board.
- Just as a country has citizens, a company has members. The members of a company are its owners, the 'equity' shareholders. The membership of large companies changes constantly, as investors buy and sell the company's shares.
- For large companies, the main issue with corporate governance is the relationship between the board of directors and the shareholders, and the way in which the board exercises its powers. The relationship between the shareholders and the board can be described as a 'principal–agent' relationship. In some companies, other stakeholders may have significant influence.
- For NHS organisations, the members are a wide and diverse range of stakeholders. Health service governance is concerned with how powers are shared and exercised by different groups to ensure that the objectives of health provision for the general public are met with the political direction being given by the DHSC, and other interest groups such as employees, suppliers and the local community being balanced and managed.

In health service governance, the idea of membership is more complex because of the range and diversity of stakeholders. Whilst an FT will have a clear membership structure, the members are not, strictly speaking, the owners of the trust. Instead, they are the recipients of the health services provided, who might be seen as 'proxy shareholders' on behalf of the general public. Further complications arise as the FT is still required to consider the views of the community it serves, regardless of whether they are members and is also required to consider the views of its other stakeholders such as employees, trade unions, local authorities, clinical commissioning groups (CCGs) and NHS England (NHSE).

CCGs also have a membership structure, comprising all of the general practices in their constituency. Even so, CCGs are also required to consider the wider views of its other stakeholders, including those organisations, which provide the services they commission. For other parts of the NHS structure (e.g. NHS trusts, Commissioning Support Units (CSUs), Accountable Care Organisations (ACOs)) there is no established membership structure but there is an equivalent variety of stakeholders. It is this variety of stakeholders and the different levels of influence that they are able to exercise within the NHS that makes health service governance an interesting and challenging subject.

The study of governance within the NHS is complicated by the overuse of the term 'governance'. The role of the governance practitioner or NHS company secretary is also made more complex (and potentially more interesting) on account of the term 'governance' being used so widely. In the NHS, there is quality governance, information governance, data governance, board governance – to name just a few.

At times, this handbook will refer to these other areas of governance to ensure that the breadth of the role of the NHS governance practitioner or company secretary is fully considered. Such references will specifically highlight the type of governance that is being referred to (e.g. quality governance).

The interests of stakeholders

Health service governance as set out by this handbook is defined as the process, practices and procedures by which power is shared and exercised by the board of directors (and the council of governors in foundation trusts (FTs) or the governing body in a CCG), and how the holders of power in the organisation should be held accountable for what they do.

Guidelines and constraints in both the public and private sector include behaving in an ethical way and in compliance with laws and regulations. This framework of law, regulation and guidance puts in place boundaries for those who exercise this power and authority to run the organisation on behalf of stakeholders. These are the groups with an interest in how an organisation acts; they include the communities in which the organisation operates, customers, the DHSC, employees, the general public, patients, sector regulators and suppliers. The aim of health service governance should be to monitor and control management to ensure that it runs the organisation in the interests of these stakeholders.

Health service governance can therefore be defined as a process for monitoring and control to ensure that management runs the organisation in the interests of stakeholders. The numerous stakeholders and the variety of their roles will be explored in Chapter 2.

Corporate comparisons

Companies in the private sector – which are mostly governed in accordance with the interests of the shareholders – provide a useful comparison with healthcare organisations. Primarily, the objective of a company in the private sector is maximising the wealth of its owners (the shareholders) subject to various guidelines and constraints. However, it can be argued that they should also be governed in the interests of all its major stakeholders, not just its owners. This argument is particularly relevant to large companies whose activities have a big impact on the economy and society, where regard must be given to other groups or individuals with an interest in what the company does.

Principles of corporate governance are therefore based on the view that a company should primarily be governed in the interests of the shareholders, and only in the interests of other stakeholder groups as a secondary consideration. The board ought to use its powers in an appropriate and responsible way and should be accountable to the shareholders.

The work of Lord Hutton and the Ownership Commission, set out in its March 2012 Report on Plurality, Stewardship and Engagement, raises interesting questions about the responsibilities of companies to consider the interests of a wider group of stakeholders. This was developed further in the Purposeful Report in February 2017, which explored the growing consensus that 'there is a public interest in securing a more meaningful change in how our wealth creation system is organised'.

The relationship between the board of directors and its variety of stakeholders, and the way in which the board exercises its powers, has been a significant distinction between corporate governance and health service governance. This distinction, however, is lessening as corporate commercial organisations are being challenged to consider a wider group of stakeholders. For example, the latest update to the UK Corporate Governance Code (UK Code) and the associated Financial Reporting Council's guide to Board Effectiveness (July 2017) (FRC Board Guide) sets out that boards must look to engage with their workforce through one, or a combination, of a director appointed from the workforce, a formal workforce advisory panel and a designated non-executive director, or other arrangements that meet the circumstances of the company and the workforce. ICSA: The Governance Institute (ICSA) and the Investment Association published *The Stakeholder Voice in Board Decision Making* in September 2017; this offers guidance on the appointment and role of directors appointed to represent the views of the workforce as well as wider guidance on stakeholder engagement.

Health service governance principles are based on the view that the organisation should be governed in such a way that balances the requirements of a wide variety of stakeholders. The board is required to use its powers in an appropriate and responsible way and is accountable in different ways to each of the stakeholders.

Why is governance important?

Regardless of sector, governance is a key issue as it regulates the power and decision-making of a small group of people who have been given a large responsibility for the stewardship of the assets of a third party.

In the context of the NHS, this stewardship involves both public assets and healthcare services. The outcome of decisions really can be a matter of life and death, as well as a matter of severe financial loss. As a result, NHS organisations have clear aims that have been set out in the NHS Constitution. They should be governed in such a way that they move towards the achievement of these aims.

Although NHS organisations and companies exist as legal persons, in reality each organisation is the organised, collective effort of many different individuals. They are controlled by boards of directors or governing bodies in the interests of their stakeholders. The interests of the board and the stakeholders ought to coincide, but in practice, they may be in conflict with each other. The challenge of good health service governance is to find a way in which the interests of a wide variety of stakeholders and the directors can all be sufficiently satisfied. This is also a challenge for companies, but the major concern rests largely on balancing the interests of the board of directors and the shareholders.

Governance and management

It is important to recognise the difference between the governance of any organisation and its management.

Powers to manage the affairs of an NHS organisation are given to the board of directors or to the governing body in the case of a CCG. The term 'board' or 'board of directors' will be used for both, with the distinguishing aspects of the governance of a CCG highlighted (see Chapter 15 for more on CCGs).

Most powers are delegated to a chief executive officer (CEO) or managing director, and further delegated to executive directors (EDs) and executive managers. The board of directors should retain some powers and responsibilities, with certain matters reserved for board decision making rather than delegated to the management team (see Chapter 9).

The board of directors should be responsible for monitoring the performance of the management team. However, the board of directors itself is not responsible for day-to-day management. It is responsible for governing the organisation. Responsibilities for governance go beyond management, and governance should not be confused with management. Even so, it is probably true to say that when a senior executive manager is 'promoted' to the board, they may consider the position of an ED to be recognition of their senior executive position. However, the promotion of an executive manager to the board creates new responsibilities for governance that are not related to management. The ED ought to think as a member of the board in performing their duties as a director, rather than as a senior executive.

This structure – where there is an effective single board that is collectively responsible for controlling the organisation or company, with no one individual having unfettered powers of decision making – is known as the **unitary board**. When an ED becomes a board member, they take on part of the collective responsibility for ensuring the achievement of corporate aims and objectives and must not solely contribute to discussions and decisions in the light of their particular executive function.

It is important to note that CCGs have not been established on the basis of a unitary board. Instead, the Good Governance Standard for Public Services (2004), upon which CCG governance is based, presupposes a form of leadership that is not based on the principle of a unitary board. This is in stark contrast to most other NHS organisations (e.g. FTs) for whom the unitary board is a core principle of governance.

The purpose of the unitary board principle is to ensure that the interests of all stakeholders are properly considered and balanced. This is explored in more detail in Chapter 7.

Principles of good corporate governance

Several concepts apply to sound corporate governance in all countries where international investors invest their money. Many of these are ethical in nature and the King III Code describes them as the 'overarching corporate governance principles'. These are:

- fairness
- accountability
- responsibility
- transparency.

King IV has now also been published and builds on the ethics of King III – see Chapter 2. These principles are directly applicable to an understanding of health service governance and are set out here with examples from both corporate and health service governance.

Fairness

Fairness refers to the principle that all shareholders should receive equal consideration. For example, minority shareholders should be treated in the same way as majority shareholders. This concept might seem straightforward in the UK, where the rights of minority shareholders are protected to a large extent by company law. In some countries, however, larger shareholders and the board of directors often disregard minority shareholder rights. There should also be fairness in the treatment of stakeholders other than shareholders.

The NHS Constitution sets out a number of rights and pledges that underpin the principle of fairness such as:

- the right to access
- the right to drugs
- the right to complain
- staff rights.

Accountability

Decision-makers who act on behalf of an organisation should be accountable for the decisions they make and the actions they take. In a company, the board of directors should be accountable to the shareholders (the company's owners). Shareholders should be able to assess the actions of the board of directors and the committees of the board and have the opportunity to query and challenge them. In an NHS organisation, a variety of stakeholders provides that level of accountability.

One problem with accountability is deciding how the board of directors should be accountable, and in particular over what period of time. According to the financial theory for companies, if the objective of a company is to maximise the wealth of its shareholders, this will be achieved by maximising the financial returns to shareholders through increases in profits, dividends, prospects for profit growth and an increasing share price. It might therefore follow that directors should be held accountable to shareholders on the basis of the returns on shareholder capital that the company has achieved. However, there is little consensus about the period over which returns to shareholders and increases in share value should be measured. Performance can be measured over a short term of one year, over a longer period of five or ten years, or even longer.

In practice, it is usual to measure returns over the short term and assess performance in terms of profitability over a 12-month period. In the short term, however, a company's share price may be affected by influences unrelated to the company's underlying performance, such as excessive optimism or pessimism in the stock markets. In the short term, it is also easier to soothe investors with promises for the future, even though current performance is not good. It is only when a company fails consistently to deliver on its promises that investor confidence ebbs away.

If company performance were to be solely judged by the return to shareholders over a 12-month period, the directors would focus on short-term results and short-term movements in the stock market price. Short-termism is easy to criticise, but difficult to disregard in practice if performance targets ignore the long term. Directors should really be looking after the underlying business of the company and its profitability over the longer term.

The problem of accountability remains, however. Even if it is accepted that company performance should not be judged by short-term financial results and share price movements, how can the board be made accountable for its contribution to longer-term success?

By way of contrast, accountability for an NHS organisation can be measured in a number of ways. These include:

- regulators: Care Quality Commission (CQC), NHS Improvement (NHSI);
- commissioners: NHS England (NHSE), CCGs, general practitioners (GPs);
- political scrutiny: DHSC, overview and scrutiny committees, Health and Wellbeing boards, Healthwatch; and
- public opinion: Friends and Family Test, patient surveys, Patient Choice agenda, national staff surveys.

Short-termism is also an issue for NHS organisations, as changes in government policy often drives the form of accountability practiced by the regulators, commissioners and political scrutiny. The views expressed by public opinion can also focus on very local issues that need to be balanced against wider healthcare changes for the public benefit.

The NHS Constitution sets out that the NHS is accountable to the public, communities and patients that it serves. The government ensures that there is always a clear and up-to-date statement of NHS accountability for this purpose (see Chapter 3).

Responsibility

The board of directors is given authority to act on behalf of the company. A further principle of corporate governance is that the board should accept full responsibility for the powers that it is given and the authority that it exercises. A board of directors should understand what its responsibilities are and should carry them out to the best of its abilities.

Accountability goes hand-in-hand with responsibility. The board of directors should be made accountable to the shareholders for the way in which it has carried out its responsibilities. Similarly, executive management should be responsible for the exercise of powers delegated to them by the board of directors and should be made accountable to the board for their achievements and performance. Within the NHS, there are a number of mechanisms for delegating responsibility, such as the scheme of delegation and standing financial instructions. The role of the board committees is to oversee and scrutinise these delegated powers, and to provide assurance to the board that responsibility is being taken appropriately by the EDs.

Transparency

Transparency means openness. In the context of corporate governance, this is a willingness by the company to provide clear information to shareholders and other stakeholders about what the company has done and hopes to achieve, without giving away commercially sensitive information. It might be useful to think of openness in terms of its opposite – being a 'closed book' and refusing to divulge any information whatsoever.

Transparency should not be confused with 'understandability'. Information should be communicated in a way that is understandable, but transparency is concerned more with the content of the information that is communicated. A principle of good governance is that stakeholders should be informed about what an organisation is doing and plans to do in the future, and about the risks involved in its business strategies.

Transparency in NHS organisations is set out by the requirements of the Freedom of Information Act 2000 (FOIA 2000) and the requirements of openness set out in the Seven Principles of Public Life (also known as the Nolan Principles). The NHS Constitution also requires that the system of responsibility and accountability for making decisions in the NHS should be transparent and clear to the public, patients and staff. The development of a 'duty of candour' is the most recent development in the NHS; this underpins the principle of transparency (see Chapter 5).

Key issues in governance

Good governance should promote the best long-term interests of the organisation. It requires an effective board of directors, with an appropriate balance of skills and experience, and well-motivated individuals as directors. The composition of the board, its functions and responsibilities, and its effectiveness, are therefore core issues in governance.

At the heart of the debate about corporate governance lie conflicts of interest (and potential conflicts of interest) between shareholders, the board of directors as a whole, individual board members, and possibly also a number of other stakeholder groups. Directors may be tempted to take risks and make decisions aimed at boosting short-term performance. Many shareholders are more concerned with long-term performance, the continuing survival of their company and the value of their investment. If a company gets into financial difficulties, professional managers can move on to another company to start again, whereas shareholders suffer a financial loss.

Similar conflicts of interest arise in health service governance, such as pressure to conceal financial or performance information, inadequate risk management processes and poor communication with key stakeholders. For example, one stakeholder group may have a particular focus on an area of service delivery while directors have to manage the wider provision of healthcare services. Directors often have to manage the competing interests of patient groups, regulators, and the financial decisions contained within government policy. Directors also have to consider their own careers within the NHS, managing the performance requirements of the regulators and any consideration of a longer-term strategy for the particular body for which they are responsible.

Transparent reporting and auditing

The board of directors or EDs could try to disguise the true performance of the organisation by giving less than honest statements or 'dressing up' publicly available information on performance, quality, safety and finances. 'Window-dressed' information makes it difficult for stakeholders to reach a reasoned judgement about the performance of an organisation, and subsequently assess whether public funding is being correctly managed and expended on key areas of service delivery. Concerns about misleading published accounts in the corporate commercial world in the 1980s and early 1990s provided an impetus to the movement for better corporate governance in the UK. Accounting irregularities in a number of companies led to a tightening of accounting standards, although the problems of window dressing are unlikely ever to disappear completely. Concerns about financial reporting in the US emerged with the collapse of Enron in 2001, which filed for bankruptcy after 'adjusting' its accounts. This was followed by similar problems at other US companies, including telecommunications group WorldCom (which admitted to fraud in its accounting), Global Crossing and Rank Xerox. It was also suggested that incomprehensible or misleading accounts contributed to the global banking crisis, with banks such as Lehman Brothers (which collapsed in 2008) possibly using questionable accounting practices to disguise the true state of their financial position.

Throughout the peak of the banking crisis of 2007–09, when Britain's financial system looked at its most vulnerable, the Co-operative Bank portrayed itself as a cut above the rest, offering ethical values untouched by the bonus culture for EDs and the high levels of debt that infected so many other banks. Yet in 2013, the Co-operative Group hit the headlines when its governance shortfalls became public, leading to significant losses resulting from a capital shortfall and controversy about its former chair Paul Flowers.

More recently, the collapse of BHS into administration in 2016, leaving 11,000 employees facing an uncertain future and 20,000 current and future pensioners facing substantial cuts to their entitlements, has raised significant concerns. According to the Work and Pensions Select Committee, BHS encapsulated many of its ongoing concerns about the regulatory and cultural framework in which business operates, including:

- the ethics of business behaviour;
- the governance of private companies;
- the balance between risk and reward;
- mergers and acquisitions practices;
- the governance and regulation of workplace pension schemes; and
- the sustainability of defined benefit pensions.

The governance issues at stake in these examples are the balancing of short- and long-term returns and the extent to which the directors in each case were aware of these situations, and if they knew about the problems why shareholders were not informed much sooner. It is now widely accepted that the directors of a company should be responsible for giving an assurance to their shareholders that they consider their company to be a going concern that will not collapse within the next 12 months.

Transparent reporting and auditing is vital for NHS organisations and it is subject to a high level of scrutiny. It must be remembered that the financial position of an NHS organisation is closely linked to its performance targets and its level of activity. While there is some guidance on how targets should be measured so correct financial data can be collated, the pressure to reach performance targets can lead to irregularities in the measurement of target data.

Exercise of board-level power

Most decision making powers in an organisation are held by the board of directors. The governance debate continues to be about the extent to which professional managers, acting as board directors, exercise those powers in the interests of their principal stakeholders (and any other organisational stakeholders), and whether the powers of directors should be restricted.

Key issues include:

- the structure of the board of directors;
- the role of independent non-executive directors (NEDs);
- the responsibilities of the board of directors; and
- the duties of directors.

Risk management

In the corporate world, investors typically expect higher rewards to compensate them for taking higher business risks. If a company makes decisions that increase the scale of the risks it faces, profits and dividends are usually expected to increase. A further issue in corporate governance is that the directors might take decisions intended to increase profits without giving due regard to the risks. In some cases, companies may continue to operate without regard to the changing risk profile of their existing businesses. When investors buy shares in a company, they have an idea of the type of company they are buying into, the nature of its business, the probable returns it will provide for shareholders and the nature of its business and financial risks. Directors, on the other hand, are rewarded on the basis of the returns the company achieves – profits or dividend growth – and their remuneration is not linked in any direct way to the risk aspects of their business. Some companies are also guilty of poor procedures and systems, so that the risk of breakdowns, errors and fraud can be high.

Good governance therefore requires an organisation to control its 'business risk' by having effective internal controls for managing operational risks. As a result, risk management is now recognised as a key ingredient of sound corporate governance.

Risk management is just as crucial in health service governance. Not only does it set out to protect public assets and the use of taxpayers' money, it also protects the quality of the healthcare services being delivered. Risk management is explored in more detail in Chapter 17.

Stakeholder engagement

Another issue in corporate governance is communication between the board of directors and the company's shareholders. Shareholders, particularly those with a large financial interest in a company, should be able to voice their concerns to the directors and expect to have their opinions heard. Small shareholders should at least be informed about the company, its financial position and its plans for the future – even if their opinions carry comparatively little weight.

In health service governance it is an explicit aspect of government policy that stakeholders are to be involved in the design and delivery of their own healthcare. Therefore, it is vital that NHS organisations provide public information about their services and future plans. Providing opportunities for the views and opinions of stakeholders to be heard is a key driver within health service governance. Better-informed boards of directors will make better healthcare decisions. In addition, the increased focus on patient choice results from research in the UK and overseas identifying that treatments are more effective if patients choose, understand and control their own care. Patient choices now include the right to choose a GP, which hospital to go to and the right to be involved in decisions about their own healthcare.

This right to choose, combined with the introduction of 'internal market' or 'quasi-market' policies, has led to a greater degree of information about the performance of individual GPs, consultants and hospitals. This has introduced the commercial concepts of marketing and market share, and a much greater awareness of costs, efficiency and accountability.

Further, the introduction of the FOIA 2000 provided a clear procedure for all public bodies to respond to requests for information about their organisations. In addition, the requirements to make NHS annual accounts, reports from regulators (such as NHSI and the CQC), national NHS surveys (staff and patient surveys) and the introduction of Quality Accounts for all providers of healthcare services, all serve to ensure a greater transparency in the relationships with NHS stakeholders.

Corporate social responsibility and the NHS

Ethical conduct is a major governance issue. There is a growing recognition that organisations need to consider social and environmental issues for commercial and governance reasons, as well as purely ethical reasons. Stakeholders expect organisations to have regard to social and environmental issues, while the financial risks from government regulation to protect the environment continue to grow. A sustainable healthcare system is achieved by delivering high quality care and improved public health without exhausting natural resources or causing severe ecological damage.

In the NHS, sustainable development is often referred to as good corporate citizenship. This means using NHS organisations' corporate powers and resources in ways that benefit, rather than damage, the social, economic and physical environment. How the NHS itself behaves can impact on people's health and on the wellbeing of society, the economy and the environment. Behaving as a good corporate citizen can save money, benefit population health and can help reduce health inequalities. Many measures that improve health also contribute to sustainable development and vice versa.

Sustainability reporting is increasingly required within NHS organisations' annual reports and Quality Accounts.

A brief history of corporate governance

To understand best the principles of health service governance it is important to understand the developments in corporate governance over time. These developments now underpin much of what currently exists in health service governance.

What seems clear from each development is that processes and systems only go so far. References are repeatedly made to behaviour and culture as the foundation stones of good governance.

The Cadbury Code

The Report of the Committee on the Financial Aspects of Corporate Governance was published in 1992 and was described as 'a landmark in thinking on corporate governance'. The report included a Code of Best Practice known as the Cadbury Code.

Whilst the terms of reference for the Committee were primarily focused on financial governance, concerns about the principles and values behind good corporate governance also meant that its findings went further than just financial governance. The Code also made recommendations relating to the structure and effectiveness of boards, internal controls and accountability to shareholders. Sir Adrian Cadbury's statement, following the review, makes interesting reading for health service governance practitioners:

> 'Corporate governance is concerned with holding the balance between economic and social goals and between individual and communal goals. The governance framework is there to encourage the efficient use of resources and equally to require accountability for the stewardship of those resources. The aim is to align as nearly as possible the interests of individuals, corporations and society.'

The significant legacies of the Cadbury Code include a voluntary system of good practice with the principles of openness, integrity and accountability at its heart and self-regulation based on 'comply or explain'. This is explored in more detail in Chapter 6.

The Greenbury Report

On the recommendation of the Cadbury Committee, a second committee was set up to review progress on corporate governance in UK listed companies. This committee issued the Greenbury Report in 1995, which focused mainly on directors' remuneration. At the time, the UK press was condemning 'fat cat' directors, particularly those in newly privatised companies.

The Greenbury Report issued a Code of Best Practice covering directors' remuneration. Its major recommendations included the following:

- The remuneration committee should be made up of entirely NEDs.
- There should be an annual remuneration report for shareholders included within the annual report and accounts.
- Remuneration (and any other benefits) should be linked to performance (both by the company and the individual director).

The Combined Code

A further committee on corporate governance, chaired by Sir Ronald Hampel, was set up in 1995 to review the recommendations of the Cadbury and Greenbury Committees. Its final report was published in 1998. The report covered a number of governance issues, such as:

- the composition of the board and role of directors;
- directors' remuneration;
- the role of shareholders (particularly institutional shareholders);
- communications between the company and its shareholders; and
- financial reporting, auditing and internal controls.

The Hampel Report also suggested that its recommendations should be combined with those of the Cadbury and Greenbury Committees into a single code of corporate governance. This suggestion led to the publication of the original 1998 Combined Code on Corporate Governance (Combined Code), which applied to all UK listed companies. Interestingly, the Hampel Report makes it clear that:

> 'Good corporate governance is not just a matter of prescribing particular corporate structures and complying with a number of hard and fast rules. There is a need for broad principles. All concerned should then apply these flexibly and with common sense to the varying circumstances of individual companies.'

The Combined Code was updated in 2003 to take account of the Higgs and Smith reports (see below), as well as in 2006 and 2008. It became the UK Corporate

DEFINITIONS AND ISSUES IN GOVERNANCE

Governance Code in 2010. Within this version (2010) a section that was addressed specifically to institutional shareholders, and dealt with the responsibilities of institutional investors for good corporate governance. This has now been replaced by a separate UK Stewardship Code (see below).

The Turnbull Guidance

A committee was set up in 1998 to provide guidance on the board's responsibilities for internal control and risk management. This committee produced the Turnbull Report. This was revised and re-named Internal Control: Guidance to Directors by the FRC in 2005, then amalgamated with the 2009 Going Concern guidance notes into the FRC Guidance on Risk Management, Internal Control and Related Financial and Business Reporting in 2014 (FRC Risk Guide).

The Turnbull Report defined an internal control system as 'the policies, processes, tasks, behaviours and other aspects of an organisation' that, taken together, help it to:

- operate effectively and efficiently: these operational controls should allow the organisation to respond in an appropriate way to significant risks to achieving the organisation's objectives (this includes the safeguarding of assets from inappropriate use or from loss and fraud and ensuring that liabilities are identified and managed);
- ensure the quality of external and internal financial reporting (financial controls); and
- ensure compliance with applicable laws and regulations, and also with internal policies for the conduct of business (compliance controls).

The Higgs Report and Guidance on Board Effectiveness (July 2018)

Corporate governance issues remained in the spotlight in the UK in 2003, with two influential reports published in that year.

The Higgs Report, commissioned by the government, considered the role and effectiveness of the chair and independent NEDs. This was updated in 2010 following a review on behalf of the FRC by ICSA. Amended guidance was issued with the title *Improving Board Effectiveness*. In a similar vein to Cadbury and Hampel, Higgs was at pains to point out that people, behaviour and culture were the key to good governance, not a process of box-ticking exercises.

As a result of the update to the UK Code during 2018, the Higgs Report and the 2010 update have been superseded by the FRC Guide (2018). The primary purpose of the FRC Guide is to stimulate boards' thinking on how they can carry out their role and encourage them to focus on continually improving their effectiveness.

The Smith Report and the FRC Guidance on Audit Committees

Further work and more detailed guidance on the role of the audit committee were commissioned by the FRC in 2003. The ensuing report was originally called the

Smith Report (after the name of the committee chair) but is now called the FRC Guidance on Audit Committees (FRC Audit Guide). It was revised in 2005, 2008, 2012 and 2016.

To assist audit committees looking to put their external audit out to tender, the FRC provided Audit Tenders: Notes on Best Practice in February 2017 (FRC Audit Tender Guide).

The Walker Report

The global financial markets and world economy were badly damaged by the banking crisis that emerged in 2007 and 2008. In the US, Lehman Brothers collapsed and other banks and brokerage firms were taken over to prevent their collapse. In the UK, the Northern Rock bank collapsed in 2007 while Royal Bank of Scotland was virtually nationalised in 2008. At the same time, the government acquired a major stake in Lloyds TSB Bank after Lloyds had agreed to take over another ailing bank, HBOS.

Recognition of governance problems in UK banks led to a review by Sir David Walker. Some of the recommendations of the Walker Report were included by the FRC in the 2010 UK Corporate Governance Code.

The Davies Report

In 2010, Lord Davies of Abersoch initiated a review into boardroom diversity at the request of the UK Government, publishing a report entitled Women on Boards in 2011.

The review rejected the imposition of a mandatory quota system, instead recommending voluntary targets and reporting requirements. In May 2011, the FRC began consulting on possible amendments to the UK Code that would require companies to publish their policy on boardroom diversity, report against it annually and to consider the board's diversity when assessing its effectiveness (among other factors). These were added to the Code in 2012. Lord Davies issued an updated report in 2015, which detailed progress that had been made and set out five next-step recommendations. The key recommendation was increasing the voluntary target for women's representation on Boards of FTSE 350 companies, to a minimum of 33%, to be achieved by 2020.

NHSI has declared that it is committed to achieving the goal of 50/50 gender balance on all NHS boards by 2020.

The UK Stewardship Code

The UK Stewardship Code was published in 2010, reviewed in 2012 and will be reviewed again in late 2018. Whereas the UK Code is concerned with governance by companies, the Stewardship Code is for institutional investors that are share owners or that manage shareholdings for other financial institutions such as pension funds. The Stewardship Code aims to enhance the quality of engagement between institutional investors and companies, so that institutional shareholders contribute positively to the governance of the companies in which they invest.

In 2016, the FRC assessed signatories to the Stewardship Code based on the quality of their stewardship Code statements. Tiering distinguishes between signatories who report well and demonstrate their commitment to stewardship, and those where reporting improvements are necessary. The tiering exercise has improved the quality of reporting against the Stewardship Code, promoted best practice and resulted in greater transparency in the UK market.

The UK Corporate Governance Code

The FRC has reviewed and amended the Combined Code regularly, and in June 2010 issued a significantly revised version under the new name of the UK Corporate Governance Code.

In September 2011, the FRC announced that it intended to consult on proposed further changes to the Code in relation to audit committees and audit re-tendering. In October 2011, the FRC announced that changes resulting from the Davies Report would also be implemented in a revised version of the UK Code. This revised version was issued in 2012, which also took account of the findings of the Walker Report. A further update to the UK Code was carried out in September 2014, which included a number of significant changes on remuneration, going concern and risk management reporting and stakeholder engagement guidance. The 2016 update to the UK Code was required in order to comply with the new EU regulations on statutory audit. The revision was accompanied by updated guidance on audit committees, revised ethical standards and revised auditing standards. The impact of the guidance for audit committees will be assessed in Chapter 19.

During 2017, the FRC then announced a fundamental review and consultation in respect of the UK Code. This was required to take account of the FRC's work on corporate culture and succession planning (*FRC: Corporate Culture and the Role of Boards* (2016)). The report addressed how boards and executive management could steer corporate behaviour to create a culture that would deliver sustainable good performance. The report looked at the increasing importance that corporate culture held in delivering long-term business and economic success, and in doing so it focused on the role of the board in shaping, monitoring and overseeing culture.

The result of the FRC review and consultation led to the re-publication of the UK Code in July 2018. The UK Code (2018) broadens the definition of governance and emphasises the importance of:

- positive relationships between companies, shareholders and stakeholders;
- a clear purpose and strategy aligned with healthy corporate culture;
- high-quality board composition and a focus on diversity; and
- remuneration which is proportionate and supports long-term success.

The UK Code (2018) is designed to set higher standards of corporate governance to promote transparency and integrity in business with a view to benefitting the economy and wider society in the long term.

The full text of the UK Code (2018) is available in the appendices to this handbook.

FRC Guidance
The FRC issues guidance and other publications to assist boards and board committees in considering how to apply the UK Corporate Governance Code to their particular circumstances. FRC papers include:

- Guidance on Board Effectiveness (FRC Board Guide);
- Guidance on Risk Management, Internal Control and Related Financial and Business Reporting (FRC Risk Guide);
- Guidance on Audit Committees (FRC Audit Guide);
- Guidance on the Strategic Report;
- Corporate Culture and the Role of Boards; and
- the UK Stewardship Code – sets out good practice for institutional investors on engaging with the companies in which they invest.

This guidance is explored in greater detail in the following chapters.

Governance and UK law
The Companies Act 2006 (CA 2006) introduced statutory duties of directors (similar to the duties that existed previously in common law and equity) and contained a requirement for quoted companies to be more accountable to shareholders by publishing a strategic business review in narrative form each year. Under new regulations in 2013, the CA 2006 now requires the remuneration report to be split into three components:

- a statement from the chairman of the remuneration committee;
- a policy report; and
- an annual report on remuneration.

It also introduces a binding shareholder vote on the policy report and the content of the annual report on remuneration (which remains subject to an annual advisory vote) is substantially different from the previous requirements. It now includes the 'single figure' for each director and a number of other new requirements.

Some aspects of corporate governance have also been transposed into UK law from the EU Directives. Amendments to the Fourth and Seventh EU Company Law Directives approved in 2006 included a requirement for quoted companies to include a corporate governance statement in their annual reports. Amendments to the Eighth Company Law Directive in 2008 required 'public interest entities' (including listed companies) to have an audit committee consisting of independent NEDs and to publish an annual corporate governance statement. The new EU

Accounting Directive, effective from 1 January 2016, introduced a wide range of amendments to the CA 2006, particularly in relation to the small companies regime, such as revised accounting thresholds and reporting exemptions. It is likely that these directives will be fully incorporated into UK law following Brexit; however, this is still to be finalised in the Brexit negotiations.

Corporate governance in other countries

The UK is seen as a leading country in the development of a corporate governance framework, but there have been similar developments in many other countries. For many countries, particularly developing countries, good corporate governance is seen as an essential basic requirement for attracting foreign investment capital. In South Africa, the King Committee developed a code of corporate governance. This was revised and strengthened in 2002, 2009 and again in 2016 (King III and IV, see Chapter 2). On an international basis, recommended principles on corporate governance were published by the Organisation for Economic Co-operation and Development (OECD) in 1999, then updated in 2004. The latest revision was in 2015, when they sought to addresses challenges such as the increasing complexity of the investment chain, the changing role of stock exchanges and the emergence of new investors, investment strategies and trading practices.

Although the US appeared to show little concern for better corporate governance throughout the 1990s, the situation changed dramatically with the collapse of Enron and other major companies in 2001. The New York Stock Exchange (NYSE) proposed recommendations for change, and statutory provisions on corporate governance were introduced in 2002 with the Sarbanes-Oxley Act. However, the adequacy of corporate governance provisions in the USA (and the UK) continues to be questioned following the banking crisis in 2007–09 and subsequent examples of poor governance such as the Co-operative Bank, Tesco and BHS.

Governance in the public and voluntary sectors

The public sector includes central government, state government (in some countries) and local government, state-run health and education services and many other regulatory and advisory bodies. While many of the principles of good corporate governance can be applied to the governing bodies of the public sector, there are also significant differences. For example, public bodies are not profit-making and are not accountable to shareholders.

The public sector has therefore adapted principles of good governance to its own specific circumstances, and to some extent the definition of 'governance' for the public sector differs in some ways from 'governance' of companies.

In the UK, the Chartered Institute of Public Finance and Accountancy (CIPFA) and Solace (the Society of Local Authority Chief Executives) published a governance framework in 2016 aimed at local government bodies called *Delivering Good Governance in Local Government*. This sets out principles of governance that local government bodies are encouraged to adopt and apply to their own particular circumstances. The framework defines governance as:

> '[H]ow local government bodies ensure that they are doing the right things, in the right way, for the right people, in a timely, inclusive, open, honest and accountable manner. It comprises systems and processes, and cultures and values, by which local government bodies are directed and controlled and through which they account to, and engage with, and, where appropriate, lead their communities.'

Interestingly, given the demands in the NHS for joint or collaborative governance arrangements, the guidance states:

> 'The development of combined authorities and devolution deals, together with elected mayors, brings about the chance to design governance structures from the bottom up. It provides the opportunity to ensure that the core principles of good governance, covering openness and stakeholder engagement, defining outcomes, monitoring performance and demonstrating effective accountability, are integrated and embedded in new structures and that mechanisms for effective scrutiny are established.
>
> New responsibilities and the development of innovative collaborative structures and ways of working provide challenges for governance such as ensuring transparency and, in particular, over managing risk. Whether working with other authorities, public sector bodies, the third sector or private sector providers, councils must ensure all joint arrangements follow the principles of good governance and are managed and reviewed with sufficient rigour.'

Nolan's Principles of Public Life

A key development for the governance of the UK public sector was the Nolan Committee on Standards in Public Life. The Committee was set up in 1995 in response to concerns that the conduct of some politicians was unethical – in particular, allegations over MPs taking cash for putting questions to Parliament.

While the Committee focused on members of parliament (MPs), its terms of reference also covered government departments and non-departmental public bodies (NDPBs). The Nolan Principles were originally intended as guidelines for individuals who were involved in public affairs and public bodies, whether as paid employees or as non-paid members of governing bodies. They are now considered to have much wider relevance and have formed the basis in the UK for developing governance guidelines for both the public sector and the voluntary sector.

The Committee on Standards in Public Life undertook a review of best practice in promoting good behaviour in public life, and in January 2013 it published its *Fourteenth Report of the Committee on Standards in Public Life. Standards matter: A review of best practice in promoting good behaviour in public life.* The report amended the definitions of the seven Nolan Principles as shown in Table 1.1. Public sector boards and their members should adhere to these Seven Principles of Public Life.

Principle	Revised description
Selflessness	Holders of public office should act solely in terms of the public interest.
Integrity	Holders of public office must avoid placing themselves under any obligation to people or organisations that might try inappropriately to influence them in their work. They should not act or take decisions in order to gain financial or other material benefits for themselves, their family, or their friends. They must declare and resolve any interests and relationships.
Objectivity	Holders of public office must act and take decisions impartially, fairly and on merit, using the best evidence and without discrimination or bias.
Accountability	Holders of public office are accountable to the public for their decisions and actions and must submit themselves to the scrutiny necessary to ensure this.
Openness	Holders of public office should act and take decisions in an open and transparent manner. Information should not be withheld from the public unless there are clear and lawful reasons for so doing.
Honesty	Holders of public office should be truthful.
Leadership	Holders of public office should exhibit these principles in their own behaviour. They should actively promote and robustly support the principles and be willing to challenge poor behaviour wherever it occurs.

Table 1.1: The Seven Principles of Public Life

Interestingly, the Good Governance Institute in its 2016 version of the Integrated Governance Handbook also encourages the adoption of two additional principles used in Scotland in relation to respect and public service. In this case, holders of public office must respect fellow members of their public body and employees of the body and the role they play, treating them with courtesy at all times. They also have a duty to act in the interests of the public body of which they are a board member and to act in accordance with the core tasks of the body.

The Standards for NHS board members

In July 2011, the Council for Healthcare Regulatory Excellence was commissioned to advise the Secretary of State (SoS) for Health and Social Care on standards of personal behaviour, technical competence and business practices for members of NHS boards and CCG governing bodies in England. These standards were issued by the Professional Standards Authority in November 2012.

The standards include implementing a transparent and explicit approach to the declaration and handling of conflicts of interest, with good practice requiring the maintenance and publication of a register of interest for all board members. Board meeting agendas should include an opportunity to declare any conflicts at the start of the meeting.

There is a distinct similarity between the Nolan Principles and the NHS board standards, as seen in Table 1.2.

Principle	Standards for NHS board members
Selflessness	Responsibility
Integrity	Integrity
Objectivity	Respect
Accountability	Professionalism
Openness	Openness
Honesty	Honesty
Leadership	Leadership

Table 1.2: The Seven Principles of Public Life and Standards for NHS

The Good Governance Standard for Public Services (2004)

The Independent Commission for Good Governance in Public Service was established by the Office for Public Management and CIPFA in partnership with the Joseph Rowntree Foundation.

The role of the Commission was to develop a common code and set of principles for good governance across all public services in the UK. In 2004, it published the Good Governance Standard for Public Services (The Good Governance Standard), a guide for everyone concerned with governance in the public services that applies to all organisations that work for the public using public money. Its application therefore extends from public sector bodies to all private sector organisations that use public money to work for the public. NHS England has advocated adherence with this standard for health service governance in CCGs.

In justifying the need for the application of good governance principles and practice in the public service sector, the Commission has commented that good governance encourages public trust and participation, whereas bad governance fosters low morale and adversarial relationships.

The Good Governance Standard builds on Nolan's Principles and consists of six main principles, each with supporting principles, together with guidelines on how these might be applied in practice. It is useful to look at these and compare them with the principles that apply to good governance in the commercial sector. There are many similarities between these principles and those that should apply in corporate governance to companies (as described earlier in this chapter).

These are general principles, and individual public sector bodies can develop their own codes of governance that are consistent with and based on these principles. The six main principles and their supporting principles are as follows:

1. Focusing on the organisation's purpose and on its outcome for citizens and users of the organisation's services.
   - Being clear about the purpose of the organisation and its intended outcomes for citizens and service users. It is suggested that the concept of 'public value' may be useful in helping organisations to identify their purpose and intended outcomes.
   - Making sure that users receive a high-quality service.
   - Making sure that taxpayers receive value for money (VFM).
2. Performing effectively in clearly defined functions and roles.
   - Being clear about the functions of the organisation's governing body. It is recommended that the governing body should describe in a published document its approach to achieving each of its stated functions. This document can then be used as a basis for measuring actual performance and achievements by the governing body. Functions could include, for example, 'scrutinising the activities and performance of the executive management' and 'making sure that the voice of the public is heard in discussions and decision making'.
   - Being clear about the responsibilities of the non-executive and the executive governors; these will differ. Many governing bodies consist of both executive and non-executive members (who may be unpaid for their services). However, they should have equal status in discussions on policy and strategy. The framework recommends that the roles of CEO and chair of the governing body should not be held by the same individual.
   - Making sure that these responsibilities are properly carried out.
   - Being clear about the relationship between the governors and the public, so that both sides in this relationship know what to expect from the other.
3. Promoting values for the whole organisation and demonstrating good governance through behaviour.
   - Putting the values of the organisation into practice. The governing body should take the lead in doing this.
   - Individual governors behaving in ways that uphold and exemplify effective governance.

4. Taking informed and transparent decisions and managing risk.
   - Being rigorous and transparent about how decisions are taken by the governing body. There should be clearly defined levels of delegation within the organisation. The governing body should not be concerned with matters that are more properly delegated to management. It should also be clear about what the objectives of its own decisions are.
   - Using good quality information, advice and support.
   - Making sure that an effective risk management system is in operation.
5. Developing the capacity and capability of the governing body to be effective.
   - Making sure that governors have the skills, knowledge and experience to perform well.
   - Developing the capabilities of individuals with governance responsibilities.
   - Striking a balance in the membership of the governing body between continuity and renewal.
   - The creation and refreshing of a governing body is similar in many respects to similar guidelines in corporate governance, although in the public sector, some governors may be elected representatives.
6. Engaging stakeholders and making accountability real.
   - Understanding formal and informal accountability relationships.
   - Taking an active and planned approach to dialogue with and accountability to the public.
   - Taking an effective and planned approach to accountability to staff.
   - Engaging effectively with institutional stakeholders. Institutional stakeholders in the public sector are very different from institutional shareholders in the corporate world. In local government, for example, institutional stakeholders include bodies representing local people. Engagement with stakeholders should help to improve the accountability of the public sector body to the public.

Charity Governance Code (2018)

The development of codes and rules for corporate governance and public sector governance has also influenced the voluntary sector. For example, the National Council of Voluntary Organisations adapted Nolan's Seven Principles of Public Life into a code of conduct for charity trustees. In addition, the Charity Commission's Statement of Recommended Practice requires larger charities to include a statement on risks in their annual report.

There are an increasing number of examples of poor governance in the voluntary and charity sector. Examples include the collapse of Kids Company amid allegations of financial mismanagement; the suicide of Olive Cooke, a victim of aggressive charity fundraising mailings; and the controversy concerning Age UK's deal to help market an EON energy tariff to older people, for which it received £6 million in commission. These exposures have led to a decline in public confidence in charities and so charities and other bodies have tried to improve their standards of governance as a way of retaining public confidence in what they are doing;

Good Governance: A code for the voluntary and community sector (2nd edition) was published in October 2010. It was revised and renamed as the Charity Governance Code (July 2017). The new code sets out seven principles, as shown in Figure 1.1.

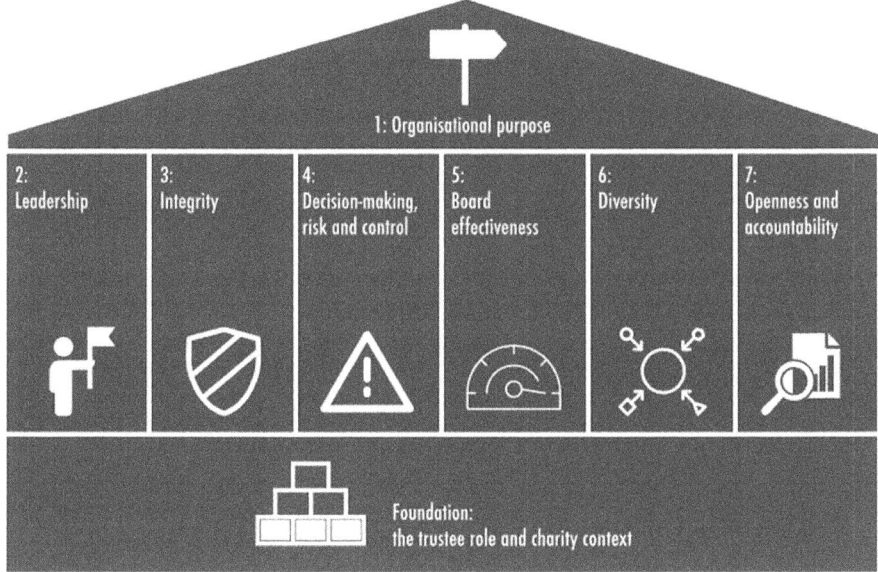

Figure 1.1: Seven principles of the Charity Governance Code

Its premise is that charity boards must be able to maintain a strategic focus, commit to board development and stay true to the organisation's charitable purposes. The code operates on an 'apply or explain' basis (see Chapter 6) and includes:

- an expectation that the board will review its own performance and that of individual trustees, including the chair, every year, with an external evaluation for larger organisations every three years
- that no trustee should serve more than nine years without good reason and that term limits are important for accountability
- boards to recruit a diverse range of trustees with the skills and experience required to lead a charity
- boards to involve stakeholders in key decisions and operating with the presumption of openness
- emphasis on the role of the chair and vice chair in supporting and achieving good governance

- increased oversight for large charities when dealing with subsidiary companies, registers of interests and third parties such as fundraising agencies or commercial ventures
- board evaluation of a charity's impact by measuring and assessing results, outputs and outcomes.

In addition, an independent regulator – the Fundraising Regulator – was established in 2016 following the Etherington review of fundraising self-regulation (2015), to strengthen the system of charity regulation and restore public trust in fundraising. Its role as regulator is to carry out the following tasks:

- Set and promote the standards for fundraising practice (the Code of Fundraising Practice and associated rulebooks) in consultation with the public, fundraising stakeholders and legislators.
- Investigate cases where fundraising practices have led to significant public concern.
- Adjudicate complaints from the public about fundraising practice, where these cannot be resolved by the charities themselves.
- Operate a fundraising preference service to enable individuals to manage their contact with charities.
- Where poor fundraising practice is judged to have taken place, recommend best practice guidance and take proportionate remedial action.

Arguments for and against governance regimes

There are different opinions about the benefits of governance, and whether these justify the costs of compliance with governance regulations. It is therefore useful to consider just what the benefits of good governance might be, and what the arguments are against having laws or codes of governance practice.

The main arguments in favour of having a strong governance regime are as follows:

- Good governance will eliminate the risk of misleading or false reporting and will prevent organisations from being dominated by CEOs or chairs.
- Stakeholders will be better protected by reducing the risks of scandals, and promoting fairness, accountability, responsibility and transparency in organisations.
- Organisations that comply with best practice in governance are more likely to achieve success. Good governance and good leadership and management often go hand-in-hand. Badly governed organisations may be very successful, and well-governed organisations may fail; however, the probability is greater that badly governed organisations will be less successful and more likely to fail than well-governed ones.
- Well-governed organisations will often develop a strong reputation and so will be less exposed to reputation risk (see Chapter 17) than organisations

that are not so well governed. Reputation risk can have an adverse impact on stakeholders such as employees, patients and suppliers.
- Good corporate governance encourages a longer-term view of success and enables longer-term planning.
- The main arguments against having a strong governance regime for organisations focus on costs, benefits and value.
- For many organisations, compliance with a code of governance is a box-ticking exercise as they adopt the required procedures and systems without considering what the potential benefits might be. The only requirement is to comply with the 'rules' and put a tick in a box when this is done. Governance requirements therefore create a time- and resource-consuming bureaucracy of governance practitioners and divert the attention of the board of directors from more important matters.
- Good governance is likely to reduce the risk of scandals and unexpected organisational failures. However, it could be argued that the current regulations or best practice guidelines are far too extensive and burdensome.
- When regulations and recommended practice become burdensome, there is an inevitable cost, in terms of both time and money, in achieving compliance. It could be argued that less regulation is better regulation. However, there has not yet been an authoritative assessment of the costs of governance compliance with the benefits of better governance systems.
- Organisations that are obliged to comply with governance regulations or best practice are at a competitive disadvantage to rival organisations from countries or regimes where governance regulation is weaker. This is one of the criticisms of widening the number of providers of healthcare beyond that of NHS organisations. If they are not subject to the same level of scrutiny and regulation, then the playing field is not level.
- The connection between good governance and good performance (due to good leadership and management) has not yet been proven or demonstrated.

Summary

- Decisions about what the company or organisation should do are taken by individuals in the company in the organisation's name. There is a gap, therefore, between the legal entity and its owners (members). This gap is 'bridged' by the individuals who act on the entity's behalf. Governance is the foundation of that 'bridge'.
- In health service governance, the idea of membership is more complex because of the range and diversity of stakeholders.
- For large companies, the main issue with corporate governance is the relationship between the board of directors and the shareholders, and the way in which the board exercises its powers.

- For NHS organisations, the members are a wide and diverse range of stakeholders. Health service governance is concerned with how powers are shared and exercised by different groups to ensure that the objectives of health provision for the general public are met with the political direction being given by the DHSC, and other interest groups such as employees, suppliers and the local community being balanced and managed.
- Much of the basis for health service governance results from guidance from outside of the NHS.
- To be a well-versed health service governance practitioner requires an understanding of history, law, specific technical knowledge, politics, health policy and a robust understanding of human behaviour.
- This diversity and complexity make for a fascinating area of work despite its connotations of checklists and tick-box exercises.
- It offers an intriguing insight into how an organisation can plan for its long-term success and then takes steps to deliver that success in a fast-paced changing external environment.
- This handbook aims to provide clarity around the scope of governance, and specifically health service governance and then to offer practical guidance on the practice of governance – enabling practitioners to 'walk the talk'.

2
Theoretical frameworks

Introduction

Chapter 2 steps back from the codes, guidance and legislation to look at the underlying fundamentals of governance and what makes 'good' governance. Over the years, governance professionals and researchers have set out to explore the theories that might underpin a robust system of corporate governance. This chapter explores a number of these theories, assesses their strengths and weakness. As each theory is explained and defined, then the approach to governance that the theory elicits will also be considered along with the applicability and relevance of these theories and approaches to health service governance.

There are a number of different theoretical frameworks to consider, including:

- agency theory;
- stakeholder theory;
- stewardship theory;
- transaction cost theory; and
- generative governance theory.

Agency theory

The most well-known framework of corporate governance come from Berle & Means (1932) who described the agency problem as one arising from the separation of ownership and control within an organisation. As early as 1776, Adam Smith raised the question when there was much discussion on how to align the interests of managers and owners. Adam Smith argued that the separation of ownership and control created poor incentives for managers to operate the firm efficiently. Consequently, corporate governance principles developed in order to address this problem.

Agency theory, therefore, is based on the separation of ownership and control in an organisation – namely, the ownership of an organisation by its shareholders and the control over the organisation's actions by its directors and senior executives. The agency relationship is a form of contract between an organisation's owners and its managers, where the owners (as principals) appoint an agent (the managers) to manage the organisation on their behalf. As part of this arrangement, the owners must delegate decision making authority to the management. This, however, gives rise to an inherent conflict of interest between the organisation's owners and managers.

- The owners (shareholders) want to increase their income and wealth over the long term. The value of their shares depends on the long-term financial prospects for the organisation. Shareholders are therefore not only concerned about short-term profits and dividends; they are even more concerned about long-term profitability.
- The managers run the organisation on behalf of the shareholders. They have an employment contract and earn a salary. If they do not own shares in the organisation, managers have no direct interest in future returns for shareholders or in the value of the shares. Unless they own shares, or unless their remuneration is linked to profits or share values, their main interests are likely to be the size of their remuneration package and their status within the organisation.

Ideally, the 'agency contract' between the owners and the managers of an organisation should ensure that the managers always act in the best interests of the owners. However, it is impossible to arrange the 'perfect' contract because any decisions managers make affect their personal welfare as well as the interests of the owners.

Agency conflicts are differences in the interests of owners and managers. They arise in several ways.

Moral hazard
This is where a manager has an interest in receiving benefits from their position in the organisation. These include all the benefits that come from status, such as a car, use of a plane, a house or flat, attendance at sponsored sporting events, and so on. A manager's incentive to obtain these benefits is higher when they have no shares, or only a few shares, in the organisation. For example, senior managers may pursue a strategy of growth through acquisitions, in order to gain more power and 'earn' higher remuneration, even though takeovers might not be in the best interests of the organisation and its shareholders.

Level of effort
This is where managers may work less hard than they would if they were the owners of the organisation. The effect of this lack of effort could be smaller profits and a lower share price.

Earnings retention
The remuneration of directors and senior managers is often related to the size of the organisation (measured by annual sales revenue and value of assets) rather than its profits. This gives managers an incentive to increase the size

of the organisation, rather than to increase the returns to the organisation's shareholders. Management are more likely to want to reinvest profits in order to expand the organisation, rather than pay out the profits as dividends. When this happens, organisations might invest in capital investment projects where the expected profitability is quite small or propose high-priced takeover bids for other organisations in order to build a bigger corporate empire.

Time horizon

Shareholders are concerned about the long-term financial prospects of their organisation, because the value of their shares depends on expectations for the long-term future. In contrast, managers might only be interested in the short term. This is partly because they might receive annual bonuses based on short-term performance, and partly because they might not expect to be with the organisation for more than a few years.

Agency costs are the costs of having an agent make decisions on behalf of a principal. In the context of corporate governance, agency costs are:

- the costs of monitoring the actions and performance of management to ensure that management is acting in their best interests;
- bonding costs that may be incurred in providing incentives to managers to act in the best interests of the shareholders (such as remuneration packages); and
- residual losses, or the cost to the shareholder which occurs when managers take decisions that are not in the best interests of the shareholders but are in the interests of the managers themselves (such as when managers pay too much for a large acquisition).

The key elements of agency theory

Agency theory is based on the view that the system of corporate governance should be designed to minimise the agency problem and reduce agency costs. One approach to reducing the agency problem is to make the board of directors more effective at monitoring the decisions of the executive management. Another approach is to design schemes of remuneration for directors and senior managers that bring their interests more into line with those of the shareholders.

Agents should also be accountable to their principals for their decisions and actions. Accountability means reporting back to the principals and giving an account of what has been achieved, and the principal having power to reward or punish an agent for good or bad performance. Greater accountability should reduce the agency problem, because it provides management with a greater incentive (obtaining rewards/avoiding punishments) to achieve performance levels that are in the best interests of the shareholders.

Agency theory may therefore be summarised as follows.

- In large companies, there is a separation of ownership from control. Professional managers are appointed to act as agents for the owners of the organisation.

- Individuals are driven by self-interest.
- Conflicts of self-interest arise between shareholders and managers.
- Managers, because they are driven by self-interest, cannot be relied on to act in the best interests of the shareholders. This creates problems in the agency relationship between shareholders and management.
- These agency problems create costs for the shareholders.
- The aim should be to minimise these costs, by improving the monitoring of management and/or providing management with incentives to bring their interests closer to those of the shareholders.

Shareholder value approach

The agency theory resulted in an approach to corporate governance that enabled the agency problem to be managed and minimised. This approach is known as the shareholder value or owner approach and is now the well-established approach to corporate governance, particularly within the UK and USA, supported by company law in advanced economies. The shareholder value approach requires a unitary board of directors (which includes independent NEDs) to govern their organisation in the best interests of its owners (the shareholders).

Under this approach, the main objective of an organisation should be to maximise the wealth of its shareholders in the form of share price growth and dividend payments, subject to conforming to the rules of society as embodied in laws and customs. The directors should be accountable to the shareholders, who should have the power to remove them from office if their performance is inadequate.

The OECD, in the introduction to its Principles of Corporate Governance, states that, from an organisation's perspective, corporate governance is about 'maximising value subject to meeting the corporation's financial and other legal and contractual obligations'.

It adds: 'This inclusive definition stresses the need for boards of directors to balance the interests of shareholders with those of other stakeholders in order to achieve long-term sustained value.'

The strength of this approach to corporate governance is its general acceptance. Many people hold the view that public companies are in business to earn profits for the benefit of their shareholders. Successful companies are perceived as those that pay dividends to shareholders and whose share price goes up. Within the broad objective of maximising shareholder values, the board of directors will also act fairly in the interests of employees, customers, suppliers and others with an interest in the organisation's affairs.

Despite its wide acceptance within corporate governance, this approach is of limited application within health service governance. As has already been established in this text, the role played by the shareholder or financial stakeholder is very limited within the NHS.

Stakeholder theory

The stakeholder theory of corporate governance was introduced by Freeman (1994) who defined stakeholders as 'any group or individual who can affect, or is affected by, the achievement of a corporation's purpose'. This evolved, in part, as a result of the recognition of the complexity of strategy and the growing recognition that, unlike as thought previously, a company wasn't just a production system where strategy was focused primarily on products and the means to produce them. Instead, there was a growing appreciation that corporations created value through the complex interaction of various networks of relationships.

Theorists began to explore other theoretical frameworks for governance and explored the corporate governance models in Japan and Germany, where corporate and institutional shareholders were required to have a monitoring role in governing corporate bodies. This is known as the two-tier structure, usually consisting of a supervisory board and a management board. This is dealt with in more detail in Chapter 7 but in essence, the management board (EDs only) is responsible for managing the organisation and the supervisory board (NEDs only) is responsible for general oversight of the organisation and of the management board. The chair of the management board (the CEO) reports to the supervisory board chair.

This theoretical framework is called the stakeholder theory and is now most often associated with Japanese and continental European practice, where law has required that half the seats on supervisory boards go to representatives of the workforce and where custom has long mandated that a company's bankers and large-block shareholders have seats on the board.

Stakeholder theory takes the view that the purpose of governance should be to satisfy, as far as possible, the objectives of all key stakeholders – customers, employees, the general public, the government, investors, local communities, and major suppliers and creditors. The board of directors should therefore consider the interests of all major stakeholders. However, some stakeholders are more important than others, so management should give priority to their interests above those of other stakeholder groups.

The focus of the stakeholder theory is articulated in two core questions formulated by Freeman (1994) was able to summarise stakeholder theory in two key questions:

i. What is the purpose of the company? This requires an articulation of the shared sense of the value the managers create and what brings its core stakeholders together. This drives the company forward and allows performance to be measured.
ii. What responsibility does management have to stakeholders? This requires an articulation of how the managers want to do business – specifically, what kinds of relationships they want and need to create with their stakeholders to deliver on the purpose of the company.

In the introduction to its principles of corporate governance, the OECD comments that an aim of government policy (public policy) should be 'to provide firms with the incentives and discipline to minimise divergence between private and social returns and to protect the interest of stakeholders'.

The OECD Principles of Corporate Governance recognise the role and rights of stakeholders. They state that a corporate governance framework should:

- recognise the rights of stakeholders that are recognised in law or through mutual agreements; and
- encourage active cooperation between organisations and stakeholders in creating wealth, jobs and the sustainability of financially sound enterprises.

Stakeholder theory states that the organisation's managers should make decisions that take into consideration the interests of all stakeholders. This means trying to achieve a range of different objectives, not just for the aim of maximising the value of the organisation for its shareholders. This is because different stakeholders each have their own (different) expectations of the organisation, which the organisation's management should attempt to satisfy.

Stakeholder theory also considers the role of organisations in society and the responsibility they should have towards society as a whole. It could be argued that some organisations are so large, and their influence on society so strong, that they should be accountable to the public for what they do. The general public are taxpayers; as such, they provide the economic and social infrastructure within which organisations are allowed to operate. In return, organisations should be expected to be 'corporate citizens', acting in ways that benefit society as a whole. This aspect of stakeholder theory is consistent with the arguments in favour of corporate social responsibility (CSR).

Stakeholder approach (pluralist approach)

The pluralist approach to corporate governance is based on stakeholder theory. This argues that the aim of sound corporate governance is not just to meet the objectives of shareholders, but also to have regard for the interests of other individuals and groups with a stake in the organisation – including the public at large. This resonates more widely with health advice governance, where the objectives of NHS organisations are influenced by a wide-ranging variety of stakeholders.

From a 'stakeholder view', governance is concerned with achieving a balance between economic and social goals and between individual and communal goals. Sound governance should recognise the economic imperatives organisations face in competitive markets and should encourage the efficient use of resources through sound investment. It should also require accountability from the board of directors to the stakeholders for the stewardship of those resources. Within this framework, the aim should be to recognise the interests of other individuals, companies and society at large in the decisions and activities of the organisation.

A problem with the stakeholder approach for corporate governance is that company law gives certain rights to shareholders, as well as placing legal duties on the board of directors towards their organisation. However, the interests of other stakeholders are not reinforced to any great extent by company law. The stakeholder approach expects that cooperative and productive relationships will be optimised only if the directors are permitted or required to balance shareholder interests with the interests of other stakeholders who are committed to the organisation. For the approach to be more applicable to corporate governance, then changes in company law would be required to introduce such an approach in practice.

A further argument against this approach is that there is a distinction between company responsibilities (stakeholder interests) and its objectives (shareholder wealth). This has some merit as shareholders have their financial holding at risk while stakeholders such as suppliers, customers and employees receive other benefits from the company and often have contractual protection if things go wrong.

At the heart of the debate is the purpose of company growth and performance – is it the production of financial profit alone or is there a wider public or social benefit?

This approach is also limited in its application to health service governance as the concept of competitive markets is limited within the NHS. While there is an increasing emphasis on a market economy within healthcare, this is still limited in reality and has now been superseded by the more collaborative approach envisioned by the Five Year Forward View (5YFV) (see Chapter 3). The concept of individual goals for stakeholders is also tempered by the overriding objective of the NHS to provide healthcare at the point of need for all. A further distinction for health service governance is that the rights of other stakeholders, such as employees, suppliers and the general public, although not well protected by company law, are protected by health law (such as the FOIA) as well as other aspects of law such as employment law, health and safety legislation and environmental law.

Enlightened shareholder approach

The enlightened shareholder approach to corporate governance says that the directors of an organisation should pursue the interests of their shareholders, but in an enlightened and inclusive way. It is a form of compromise between the agency view and the stakeholder view.

The directors should look to the long term, not just the short term, and they should have regard to the interests of other stakeholders in the organisation, not just the shareholders. Managers should be aware of the need to create and maintain productive relationships with a range of stakeholders having an interest in their organisation.

A criticism of the enlightened shareholder view is that most shareholders do not fit the image of enlightened investors. Most shares in public companies are owned by institutional investors, who themselves may be relatively unaccountable to their beneficiaries. When companies become a target for a takeover bid, speculative investors such as hedge funds may acquire large but short-term shareholdings, with a view to making a quick profit from their investment. However, the role of institutional investors in corporate governance is likely to evolve in the future, with institutions expected to be more proactive in promoting the rights and interests of shareholders.

This approach is of greater application to health service governance as it does address the need to balance the competing needs of the different stakeholders. Its limitation, however, is in its lack of clarity on how to balance diverse and/or differing stakeholder interests. This is still largely a shareholder-driven approach to governance and is limited in its application to health service governance.

The King Code: an integrated approach

The King Code or King Report was first introduced in 1994 and was developed by the Institute of Directors in South Africa. A revised Code (King II) was published in 2004, with a further revision (King III) published in 2009 and King IV in 2016. These codes reject an enlightened shareholder approach to governance in favour of a 'stakeholder-inclusive' approach.

This approach is explained in some detail in the introduction to King III. The enlightened shareholder model and the stakeholder-inclusive model both take the view that the board of directors should consider the interests and expectations of stakeholders other than shareholders; however, the two models differ significantly in their emphasis.

- In the 'enlightened shareholder' approach, the legitimate interests and expectations of stakeholders only have an instrumental value. Stakeholders are only considered in as far as it would be in the interests of shareholders to do so.
- In the case of the 'stakeholder-inclusive' approach, the board of directors considers the legitimate interests and expectations of stakeholders on the basis that this is in the best interests of the organisation, and not merely as an instrument to serve the interests of the shareholder.

The King Code, therefore, states that a board of directors should consider what is best for the organisation; in doing so, it should have regard to the legitimate interests and expectations of all stakeholders. It should then integrate these or decide how they should be traded off against each other, on a case-by-case basis, with the aim of making decisions that are in the best interests of the organisation.

The shareholder does not have any predetermined precedence over other stakeholders. The 'best interests of the organisation' are defined not in terms of maximising shareholder wealth, but 'within the parameters of the organisation as a sustainable enterprise and the organisation as a corporate citizen'.

Stewardship theory

Stewardship theory has its roots in psychology and sociology and is based on the premise that managers and board members are motivated by more than increasing their personal wealth. It is concerned with the behaviour of executives and directors who act as stewards to protect and maximise shareholders' wealth: in so doing, the stewards maximise their own potential. In this theory, stewards are executives and directors within an organisation, working for the shareholders, who protect and make profits for the shareholders. Unlike agency theory, stewardship theory stresses not the perspective of individualism, but the role of top management acting as stewards, integrating their goals as part of the organisation. The stewardship theory suggests that stewards are satisfied and motivated when organisational success is attained.

This theory also sees the need to engage with a range of interests but prioritises a positive connection between public bodies and civil society. The key role of those who govern is to create a framework of shared values, then to engage with key stakeholders and a suitably skilled and autonomous workforce – all of whom benefit from helping the organisation to achieve its goals.

Whereas agency theory assumes that being a manager or employee suppresses an individual's own aspirations, stewardship theory requires organisational structures that empower the steward and offers maximum autonomy built on trust. It stresses the position of employees or executives to act more autonomously so that the shareholders' returns are maximised.

Unlike most theories of corporate governance and agency theory which focus on individuals working purely for self-interest at the expense of owners. The stewardship theory rejects this notion. In stewardship theory, the manager places the firm ahead of their personal interest. The stewards are involvement-oriented and trustworthy. For this theory to work well, the manager needs to be given a clear and unambiguous role and the organisational structure should give and support acceptable authority, worth and power to the management.

Interestingly stewardship theory would promote the combining of the role of the CEO and the Chair as this reduces costs and enables them to be a better steward for the company.

Stewardship theory can also be seen in the behaviour of executives and directors when decisions are made to maximise financial performance, as well as shareholders' profits, in order to protect their reputations as decision-makers in organisations. In other words, executives and directors are also managing their careers in order to be seen as effective stewards of their organisation.

Policy governance approach

The policy governance approach was first developed by John Carver in the 1970s and is a model that may allow the stewardship theory to be put into practice. The approach distinguishes sharply between the role of 'owners' and 'operators'.

According to John Carver, this approach sees boards act as 'owner representatives' who set objectives but fully delegate the running of the organisation to operators through the CEO as the main point of contact. A framework of policies limits the freedom of the management, ensuring that the effectiveness of an activity is not prioritised over its being ethical or prudent. However, by setting clear and unambiguous roles, the manager as steward is best placed to put the company above their own self-interest.

Under this approach, corporate governance will enable the board (owner representatives) to:

- cradle the vision and explicitly address fundamental values;
- force an external focus;
- enable an outcome-driven organising system;
- force forward thinking;
- enable proactivity;
- facilitate diversity and unity in board composition and opinion;
- describe relationships to relevant constituencies;
- delineate the board's role in common topics (ensuring the board's specific contribution to any topic is clear);
- determine what information is needed; and
- balance over-control and under-control.

Experts in the model argue boards should govern with an emphasis on:

- outward vision rather than an internal preoccupation;
- encouragement of diversity in viewpoints;
- strategic leadership more than administrative detail;
- clear distinction of board and chief executive roles;
- collective rather than individual decisions;
- future rather than past or present; and
- proactivity rather than reactivity.

Carver also cautions against excessive intrusion into the operational details but balances this with stating that boards remain accountable to their owners for all operational details and must therefore control them – the question is how to make this practical.

A further criticism of this approach points out that delegation, the granting of authority to the CEO, can become an 'abdication' of the board's responsibility to control all organisational actions. However, delegation accompanied by careful monitoring to ensure it achieves the results intended can be an exercise of the 'due diligence' expected of the board.

The policy governance approach requires a clear direction from boards in setting the objectives of the organisation. These objectives need to be established in direct correlation with the wishes of the owners (or beneficiaries) of the organisation. Having established clear objectives, the board then fully delegates the running of the organisation to the management team via the CEO as the main point of contact.

This form of governance can be seen clearly in charitable trusts where the trustees act as the representatives of the owners, and the CEO is held to account at the board meetings of the trustees. In this approach, it would be unusual for members of the management team also to act as a trustee. The trustees are responsible for establishing a framework of policies within which the CEO and their management team operate, ensuring that the effectiveness of an activity is not prioritised over its being ethical or prudent.

This approach has been adopted by some foundation trusts within the NHS, although they differ from the trustee model outlined earlier in that their EDs are also voting members of the foundation trust board. One of the advantages of this approach is the direct focus on the objectives of the organisation with a clear set of policies within which the CEO and team may operate. The success or otherwise of this approach for health service governance lies in the extent to which the board can define the objectives for the organisation and balance the competing interests of the diverse variety of the stakeholders.

Transaction cost theory

Transaction cost theory is a variation on the agency understanding of governance assumptions. It describes governance frameworks as being based on the net effects of internal and external transactions, rather than as contractual relationships outside the firm (i.e. with shareholders).

Transaction cost theory and agency theory essentially deal with the same issues and problems. Where agency theory focuses on the individual agent, transaction cost theory focuses on the individual transaction.

- Agency theory looks at the tendency of directors to act in their own best interests, pursuing salary and status. Transaction cost theory considers that managers (or directors) may arrange transactions in an opportunistic way.
- The corporate governance problem of transaction cost theory is, however, not the protection of ownership rights of shareholders (as is the agency theory focus) rather the effective and efficient accomplishment of transactions by firms.

Transaction cost theory provides a different basis for explaining the relationship between the owners of an organisation and its management. Although it is an economic theory, it attempts to explain companies not just as economic units, but as organisations consisting of people with differing views and objectives.

The operations of an organisation can be performed either through market transactions or by carrying out work in-house. For example, an organisation could obtain its raw materials from an external supplier or it could make the materials itself. Similarly, an organisation could hire self-employed contractors to carry out activities or it could hire full-time employees. In economic terms, a firm's decision about whether to arrange transactions in the open market or whether to do the work in-house (itself) should depend on which is cheaper. When a firm does work in-house, it needs a management structure and a hierarchy of authority with senior management at the top. According to transaction cost theory, the structure of a firm and the relationship between the owners of a firm and its management depends on the extent to which transactions are performed in-house.

Total costs are defined as the sum of production costs and transaction costs.

- Production costs are the costs that would be incurred by the organisation in an ideal economic market. In an ideal economic market, production costs are minimised.
- Transaction costs are additional costs incurred whenever the perfect economic market is not achieved. For example, an organisation might buy goods from a supplier who is not the cheapest available, because it is not aware of the existence of the cheapest supplier. An organisation might sell goods on credit to a customer, not knowing that money owed will become a bad debt.

Transaction costs are sometimes higher when a transaction is arranged in the market, and sometimes higher when the transaction is carried out in-house. Carrying out activities in-house rather than arranging contracts externally is referred to as vertical integration. Total costs are minimised when transaction costs are minimised. This should determine the optimal size of the firm and the size of the management hierarchy in the firm.

The way in which an organisation is organised, and the extent to which it is vertically integrated, also affect the control the organisation has over its transactions. As a general rule, it is in the interests of an organisation's management to carry out transactions internally, rather than in the external market. Performing transactions internally:

- removes the risks and uncertainties about prices of products and product quality; and
- removes all the risks and costs of dealing with external suppliers.

Traditional economic theory is based on the assumptions that all behaviour is rational and that profit maximisation is the rational objective of all businesses. Transaction cost economics changes these assumptions by attempting to allow for human behaviour and the fact that individuals do not always act rationally. The theory is based on two assumptions about behaviour:

- bounded rationality
- opportunism.

Bounded rationality
Human beings act rationally, but only within certain limits of understanding. For example, the managers of an organisation will, in theory, act rationally in seeking

to maximise the value of the organisation for its shareholders, but their bounded rationality might make them act differently.

Business is very complex, and large businesses are much more complex than small businesses. However, in any business, there is a limit to the amount of information that individuals can remember, understand and deal with. No one is capable of assessing all the possible courses of action and no one can anticipate what will happen in the future. In a competitive market, no one can anticipate with certainty what competitors will do.

Playing chess has been used as an example of bounded rationality. The game is very complex and there are many different possible moves. The actions of the opponent in a game of chess cannot be predicted, so it is impossible to predict what the opponent will do in response to a particular move. The same problem applies to managing an organisation. It is impossible to predict with certainty what will happen, because there are too many factors and too many possibilities to consider.

When individuals reach the boundaries of their understanding because a situation is too complex or too uncertain, there is a greater tendency to carry out transactions in-house and to have vertical integration.

Opportunism

Transaction cost theory also assumes that individuals will act in a self-interested way and 'with guile'. They will not always be honest and truthful about their intentions. Opportunism is defined as 'an effort to realise individual gains through a lack of candour or honesty in transactions'. For example, an individual might try to take advantage of an opportunity to gain a benefit at the expense of someone else.

Managers are opportunistic by nature. Given the opportunity, they will take advantage of any way of improving their own benefits and privileges. A problem with opportunism is that external parties (such as contractors and suppliers) cannot always be trusted to act honestly. As a result, there may be a tendency for an organisation to carry out transactions itself, rather than to rely on external suppliers.

However, there is also a risk that by taking control of transactions internally, managers will have opportunities to take decisions and actions that are in their personal interests. This self-interested behaviour needs to be controlled. In this respect, transaction cost theory has similarities with agency theory. Although they are based on different assumptions, both agency theory and transaction cost theory support the need for controls over corporate governance.

This approach also has limited relevance for health service governance as there is little opportunity for decision making about in-house or external transactions as there are usually dictated centrally by DHSC policy. The theory also relies on a competitive market, which makes it less relevant for health service governance. However, there are some echoes of health service governance in the explanations of bounded rationality and opportunism as a way of understanding how health service organisations might operate.

Generative governance theory

A new approach has recently emerged from the experience of not-for-profit boards in the US, described by Richard Chait, William Ryan and Barbara Taylor as 'governance as leadership' or generative governance.

They set out three modes in which the board should be effective:

- fiduciary
- strategic
- generative.

The main contribution of this tri-modal model is to emphasise the role of 'generative thinking' in producing a sense of what knowledge, information and data mean. This requires an active process of dialogue and engagement between the board, staff and service users.

The fiduciary mode is where boards are concerned primarily with the stewardship of tangible assets that makes up the core of governance. The fiduciary work is intended to ensure that nonprofit organisations are faithful to their mission, accountable for performance, and compliant with the relevant laws and regulations. Without this, the organisation, including its stakeholders, could be harmed.

The strategic mode is where boards develop strategy with management to set the organisation's priorities and course, and to deploy resources accordingly. Without this, there is little power or influence and governance would primarily be about staying on course rather than setting the course.

The generative mode is where boards, along with executives, frame problems and make sense of ambiguous situations – which in turn shapes the organisation's strategies, plans and decisions.

This theory of governance claims that most organisations lack the frameworks and practices for this work.

The governance as leadership approach

The governance as leadership or 'generative' approach relies on the interplay of three key roles for boards. This requires an active process of dialogue and engagement between the board, staff and service users.

The approach requires boards to understand their stewardship role in respect of the public assets of their organisation, to be accountable for performance and to ensure compliance with the relevant laws and regulations. At the same time, boards need to work with the executive management to set the organisation's priorities for the future and to deploy resources accordingly. None of this seems significantly different to the approaches already outlined and relies on the key relationship between the board and the executive management team.

The final aspect to this approach is what distinguishes it from the others, however, and relies on sharing knowledge, experiences, information and the analysis of organisational data. This final role for the board is to lead, along with executives, on framing problems and making sense of ambiguous situations – which in turn shapes the organisation's strategies, plans and decisions. This third role is of significant importance for health service governance as it provides an opportunity to manage the competing interests of a diverse stakeholder base.

Summary

- Governance can be defined as a system that allows organisations to be effective in the delivery of their strategic objectives.
- In order to understand the underlying differences between health service governance in the NHS and corporate governance in the private sector it is useful to consider the theoretical frameworks for corporate governance that have been set out in this chapter.
- There are different frameworks and approaches to corporate governance, which vary according to the extent to which the interests of stakeholders other than the organisational shareholders are recognised. The underlying framework and approach taken by the directors of an organisation affects decision making at a strategic level.
- A stakeholder in an organisation is someone who has an interest or 'stake' in it and is affected by what the organisation does. A stakeholder, in turn, has an influence on what the organisation does. Each stakeholder or stakeholder group may expect the organisation to behave or act in a particular way with regard to the stakeholders' interests. A stakeholder can also expect to have some say in some of the decisions an organisation makes and some of the actions it takes.
- The importance of good governance is often only highlighted in circumstances where an organisation has failed or is in crisis. It is often seen in organisations where there is a wide separation between stakeholder interests and management. For example, the separation between NHS stakeholders and Parliament is vast; it is only through the health service governance regimes of the individual parts of the NHS that stakeholders can exercise the relatively limited powers they have to hold the boards of directors to account.
- While corporate governance may be restricted by company law to observe the primary role of shareholders, thus endorsing the primacy of agency theory for corporate governance, there are increasingly challenges to this theoretical framework as the only means of explaining governance.
- All of these theoretical frameworks and approaches can be considered in respect of health service governance and indeed, no one approach should be

seen as providing the only approach to governance. It is more likely that the interplay of a number of these approaches will frame the development of good health service governance that is not bound by the company legislation that enshrines the legal rights of shareholders.

3
Definitions and issues in Health Service Governance

Introduction

Chapter 3 offers further clarity on the distinctions of health service governance and then goes onto explore why it matters and what the outcomes of poor health service governance are likely to be. The foundations of health service governance are based in the NHS Constitution, which is summarised in this chapter along with the main drivers from the 5YFV.

Defining health service governance

It is essential that there is a good understanding of what health service governance is, and what it is intended to achieve.

The NHS often faces times of uncertainty with short- and long-term policy competing for attention. This is particularly true with the significant changes introduced by the 5YFV, the introduction of Sustainability and Transformation Partnerships (STPs) and the development of new models of care (covered in Chapter 16). Good governance is vital for NHS organisations as they face another series of major changes and will be key to ensuring that there is effective leadership, responsible stewardship of public assets and services, and public accountability.

Health service governance is not a product in itself. Instead, it is foundational to the delivery of 'high quality for all' as envisaged in 2008's Darzi report (covered in more detail later).

Health service governance – a definition

There have been numerous attempts to define corporate governance. The classic definition has been provided by the UK Code and it can be adapted for health service governance as follows:

> 'Health service governance is the system by which NHS organisations are directed and controlled. Boards of directors or governing bodies are responsible for the governance of their organisations. The stakeholders' role in governance is to appoint the directors and the auditors and to satisfy themselves that an appropriate governance structure is in place. The responsibilities of the board or governing body include setting the organisation's strategic aims, providing

the leadership to put them into effect, supervising the management of the business and reporting to stakeholders on their stewardship. The actions of the board or governing body are subject to laws, regulations and the stakeholders in general meeting.'

Governance can, therefore, be defined as a system that allows organisations to be effective in the delivery of their strategic aims. The strategic aims for the NHS are set out in the NHS Constitution, which attempts to clarify the expectations of the taxpayer into rights and pledges that should be delivered (see later in this chapter). As a consequence, health service governance has to create a system that enables effective delivery of those healthcare rights and pledges, tailored for the local communities in which it is delivered by the individual parts of the NHS. The NHS Constitution provides an overriding strategy that is then underpinned at a local level by each NHS organisation as it actively considers its own specific local strategy.

Why does health service governance matter?

The importance of good governance is often only highlighted in circumstances where an organisation has failed or is in crisis. It tends to be seen in organisations where the separation between stakeholder interests and management is wider. This is a significant risk for NHS organisations; government spending on healthcare for 2018/19 was budgeted at £114 billion and yet the recipients of the healthcare provided are often very distant from the holders of the healthcare budget. Health service governance in NHS organisations therefore must be resilient enough to hold NHS organisations to account for the responsibility of managing this expenditure. The separation between NHS stakeholders and Parliament is vast, and it is only through the health service governance regimes of the individual parts of the NHS that NHS stakeholders can exercise the relatively limited powers they have to hold the boards of directors to account.

The consequences for the NHS when health service governance goes wrong are often catastrophic for the patients and families involved, as well as very public. Sadly, there have been a number of cases where the poor health service governance has led to tragedy (e.g. Mid Staffordshire NHS Foundation Trust, University Hospitals of Morecambe Bay NHS Foundation Trust, Southern Health NHS Foundation Trust and Shrewsbury and Telford Hospital NHS Trust).

While poor governance within the NHS is unlikely to lead to its complete disappearance (unlike a corporate body), it is likely to lead to the continual pressure to move towards greater centralisation of control by the government. Political opinions will differ as to whether this is in the best interests of the recipients of a publicly funded healthcare system. Lessons in good practice have generally resulted from such misconduct and poor decision making. However, it is the reputation of the NHS and patient care that consequently suffer repeatedly in the meantime.

The following summary of the scandal at Mid Staffordshire NHS Foundation Trust describes the consequences of poor governance.

Mid Staffordshire NHS Foundation Trust

Mid Staffordshire NHS Foundation Trust was at the centre of one the largest healthcare scandals in recent times. The Healthcare Commission (now CQC) had been first alerted by the high mortality rates in patients admitted as emergencies. When the FT failed to provide what the Commission considered to be an adequate explanation, a full-scale investigation was carried out between March and October 2008. Subsequent reports and inquiries led to full public inquiry chaired by Robert Francis QC. His final report was published on 6 February 2013, making 290 recommendations and calling for a 'fundamental culture change' across the health and social care system to put patients first at all times. It called for action across six core themes:

- culture
- compassionate care
- leadership
- standards
- information
- openness, transparency and candour.

Robert Francis QC commented:

> 'Whilst the executive and non-executive board members recognised the problems, the action taken by the board was inadequate and lacked an appropriate sense of urgency. The trust's board was found to be disconnected from what was actually happening in the hospital and chose to rely on apparently favourable performance reports by outside bodies such as the Healthcare Commission, rather than effective internal assessment and feedback from staff and patients. The trust failed to listen to patients' concerns, the board did not review the substance of complaints and incident reports were not given the necessary attention.'

The consequences for Mid Staffordshire NHS Foundation Trust were that on 1 November 2014 the services previously managed by Mid Staffordshire NHS Foundation Trust were transferred to the management of University Hospitals of North Midlands NHS Trust and the Royal Wolverhampton NHS Trust. Both the County Hospital (formerly Stafford Hospital) and Cannock Chase Hospital remain open.

The scandal gave rise to a number of publications and recommendations, which have been summarised below:

Patients First and Foremost (March 2013) was a radical plan to prioritise care, improve transparency and to ensure clear action and clear accountability where poor care was detected. The key changes included the following:

- The CQC appointed three Chief Inspectors of hospitals, adult social care and primary care.
- The Chief Inspector of Hospitals began a first wave of inspections of 18 trusts.
- The CQC consulted on a new system of ratings with patient care and safety at its heart and on a new set of fundamental standards that must underpin all care in the future: the inviolable principles of safe, effective and compassionate care.
- Legislation to introduce a responsive and effective failure regime looking at quality as well as finance.

Transforming Participation in Health and Care (September 2013) offered guidance to commissioners on involving patients and the public in decisions about their care and their services.

Hard Truths – The Journey to Putting Patients First (January 2014) provided a detailed response to the 290 recommendations the inquiry made across every level of the system. The NHS Constitution was revised as a result of the Francis Report. Some of the key actions that followed the publication of Hard Truths included the following:

- All hospitals to clearly set out how patients and their families can raise concerns or complain, with independent support available from local Healthwatch or alternative organisations.
- Trusts to report on complaints data and lessons learned quarterly, and the Ombudsman to significantly increase the number of cases considered.
- The passing of the Care Act 2014 which led to a statutory and professional duty of candour, a new fit and proper person's test and the introduction of a new criminal offence applicable to care providers that supply or publish certain types of false or misleading information. This is covered in more detail later.
- All arm's-length bodies and the Department of Health (now DHSC) were to sign a protocol to minimise bureaucratic burdens on trusts by aligning their regulatory requirements.

The Keogh Review into the Quality of Care and Treatment Provided by 14 Hospital Trusts in England led to 11 hospitals being placed into 'special measures' to put them back on a path to recovery and then to excellence.

The Cavendish Review: An Independent Review into Healthcare Assistants and Support Workers in the NHS and Social Care Settings (July 2013) set out how the training and support of healthcare and care assistants could be improved so that patients receive compassionate care in both NHS and social settings.

A Promise to Learn – A Commitment to Act: Improving the Safety of Patients in England (August 2013) described a partial loss of focus on quality and safety as primary aims, inadequate openness to the voices of patients and carers, insufficient skills in safety and improvement, inadequate staffing for patients' needs, and a very unhelpful complexity and lack of clarity and cooperation amongst regulatory agencies.

A Review of the NHS Hospitals Complaints System: Putting Patients Back in the Picture (October 2013) focused on four areas for improvement: quality of care; how complaints were handled; independence in the complaints procedures; and whistleblowing.

Common themes in poor governance

Aspects of poor governance include:

- a board of directors that fails to perform its duties properly, perhaps because it is dominated by one or more individuals, or because it fails to carry out its appointed tasks;
- a poor relationship between the board and the main stakeholders;
- failure to deliver the appropriate returns or services required by either statute or by regulators;
- ineffective systems of risk management, and exposure to errors and fraud due to inadequate internal control systems;
- inappropriate remuneration and reward systems for directors and senior executives;
- misleading performance reporting to regulators and stakeholders; and
- unethical business practices.

Therefore, a key issue in governance continues to be the relationship between the board of directors, its main stakeholders (such as patients, staff and the DHSC) and other important stakeholders. The following quote from the NHS Providers and DAC Beachcroft LLP publication *The Foundations of Good Governance: A Compendium of Best Practice* is illuminating:

> 'Governance is sometimes regarded as an obscure subject, not necessarily visible in its own right, but it becomes a high-profile reputation issue when it is found lacking. At its core, delivering good governance is about strong, dynamic leadership and it should not be the preserve of "governance specialists" or experts, nor should it be driven by compliance with processes alone. Corporate governance is about leadership and is the system by which all board-led organisations across the public and private sectors are directed and controlled including NHS foundation trusts and NHS trusts.'

The NHS Constitution

The NHS Constitution for England is a formal constitution, which lays down in one document the objectives of the NHS, the rights and responsibilities of the various parties involved in healthcare in England and the guiding principles that govern the service.

The following are required by law to take account of the NHS Constitution in their decisions and actions:

- the Secretary of State for Health and Social Care;
- all NHS bodies, including CCGs, NHS trusts and NHS FTs;
- all private and voluntary sector providers supplying NHS services; and
- local authorities in the exercise of their public health functions.

The Constitution was first published on 21 January 2009 and was one of a number of recommendations in Lord Darzi's 2008 report *High Quality Care for All*. This set out a ten-year plan to provide the highest quality of care and service for patients in England. These rights and responsibilities had previously evolved in common law, through UK or EU law, or were policy pledges by the NHS and government. They have now been written into the Constitution. Under the Health Act 2009, all providers and commissioners of NHS care are under a legal obligation to have regard to the NHS Constitution in all their decisions and actions. The Constitution enables the NHS to remain true to fundamental principles and values which are as relevant now as they were when the NHS was founded, and which continue to enjoy strong support from the public.

There are legally binding requirements for revising and updating the Constitution, which guarantee that the principles and values that underpin the NHS are subject to regular review and recommitment. These requirements also mandate that any government which seeks to alter the principles or values of the NHS – or the rights, pledges, duties and responsibilities set out in the Constitution has to engage in a full and transparent debate with the public, patients and staff. The latest version of the Constitution was published in July 2015.

To accompany the updated NHS Constitution, the DH (now DHSC) also published a Handbook to the NHS Constitution, which explains the rights, pledges and responsibilities set out in the NHS Constitution in more detail. An addendum published in September 2017 also set out how the NHS Constitution applied to public health services, local authorities and Public Health England (PHE). A consolidated version of the Handbook was published in January 2019.

The Constitution is structured as follows:

- **Values** – six values that should underpin everything NHS service providers do.
- **Principles** – seven principles that guide the NHS in all that it does.
- **Rights and responsibilities** – some required by law.
- **Pledges** made by the NHS about the way it will work with patients, the public and its staff.

Values of the NHS
1. Working together for patients.
2. Respect and dignity.
3. Commitment to quality of care.

DEFINITIONS AND ISSUES IN HEALTH SERVICE GOVERNANCE

4. Compassion.
5. Improving lives.
6. Everyone counts.

Principles of the NHS

1. The NHS provides a comprehensive service, available to all.
2. Access to NHS services is based on clinical need, not an individual's ability to pay.
3. The NHS aspires to the highest standards of excellence and professionalism.
4. The patient will be at the heart of everything the NHS does.
5. The NHS works across organisational boundaries and in partnership with other organisations in the interest of patients, local communities and the wider population.
6. The NHS is committed to providing best value for taxpayers' money and the most effective, fair and sustainable use of finite resources.
7. The NHS is accountable to the public, communities and patients that it serves.

Rights, responsibilities and pledges

The Constitution grants patients 'rights', which are intended to be legally enforceable and also makes other non-binding 'pledges'.

The rights and pledges cover the seven key areas of the NHS Constitution:

1. access to health services;
2. quality of care and environment;
3. nationally approved treatments, drugs and programmes;
4. respect, consent and confidentiality;
5. informed choice;
6. involvement in your healthcare and in the NHS; and rights; and
7. complaints and redress.

The NHS Constitution also recognises that patients and the public can make a significant contribution to their own, and their family's good health and wellbeing. The Constitution sets out key responsibilities as follows:

- Take personal responsibility for your own and your family's good health and wellbeing.
- Register with a GP practice – the main point of access to NHS care as commissioned by NHS bodies.
- Treat NHS staff and other patients with respect and recognise that violence, or the causing of nuisance or disturbance on NHS premises, could result in prosecution. Abusive and violent behaviour could result in a patient being refused access to NHS services.
- Provide accurate information about your health, condition and status.

- Keep appointments or cancel within reasonable time. Receiving treatment within the maximum waiting times may be compromised otherwise.
- Follow the course of treatment agreed upon and talk to your clinician if this is difficult.
- Participate in important public health programmes such as vaccination.
- Ensure that those closest to a patient are aware of their wishes about organ donation.
- Give feedback – both positive and negative – about your experiences and the treatment and care received, including any adverse reactions. Feedback will help to improve NHS services for all.

Staff rights, pledges, and expectations

In a similar way, the Constitution applies to all staff doing clinical or non-clinical NHS work – including public health – and their employers. It covers staff wherever they are working, whether in public, private or voluntary sector organisations. Whilst staff have extensive legal rights, embodied in general employment and discrimination law, the Handbook to the NHS Constitution Handbook sets out the legal rights, other rights, pledges, and expectations that staff and employers can expect.

In addition to the legal rights, there are a number of pledges that the NHS is committed to achieve. Pledges go above and beyond the legal rights. They are not legally binding, but represent a commitment by the NHS to provide high-quality working environments for staff. The NHS pledges to do the following:

- Provide a positive working environment for staff and promote supportive, open cultures that help staff do their job to the best of their ability.
- Provide all staff with clear roles and responsibilities and rewarding jobs for teams and individuals that make a difference to patients, their families and carers and communities.
- Provide all staff with personal development, access to appropriate education and training for their jobs, and line management support to enable them to fulfil their potential.
- Provide support and opportunities for staff to maintain their health, wellbeing and safety.
- Engage staff in decisions that affect them and the services they provide, individually, through representative organisations and through local partnership working arrangements. All staff will be empowered to put forward ways to deliver better and safer services for patients and their families.
- Have a process for staff to raise an internal grievance.
- Encourage and support all staff in raising concerns at the earliest reasonable opportunity about safety, malpractice or wrongdoing at work, responding to and, where necessary, investigating the concerns raised and acting consistently with the Employment Rights Act 1996.

DEFINITIONS AND ISSUES IN HEALTH SERVICE GOVERNANCE

The Constitution is clear that all staff have responsibilities to the public, their patients and their colleagues. These responsibilities are as follows:

- To accept professional accountability and maintain the standards of professional practice as set by the appropriate regulatory body applicable to the profession or role.
- To take reasonable care of health and safety at work for themselves, their team and others, and to co-operate with employers to ensure compliance with health and safety requirements.
- To act in accordance with the express and implied terms of the contract of employment.
- Not to discriminate against patients or staff and to adhere to equal opportunities and equality and human rights legislation.
- To protect the confidentiality of personal information that they hold.
- To be honest and truthful in applying for a job and in carrying out that job.

Overall, the NHS Constitution is a key strategic document for understanding the parameters by which all of the individual parts of the NHS are required to function. In addition to this and in the light of the current financial, access and quality demands being placed on the NHS the other key document which is driving the strategic direction is the Five Year Forward View.

The Five Year Forward View and the 2018 funding settlement

Following the introduction of the new structure under the Health and Social Care Act 2012, the findings of the Francis Review and the Nicholson Challenge (saving £15–20 billion through efficiency savings from 2011 to 2014 as introduced by the then leader of the NHS, Sir David Nicholson), the NHS faced a major crisis relating to both the quality and safety of treatment and the ongoing funding of the NHS to meet the growing demands and activity. The 5YFV, published in October 2014 by the NHS leadership bodies (NHSE, NHSI, PHE, Health Education England (HEE) and the CQC), set out three underpinning principles for change for the NHS, namely closing three gaps in healthcare:

- the health and wellbeing gap;
- the care and quality gap; and
- the funding and efficiency gap.

The 5YFV built on the findings of the Dalton Review commissioned by the Secretary of State in February 2014 to explore options for providers of NHS care and to 'reduce variations in clinical standards, financial performance and patient safety'. The principle guiding the Dalton Review was that all patients should expect to receive the same high standards of care, no matter where or in what setting. The review aimed to encourage boards to explore how new organisational models could help safeguard an organisation's ability to provide safe and high-quality care. It made recommendations for boards and national bodies, in order for the necessary changes to be made quickly and easily. New organisational models explored by the review included those in Table 3.1.

Model type	Description
Collaborative	Bring together two or more organisations voluntarily to pool resources and achieve better outcomes (e.g. federation or joint venture)
Contractual	More formalised agreements with performance and quality standards agreed as part of the arrangement (e.g. service level chains and management contracts)
Consolidation	Change of ownership with new organisation coming into being potentially providing different services (e.g. integrated care organisations, mergers & acquisitions, multi-site trust and foundation groups)
Other options	Buddying, informal partnering and clinical/strategic networks, mutual social enterprises

Table 3.1: Organisational models

Led by the then Salford Royal NHS Foundation Trust CEO Sir David Dalton, (Sir David is now CEO of NHS Improvement) the review also identified five key themes for the pace of transformational change that is required within the NHS as follows:

1. One size does not fit all.
2. Quicker transformational and transactional change is required.
3. Ambitious organisations with a proven track record should be encouraged to expand their reach and have greater impact.
4. Overall sustainability for the provider sector is a priority.
5. A dedicated implementation programme is needed to make change happen.

In the future, it suggested, organisations are likely to operate more than one organisational form for their service portfolio. It recommends that trust boards consider whether a new organisational form may be most suited to support the delivery of safe, reliable, high-quality and economically viable services.

The Dalton Review did not set out any of the governance detail required for these new models or organisational forms, nor did it set out a clear governance framework for boards and governing bodies to proceed with such transformation. Instead, it stated that a procurement framework must be developed to allow credentialed organisations to register for management contract and/or acquisition opportunities with stronger trusts acting as 'system architects', which would be encouraged to develop innovative organisational models and to codify and spread their success elsewhere.

The Dalton Review saw the overall sustainability of the provider sector as a priority and encouraged the DH (now DHSC) and system regulators to create a single, unified process with standardised documentation to support future transactions as providers moved towards new models of care. It was clear, however, that trust boards and CCG governing bodies were to be responsible for ensuring the sustainability of the local health economy as opposed to their individual organisation.

The 5YFV picked up on these themes and was equally committed to exploring new models of care; consequently, less focus was placed on providers achieving FT status as it had become apparent that the FT process alone could not meet the significant challenges faced by the NHS sector. Indeed, it might be said that the FT process itself set provider trusts working competitively against each other and did not encourage collaboration and working across the health economy.

Between January and September 2015, 50 vanguards were selected to take a lead on the development of new care models which would act as the blueprints for the NHS in future and the inspiration to the rest of the health and care system.

In terms of closing the funding and efficiency gap, the 5YFV forecast that the NHS would have a £30 billion gap in funding by 2020/21 if current demand trends continued, the NHS received flat real term funding and no further efficiencies were delivered. It went on to project that the NHS would need in the range of £8 billion to £21 billion real-term growth annually by 2020/21, depending on demand and efficiency assumptions.

The 5YFV also called for a radical programme of health prevention and public health measures, alongside a review of the provision of social care and its associated funding, particularly for frail older people.

Carter Review (2016)

In June 2014, Lord Carter was asked to carry out a review by the Secretary of State as part of the aim to make the NHS safer and more efficient to ensure that the NHS would get the best value from its £102 billion annual budget and to help the NHS implement a seven-day service. Lord Carter's final report (February 2016) concluded that addressing unwarranted variation in use of resources across acute non-specialised hospitals could save up to £5 billion by 2020/21. The review recommended key measures, such as moving to e-rostering systems; adopting 'model hospital' standards; prioritising the role of procurement; and working more closely with neighbouring hospitals. NHSI was tasked with implementing the recommendations and Lord Carter was appointed as a NED of NHSI. These recommendations also formed part of the sustainability and transformation planning process that was underway under the 5YFV.

Delivering the Five year Forward view

In December 2015, *Delivering the Forward View: NHS Planning Guidance: 2016/17–2020/21* outlined a new approach to help ensure that health and care services were built around the needs of local populations. To do this, every health and care system in England was required to produce a multi-year sustainability and transformation plan (STP), showing how local services would evolve and become sustainable over the next five years – ultimately delivering the 5YFV vision of better health, better patient care and improved NHS efficiency. These sustainability and transformation plans led to the development of STPs.

The King's Fund was clear, however, that fundamental changes to how health services were commissioned, paid for and regulated would be required to deliver the vision of the 5YFV.

As a result, local health and care systems came together in January 2016 to form 44 'footprints' which were required to deliver plans based on the needs of local populations to drive genuine and sustainable transformation in patient experience and health outcomes of the longer term. The footprints were locally defined, based on natural communities, existing working relationships and patient flows, and they were supposed to take account of the scale needed to deliver the services, transformation and public health programmes required, along with how they would best fit with other footprints. All sustainability and transformation plans were delivered in June 2016 with an intended implementation date of autumn 2016 onwards.

In order to support the extent of transformation required, the King's Fund argued for a sustainability transformation fund (STF) to provide financial support through the transition, which was established under the jurisdiction of NHSE for each year of Parliament with the value of the fund in 2016/17 at £2.1 billion rising to £3.4 billion by 2020/21. Access to the STF was conditional on providers agreeing to financial control totals for 2016/17 that allowed provider trusts to return to aggregate financial balance. These control totals were part of the new financial oversight regime that NHSI put in place for 2016/17 onwards and were annual financial targets that had to be achieved to unlock access to national funding and other financial benefits.

In October 2018, NHSE and NHSI then wrote in a joint letter to STPs and Integrated Care Systems (ICSs) requiring them to develop and agree a further five-year plan by the autumn of 2019. The five-year plan would include a one-year operational plans for 2019–20 – known as the 'transitional year' – with the new five-year plans replacing those which were previously drawn up and were based on the previous five-year funding settlement to 2020–21. The letter confirmed that control totals were no longer seen as the best way to manage provider finances and that the intention would be to return to the requirement to break even. The five-year plans will be aggregated to develop a national NHS 10-year plan in response to the government's commitment to increase the NHSE budget by £20.5 billion in real terms by 2023–24. This plan was published on 7 January 2019 as the NHS Long-Term Plan (LTP).

The NHS Long Term Plan (LTP)

The plan builds on the policy platform laid out in the 5YFV, which described how integrating care was essential to meet the needs of a changing population. The funding increase amounts to 3.4% average real-terms annual increase in NHSE's budget between 2019/20 and 2023/24 as set out in Figure 3.1. The funding settlement only applies to NHS spending and does not include wider DHSC areas such as capital, education and training. In addition, the governmental spending review and green papers expected later in 2019 will also need to consider local authority public health spending, wider improvements in population health as well as social care and prevention.

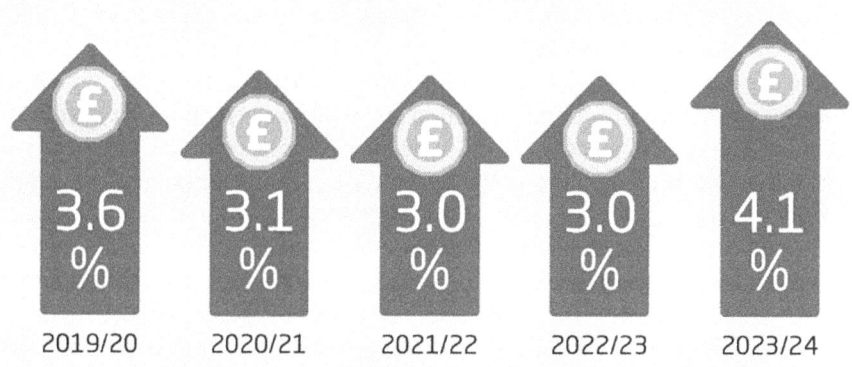

Figure 3.1: NHS funding 2019/20 to 2023/24

The plan prioritises the drive towards integrated care and population health with an uplift for primary medical and community health services. It includes a set of clinical priorities, which focus on children and young people, cancer, cardiovascular disease, stroke, diabetes, respiratory disease and mental health.

STPs and ICSs are required to develop and implement their own strategies for the next five years, and these need to be published by autumn 2019.

These strategies will set out how they intend to take the ambitions that the LTP details and work together to turn them into local action to improve services and the health and wellbeing of the communities they serve – building on the work they have already been doing.

Interestingly, the LTP does not require any changes to the law in order to be implemented but has asked that the NHS make consensus proposals for how primary legislation might be adjusted to better support delivery of the agreed changes set out in the LTP. So, for the time being it would seem that new models of care will continue to develop along informal and consensual lines with the associated governance implications that are set out in Chapter 5.

The LTP is clear, however, that amendments to primary legislation could significantly accelerate progress on service integration, on administrative efficiency, and on public accountability and that Parliament and the Government would be open to considering changes to: 'create publicly-accountable integrated care locally; to streamline the national administrative structures of the NHS; and remove the overly rigid competition and procurement regime applied to the NHS'.

Summary

- The specific governance arrangements and the issues that arise for the various forms and models of NHS organisation are set out in detail in the respective chapters, for example, Chapter 14, Foundation Trusts, Chapter 15, Clinical Commissioning Groups etc.
- The underlying principles for health service governance, however, remain the same regardless of form and all healthcare bodies are bound to act within the constraints of best practice, both in the process, practices and procedures by which power is shared and exercised by those who make up the controlling mind of the organisation – and in how the holders of power in the organisation should be held accountable for what they do.
- Health service governance is key to ensuring that there is effective leadership, responsible stewardship of public assets and services and public accountability.
- Whilst this chapter establishes the background and context for the NHS as a whole, the general direction of travel towards more collaboration and creating new organisational structures for the delivery of care gives rise to some interesting governance issues. These issues will be addressed in more detail in Chapter 5.
- However, the issues fall under the four pillars of governance set out in the preceding chapter, namely – fairness, accountability, responsibility and transparency.
- So, for example, STPs are not statutory bodies, rather they are collective discussion forums that aim to bring together health and care leaders to support the delivery of improved health and care based on the needs of local populations. As a consequence, consideration needs to be given as to how they are governed so as to support these four principles.
- In the absence of any legislative changes, the STPs do not replace the existing local bodies or change local accountabilities. The same can be said of the NHS Assembly, which will provide a national forum for debate on national policy.
- Whether you credit the phrase 'with great power comes great responsibility' to Voltaire in nineteenth-century France, Franklin D. Roosevelt in 1945 or to

the uncle of the comic book character Spider-Man, the intention remains the same. Those who exercise power must be held to account for the decisions they make. Health service governance provides a framework of law, regulation and guidance to put in place boundaries for those who exercise this power and authority with regard to the world's largest publicly funded health service.

4
The structure of the NHS

Introduction

Chapter 4 explores the NHS landscape in all its complexity. The way in which these distinctive parts work together provide a governance framework for the delivery of the NHS Constitution whilst each distinctive part also has its own governance arrangements. The regulatory system is outlined as well as the structures that are in place to support local accountability. This chapter will then describe how all the many parts work together while later chapters will explore the governance arrangements for the individual parts (e.g. foundation trusts, clinical commissioning groups etc).

The NHS

Health service governance is the governance that is applied to National Health Service (NHS) organisations. Therefore, it is useful to clarify the structure and guiding principles of the NHS.

The NHS is the shared name of three of the four publicly funded healthcare systems in the United Kingdom (UK). They provide a comprehensive range of health services, the vast majority of which are free at the point of use to residents of the UK.

The NHS in England was created by the National Health Service Act 1948 (NHS Act 1948), which created an NHS for both England and Wales. Responsibility for the NHS in Wales was passed to the Secretary of State for Wales in 1969, leaving the Secretary of State for Social Services solely responsible for the NHS in England. In January 2018, the cabinet reshuffle saw these two being combined again under the new name of the Department of Health and Social Care (DHSC).

The English NHS is the only system officially called the NHS, the others being NHS Scotland and NHS Wales. The Northern Irish equivalent to the NHS is called Health and Social Care (HSC). Each system operates independently and is politically accountable to the relevant government: the Scottish Government, the Welsh Government, the Northern Ireland Executive or the UK Government (for the English NHS).

Despite their separate funding and administration, there is no discrimination when a resident of one country of the UK requires treatment in another – although

THE STRUCTURE OF THE NHS

a patient will often be returned to their home area when they are fit to be moved. The financial and administrative consequences are dealt with by the organisations involved and no personal involvement by the patient is required.

The NHS has agreed a formal Constitution, which lays down in one document the objectives of the NHS, the rights and responsibilities of the various parties involved in healthcare in England (patients, staff and trust boards) and the guiding principles that govern the service. This was set out in more detail in the previous chapter. In summary, the guiding principles of the NHS are as follows.

- The NHS provides a comprehensive service, available to all irrespective of gender, race, disability, age, sexual orientation, religion, belief, gender reassignment, pregnancy and maternity or marital or civil partnership status.
- Access to NHS services is based on clinical need, not an individual's ability to pay (except in exceptional circumstances sanctioned by Parliament).
- The NHS aspires to the highest standards of excellence and professionalism to provide high-quality care that is safe, effective and focused on the patient experience.
- The NHS aspires to put patients at the heart of everything it does.
- The NHS works across organisational boundaries and in partnership with other organisations in the interest of patients, local communities and the wider population. The NHS is an integrated system of organisations and services bound together by the principles and values reflected in the Constitution.
- The NHS is committed to providing best value for taxpayers' money and the most effective, fair and sustainable use of finite resources.
- The NHS is accountable to the public, communities and patients that it serves.

The DHSC is the government department responsible for policy in health and social care matters. It is responsible for the NHS in England, along with a few elements of the same matters that are not otherwise devolved to the Scottish, Welsh or Northern Irish governments. The DHSC then delegates powers to the various authorities and boards established to oversee and scrutinise the provision of healthcare. This structure was altered radically in 2013 by the Health and Social Care Act 2012 (HSCA 2012).

The Statement of Accountability

The Statement of Accountability describes how the NHS in England currently works and who is responsible for its different parts. It is required by the NHS Constitution. In May 2013, a revised Statement of NHS Accountability for England was published in A Guide to the Healthcare System in England, to bring it into line with the revisions made to the NHS Constitution in April 2013. Despite the transformational changes being required through the 5YFV (see Chapter 16), the Statement of Accountability has not yet been updated as there is no new legislation to enable these new models or governance arrangements.

The NHS is a system of organisations responsible for organising and providing a comprehensive health service. The funding for running the NHS is granted to the DHSC by Parliament out of national taxation. There is therefore a continuous thread of accountability to the government running throughout the NHS.

The Secretary of State for Health and Social Care is accountable to Parliament, and through Parliament to the voters, for the promotion of a comprehensive health service and for the use of public money. Any decision taken by ministers about health policy can be scrutinised by Members of Parliament. The Health Select Committee and the Public Accounts Committee provide a scrutiny function holding the government to account for the delivery of health policy and effective use of resources. Other Select Committees perform similar functions in other policy areas. It is the role of the DHSC to support the Secretary of State in discharging their duties.

The Secretary of State for Health and Social Care is a politician and is the Cabinet minister responsible for health in England. They have a duty to promote a comprehensive health service in England and ministerial responsibility to Parliament for the provision of the health service. The Secretary of State has a number of further legal duties, particularly in relation to improving the quality of services and reducing health inequalities. They must also keep the performance of the health service under review and lay before Parliament a published report on this performance annually. They are responsible to Parliament for the provision of the health service and they work through the DHSC to provide strategic direction for the NHS (as well as the wider health and care system). They hold all of the national bodies to account for their operational and financial performance, thereby ensuring that the different parts of the system work properly together. They take decisions on national health, public health and social care policy, advised by the civil servants who make up the DHSC.

The DHSC's purpose is to help people live better for longer. It leads, shapes and funds health and care in England, making sure people have the support, care and treatment they need, with the compassion and dignity they deserve. The DHSC, on behalf of the Secretary of State, acts as 'system steward' – it is the only body with oversight over the whole health and care system, and it works to ensure the system operates effectively to meet the needs of people and their communities. This stewardship role has several main aspects. These are as follows:

- Setting national priorities that reflect what patients, service users and the public value. The DHSC sets ambitions and priorities for the NHS and health care system, through the outcomes frameworks and the Mandate (explained later). It also supports the delivery of ministerial ambitions, priorities and policies; and does this through obtaining information and intelligence, and appropriate monitoring.
- Securing and allocating resources to meet priorities and deliver services. The DHSC secures and distributes resources for the NHS, and the health and care system, by securing public funding for the NHS, public health and

social care from HM Treasury through the Spending Review process. It is an important stakeholder and shareholder in NHS provider organisations and is a key source of funding for capital investment. It can also secure additional sources of funding (e.g. through existing prescription and dental charges, and directly allocates resources to local authorities for public health).
- Sponsoring national health and care system bodies by supporting them and holding them to account for the delivery of their role. 'Sponsorship' means the DHSC ensuring organisations are delivering their functions, meeting their statutory duties, and using public money efficiently and effectively. The specifics of the relationships between the DHSC and its sponsored bodies are set down in 'framework agreements'.
- Fostering relationships, collaborating with patient organisations, and ensuring the system works well together. This involves ensuring all health and care bodies, and other bodies, work effectively together and with common purpose, whilst recognising their own unique roles and autonomy in deciding how to carry out their defined functions. The DHSC also works with other government departments on health matters.
- Creating and updating the policy and legislative frameworks within which the health and care system operates. It oversees an effective regulatory framework that ensures all organisations and professionals meet essential standards of quality and safety.
- Accounting to Parliament and the public for the effectiveness of the health and care system. This includes supporting ministerial accountability to Parliament and the public for the effectiveness of the health and care systems, the effective use of resources voted by Parliament, and the discharge of Secretary of State's legal duties. Ultimately, the Secretary of State has powers to remove the chairs of the major national health bodies from office and (in the case of significant failure to exercise their functions properly) powers of direction, which could force an organisation to undertake or cease a particular course of action. Failure to comply with such a direction could result in the function being carried out by another body. The DHSC is accountable to Parliament and the public. It does not lead on the day-to-day running and organisation of health services.

Whilst the DHSC remains responsible for the health and care legislative framework and ministers continue to be ultimately accountable, most day-to-day operational management in the NHS takes place at arm's length from the DHSC since HSCA 2012. With the exception of the remaining special health authorities, all organisations in the NHS have their own statutory functions conferred by legislation, rather than delegated to them by the Secretary of State.

The Statement of Accountability sets out a number of areas of focus within the NHS structure, namely:

- providing care;
- commissioning care;

- improving public health;
- empowering people and local communities;
- supporting the health and care system;
- education and training; and
- safeguarding patients' health.

The individual parts of the NHS that make up this NHS structure are set out in Figure 4.1, which shows the main organisations that now make up the healthcare system in England.

Providing care

The provision of healthcare by the NHS is divided into two sections: primary and secondary care.

Primary care

Providers of 'primary care' are the first point of contact for physical and mental health and wellbeing concerns in non-urgent cases. These include GPs, dentists, opticians and pharmacists (for medicines and medical advice). For urgent cases, patients can visit a provider of urgent care, such as an accident and emergency department. Health care professionals within GP practices aim to resolve problems locally, including through services provided by the practice. If a condition requires more specialised treatment, or further investigation, patients may be referred to another healthcare provider. These could be based in a hospital, or in the community. Patients are entitled (where possible) to choose between different types of care and providers of their care. They should be supported to make the choice that is best for them.

Community-based care is becoming the preferred means of providing care for the majority of longer-term and mild to moderate conditions. This enables people to keep their normal routine, staying close to family and friends. Hospital services remain a key part of the NHS, such as for specialised, surgical or emergency care.

Secondary care

Providers of secondary care are those bodies that provide acute healthcare. This can be either elective care or emergency care. Elective care means planned specialist medical care or surgery, usually following referral from a primary or community health professional such as a GP. Most of these services are provided by 'NHS bodies', which are part of the public sector.

There are, however, also many other types of organisation involved in providing NHS care, including providers from the independent sector or voluntary sector. For example, pharmacies tend to be independent sector organisations, and most GPs and dentists have traditionally worked as contractors for the NHS, either individually or in partnerships. The third sector includes organisations such as local community groups, voluntary groups, registered charities, social enterprises

THE STRUCTURE OF THE NHS 65

and co-operatives. All organisations contracted to provide NHS services must meet the NHS's required levels of care. Not all provider organisations, however, will have a board as such; for example, GP practices are unlikely to have boards. Every organisation, however, will have a person or people who are legally accountable for the service they are providing.

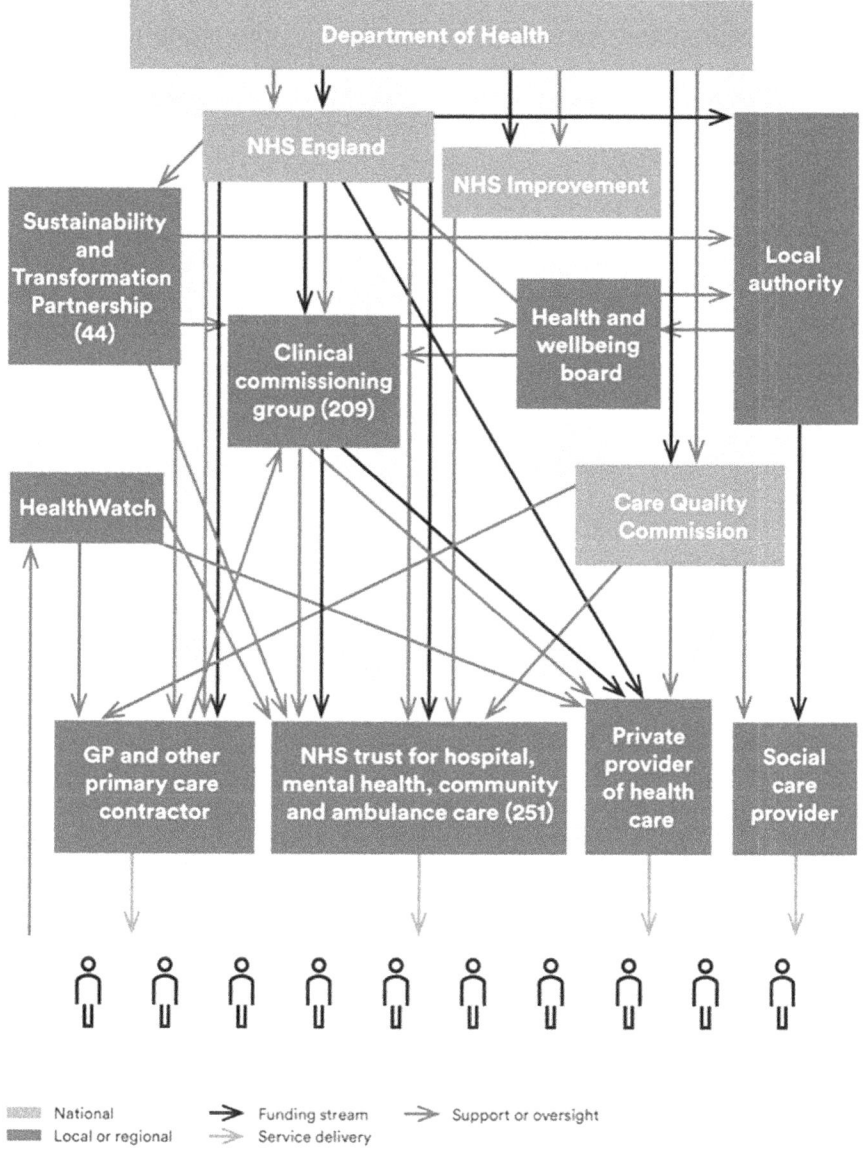

Figure 4.1: The NHS structure

The majority of NHS services, such as hospitals, belong to either an NHS trust or FT. Until recently it has been the government's ambition that all NHS trusts would ultimately become NHS FTs. Each trust can have multiple sites, meaning one or more hospitals often belong to a single trust. However with the developments of new care models and the proposed transformation work of the Sustainability and Transformation Partnerships (STPs) (see Chapter 16) this may not now be the case and non-FTs (NHS trusts) may well find themselves involved in joint ventures, mergers & acquisitions or other collaborative models of working (see Chapter 16). The secondary care sector is regulated by NHSI, which is the operational name for the organisation that brings together Monitor and the NHS Trust Development Authority.

As of September 2018, there were 150 FTs with a number of mergers & takeovers completed resulting in a remaining 77 NHS trusts. There are still further mergers and acquisitions under consideration. NHSI has incorporated Monitor's role to 'authorise' new FTs. In order to become an FT, NHS trusts had to demonstrate that they were well led and able to provide good quality services for patients on a sustainable basis, achieving an overall rating of 'Good' or 'Outstanding' from the Chief Inspector of Hospitals. There is more information on these ratings in the section below on the CQC. The STP process, which was covered in more detail in Chapter 3, will incorporate similar standards for NHS trusts, but may require these trusts to become part of an FT or a different type of organisation as set out in the Dalton Review in December 2014.

Foundation trusts

In NHS FTs, the board of directors is directly accountable to their local population through their membership and council of governors. The public, patients, service users, their families and carers, and staff can join their local FT as members. Members elect governors to represent them. In an FT, the council of governors oversees the organisation's board, holding the board to account for the performance of their organisation. These are covered in more detail in Chapter 14.

NHS trusts

In NHS trusts, the board is accountable to the Secretary of State for Health and Social Care via NHSI. The services and hospitals that are currently NHS trusts are included within the 5YFV STPs. Such trusts will be required to become part of the footprints within their respective STPs, which may or may not include FT status (see Chapter 16).

Commissioning care

The NHS is funded by taxation with a fixed budget available to spend on services for the whole population. The challenge faced by the NHS is how to spend that budget in a way that results in the best possible outcomes for individual patients and delivers value for money for the public. This planning and purchasing of NHS services is undertaken by organisations (or individuals) known as commissioners. They are responsible for assessing the reasonable needs of their populations and using their buying power as purchasers to secure services that are affordable and of the highest quality. They can buy services from any provider that meets NHS standards of care and prices. As part of their role, commissioners have to work together with providers to determine the services needed for local areas.

Clinical commissioning groups

Given the complexity and scale of the healthcare system, it is more efficient to plan and commission healthcare at a population level, such as for a town and its surroundings or a metropolitan borough. All GP practices are required to be a member of CCG. In order to plan their commissioning decisions, local authorities and CCGs (coming together through health and wellbeing boards (HWBs)) use Joint Strategic Needs Assessments (JSNAs), and Joint Health and Wellbeing Strategies (JHWSs) to agree local priorities for local health and care commissioning. CCGs are held to account by their regulator NHSE which has a statutory duty (under the HSCA 2012) to conduct an annual assessment of every CCG. The framework for this and further detail on the structure and governance arrangements for CCGs can be found in Chapter 15.

NHS England (NHSE)

As it is not appropriate to commission some services locally, NHSE (known in HSCA 2012 as the NHS Commissioning Board) commissions these services, which are more appropriate to commission at a national level. These include specialised services (such as those for rare diseases), offender healthcare and some services for members of the armed forces. NHSE is also responsible for commissioning primary care, including GP services.

In addition to commissioning services itself, NHSE also has responsibility for ensuring the overall system of commissioning NHS-funded services works well. This involves working on plans to improve commissioning for specific conditions (such as dementia) or patient groups (such as children's services). NHSE provides information and resources for CCGs and holds them to account for how they carry out their commissioning activities and improve the healthcare outcomes that matter locally.

NHSE is an executive non-departmental public body. It works under its mandate from the government to improve the quality of NHS care and health outcomes, reduce health inequalities, empower patients and the public and promote innovation. Its key responsibilities include:

- authorisation and oversight of CCGs and support for their ongoing development;
- the direct commissioning of primary care, specialised health services, prison healthcare and some public health services (including, for a transitional period, health visiting and family nurse partnerships); and

- developing and sustaining effective partnerships across the health and care system.

NHSE was originally established with 27 area teams but has now been integrated into five regional teams: London; Midlands and East; North; South East and South West, each maintaining a local presence. The regions cover healthcare commissioning and delivery across their geographies and provide professional leadership on finance, nursing, medical, specialised commissioning, patients and information, human resources, organisational development, assurance and delivery. The regional teams work closely with organisations such as CCGs, local authorities, HWBs as well as GP practices. As closer working with NHSI continues, the regional teams will be integrated under the leadership of one regional director working for both organisations, and a move to seven regional teams.

NHSE is one single organisation with senior clinical leadership at all levels operating to a common model. It has one board, composed of:

- the chair of the board (appointed by the Secretary of State);
- eight other members (appointed by the Secretary of State) who, together with the chair, are the non-executive members of the board; and
- the chief executive and three other executive members.

In the 5YFV, NHSE set out its vision for the future. This is set out in more detail in Chapter 16. Overall, the NHSE has been set the objective of ensuring that any proposals for major service change meet four tests:

1. strong public and patient engagement;
2. consistency with current and prospective need for patient choice;
3. a clear clinical evidence base; and
4. support for proposals from clinical commissioners.

If the relevant local authority does not consider the proposed changes to be in the best interests of the local population, they can refer the matter to the Secretary of State.

NHSE is operationally independent from the DHSC, with the SoS setting out what the government expects from NHSE in the Mandate. The Mandate, a legally binding annual publication by the SoS setting out NHSE's objectives, highlights the areas of health and care where the government expects to see improvements in the NHS and contains a number of objectives which NHSE must seek to achieve. The Mandate is intended to provide the NHS with stability to plan ahead; it is set for a number of years at a time. The SoS refreshes it every year, albeit not during the year without the agreement of NHSE (except in exceptional circumstances or after a General Election). It is the main way in which the SoS holds NHSE to account for the NHS commissioning system. The Mandate 2016/17 set out objectives to 2020, which centred on the 5YFV and seven-day working in the NHS. This mandate was refreshed for 2018/19. It also sets an overarching objective for

NHSE to improve outcomes for people using the NHS, in particular to improve against all indicators (or measures) in the NHS Outcomes Framework. The NHS Outcomes Framework sets out the outcomes and corresponding indicators used to hold NHSE to account for improvements in quality. It was developed in partnership between clinicians and stakeholders. NHSE then follows a similar approach in the CCG Improvement and Assessment Framework (CCG IAF) which is used as a central framework for public accountability of the NHS. The CCG IAF has also been designed to supply performance indicators for adoption in STPs as markers of success. More detail on the reporting requirements and assurance role of NHSE is contained in Chapter 18.

During 2018, the trust oversight role of NHSI (not the market regulation role of Monitor) was combined with NHSE's role again via a legal workaround rather than legislative change. The organisations cannot have the same Chair and CEO so instead cross-representation on their respective boards has been created through the creation of associate (non-voting) NEDs. Joint senior appointments are being made, and the regional structures of the two organisations are progressively being merged as seven new joint regional offices are developed. Interestingly this will begin to blur the commissioner/provider split at a national level, but further information will be needed as to the new regional offices will relate to STPs, ICSs and local systems.

Commissioning support units (CSUs)

CSUs provide commissioning support services to NHS commissioners, including local CCGs, NHSE, acute trusts and local government.

Commissioning support is NHS money spent on non-clinical services. While CSUs do not provide direct patient care or treatment, the five CSUs across England play a key role in helping commissioners to improve patient care and achieve savings, releasing resources for reinvestment in frontline clinical services. The units are designed to provide commissioning support services that enable clinical commissioners to maximise resources and focus their clinical expertise and leadership on securing the best outcomes for patients and driving up quality of NHS patient services.

CSU specialist support services include:

- contract management and negotiation;
- business intelligence;
- information governance;
- financial management;
- human resources (HR), estates and IT;
- healthcare procurement and market management;
- non-clinical purchasing;
- communications and patient engagement; and
- bespoke services such as individual funding request management, infection prevention, governance and quality.

CSUs are not geographically defined. In some cases, customers are local or regional clinical commissioners, and in others, they include CCGs in other parts of England. Some CSUs also provide services to NHSE, local government, and acute trusts. In addition to specialist business support services, CSUs work in partnership with NHSE, commissioners, acute and community health and social care providers to develop new services and improve existing services through innovation in technology, data intelligence, clinical pathway design, patient experience initiatives and patient information campaigns.

Currently governed by NHSE, CSUs were planned to become autonomous organisations in 2016 as fully established, self-sustaining entities in a competitive market. There is at present no update on progress to achieve this. CSU's are managed by an executive team, which reports to the CSU's managing director. The managing director is directly accountable to NHSE.

Local authorities

Local authorities (or councils) have a wide range of duties and responsibilities regarding the health of their populations. These extend beyond the NHS into both public health and social care. Since 1 April 2013, local government has led the public health system at local level. The changes under the HSCA 2012 also mean that local authorities in England have a statutory duty to take steps to improve the health of the people in their area as well as other public health functions and in order to improve their work, CCGs and local authorities have, for example, the freedom to commission services together. The relevant local authorities are:

- county councils;
- unitary authorities, including metropolitan district councils;
- London boroughs and the Common Council of the City of London; and
- the Council of the Isles of Scilly.

With these new functions comes the responsibility for a range of services that were previously commissioned and provided by NHS bodies. This does not mean that local authorities are now NHS bodies. However, when they are undertaking their public health functions, they are an important part of the comprehensive health service and, like NHS bodies, must have regard to the NHS Constitution.

Local authorities also commission social care for their local populations based on local criteria and national minimum standards. Unlike NHS care, state funded social care is means tested. The DHSC has responsibility for national adult social care policy and has committed to changing how care is paid for (subject to legislation), with the overall aim of a sustainable and fair partnership between the government and individual for care costs. The Adult Social Care Outcomes Framework defines national priorities for the social care sector and includes indicators that enable the public and other stakeholders to assess the performance of services. The Department for Education has responsibility for national children's social care policy.

Upper tier and unitary local authorities in England have, by law, powers to review and scrutinise any matter relating to the planning, provision and operation of the health service (including public health) in its area. This enables scrutiny of the quality of services provided locally and proposals put forward for significant changes to those services, such as re-organising stroke care in an area. Every upper tier and unitary local authority area in England has arrangements with a Local Healthwatch organisation to support patient and public involvement activities in its area.

Local authorities also have the responsibility for improving the public health of the people in their area. This includes the planning and provision of public health services, such as smoking cessation, and considering the public health effects through the planning of other linked services, such as education, housing, social care and transport. Local authorities are supported in this work by PHE.

One of the criticisms of a number of STPs is that they have not included the local authorities sufficiently for this engagement to occur and consequently this is having an impact on the ability of the STP to deliver. Indeed, a number of STPs have adopted a local brand for system working other than the STP, which is more appealing to local partners and the public. For example, the Coventry and Warwickshire STP has now been renamed the Better Health, Better Care, Better Value programme.

Figure 4.2 sets outs how the money flows within the NHS.

Improving public health

Whilst responsibilities for improving health lie with both providers and commissioners, PHE has a key responsibility in this area with regard to local authorities.

Public Health England (PHE)

PHE is an operationally independent executive agency of the DHSC, which supports local authorities in their duty to improve public health and has national responsibility for protecting the public against major health risks. NHSE also commissions some national public health services. PHE makes comparative data available to help drive improvements and reports annually on progress against the public health outcomes set out in the Public Health Outcomes Framework.

The CEO of PHE is responsible for the leadership and management of PHE and the delivery of its objectives and is accountable to the SoS. The CEO is appointed by the DHSC Permanent Secretary through fair and open competition in line with the Civil Service Commission Recruitment Principles. The CEO has an unfettered right of access to the Secretary of State and Minister with responsibility for public health to raise any matters or concerns and to respond personally to any issues they wish to raise.

72 HEALTH SERVICE GOVERNANCE HANDBOOK

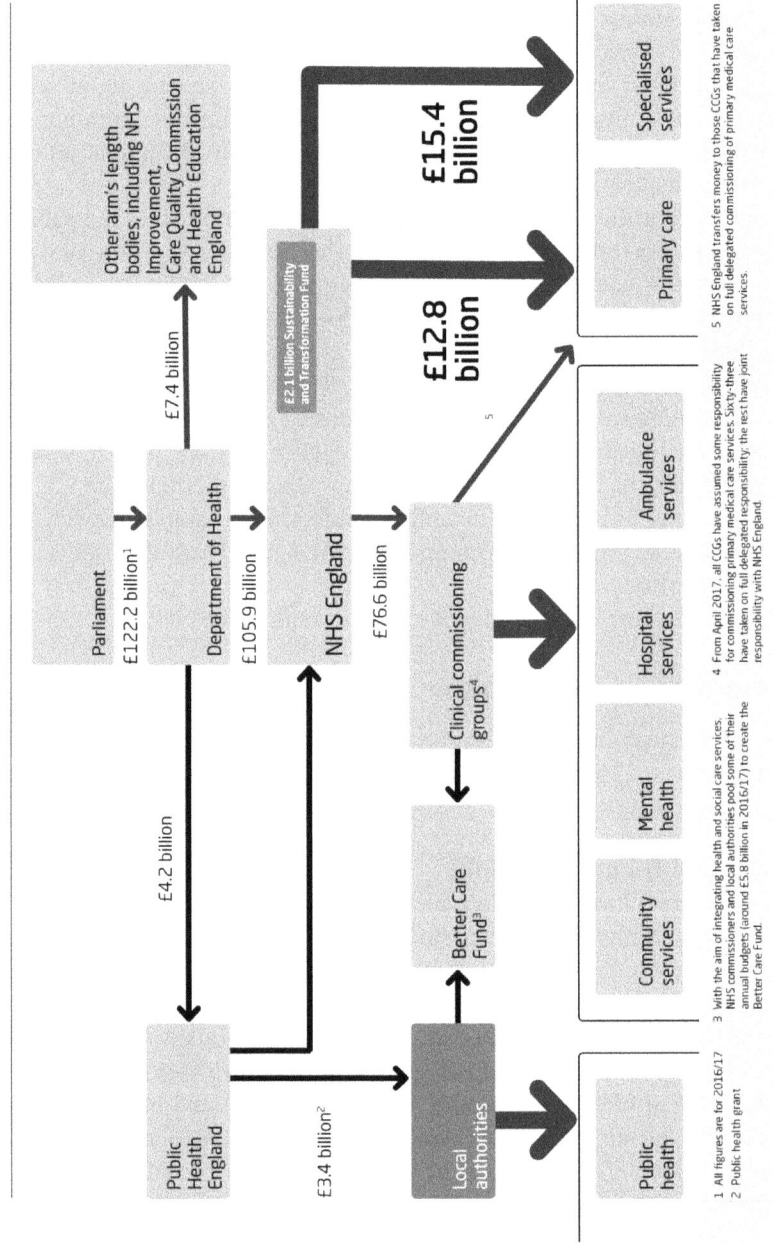

Figure 4.2: Money flow in the NHS (2016/2017)

The CEO is supported by an Advisory Board, of which the non- executive Chair and non-executive members are appointed by the Secretary of State. Appointments are transparent, made on merit and managed in a way that complies with the Commissioner for Public Appointments' Code of Practice for Ministerial Appointments to Public Bodies.

Empowering people and local communities

There are a number of ways in which the NHS structure makes provision for the engagement of the public and local communities.

Overview and Scrutiny Committees

The public's opinion can influence local health services through the overview and scrutiny committees of local authorities. Overview and scrutiny committees (OSCs) are made up of elected local councillors, supported by council officials. They allow democratically elected community leaders to voice the views of their constituents and require local NHS bodies to listen and respond.

OSCs have the power to scrutinise the operation and planning of local health services. All councillors, except for leaders and cabinet members, are able to be members of overview and scrutiny committees. They review the policies made by the council and its partners. They can refer decisions back to the cabinet or decision-maker for reconsideration if they have concerns. This power of scrutiny includes the right to scrutinise and make reports to NHS bodies, require officers of NHS bodies to attend scrutiny committee meetings when requested (often called the Health Overview and Scrutiny Committee (HOSC)), ask for information about the planning and provision of services from NHS bodies and require them to respond to their recommendations. Where scrutiny committees have concerns about substantial changes being proposed by NHS bodies, if they were not considered to be in the interests of local health services, they can refer decisions back to the NHS. If these are not satisfactorily resolved, they can be referred to the Secretary of State.

As such, the HOSC has held NHS bodies to account for the quality of their services through these powers. Under HSCA 2012, local authorities were no longer required to have overview and scrutiny committees to discharge health scrutiny functions but they continue to have such functions, which they are able to discharge in various ways. For example, local authorities may choose to continue to operate their prior HOSCs, or may choose to put in place other arrangements such as appointing committees involving members of the public. HSCA 2012 also provided that the requirements for an NHS body to consult the local authority overview and scrutiny committee and to require officers of NHS bodies to attend before the committee to answer questions will also potentially include CCGs, NHSE and other providers of health services, including independent sector providers.

If there is a HOSC, then it should be involved early on in discussions about any reconfiguration of health services and should take a view about whether changes are in the interests of local health services. For example, it can examine the proposal in the light of councillors' knowledge of their local area and make recommendations about how the people who use services, particularly vulnerable groups, can be informed about changes to services. It should also assess the impact of such changes after implementation.

Instead of the HOSC, the HWBs created by HSCA 2012 were set up to operate differently from these existing local authority scrutiny committees. This was because, for the first time, officers (such as the director of adult social services, the director of children's services and the director of public health), CCGs and the local Healthwatch will have the same statutory status as councillors.

Although local authorities are no longer required to have such committees as the means by which they discharge their scrutiny function, in practice most have retained them. The last guidance from Government on scrutiny was issued in 2006. The role of scrutiny has changed significantly since then and the Government has committed to publishing new guidance but the timetable for this continues to be delayed. This guidance will consider the increased scrutiny of external bodies, most notably health bodies given that councils are delivering services through increasingly varied partnership arrangements – including contracting to private companies, creating arms-length bodies or working with other public bodies.

Health and wellbeing boards (HWBs)

HWBs were established by the HSCA 2012 and are formally constituted council committees. They were established to encourage work to improve local health and wellbeing outcomes, including (where appropriate) more joined-up working across the NHS, public health, social care and other services.

The boards have very limited formal powers. They are constituted as a partnership forum rather than an executive decision-making body. In most cases, HWBs are chaired by a senior local authority elected member. The board must include a representative of each relevant CCG and local Healthwatch, as well as local authority representatives. The local authority has considerable discretion in appointing additional board members. Most have chosen not to invite providers to become formal members, though many engage with providers in other ways.

HWBs assess the current and future health and social care needs of the local community through JSNAs. JSNAs are based on a principle of analysing the available evidence on the local community's health and social care needs. This includes engaging and working with a wide range of local stakeholders such as patient groups, voluntary organisations and the public. Using the JSNA, HWBs jointly agree strategic priorities for local health and social care services in JHWSs. Taken together, JSNAs and JHWSs are intended to form the basis of commissioning plans across local health and care services (including public health and children's services) for CCGs, NHSE and local authorities. Boards are under a statutory duty to involve local people in the preparation of JSNAs and the development of JHWSs.

A progress report published in April 2017, *The Power of Place*, a fourth review of the state of health and wellbeing boards concluded that the context in which HWBs now operate is much more pressured and politically turbulent, with the most significant organisational development being the establishing of STPs across 44 geographical footprints in England. Most STPs cover several HWBs and as a consequence there was a wide spread perception that the STP process had by-passed many HWBs.

The report also reviewed the drivers of and barriers to effect of HWBs; it identified five factors as particularly important. They are as follows:

- A focus on place: 'the role of the HWB is to have a strong message about what the local vision and priorities are and to have the confidence to argue for what is needed.'
- Committed leadership: 'the value of the HWB being chaired by the council leader or by a cabinet member with a role or breadth of interest and influence that extends beyond health and care.'
- 'Collaborative plumbing': 'the HWB board is able to exploit its members' other roles to understand and informally influence developments associated with the STP.'
- A geography that works: 'the role of an effective board is to make the geography work.'
- A director of public health who understands the role of the HWB: 'helping to shape the development of the HWB and its work programme'.

HWBs in their entirety remain accountable to communities, service users and overview and scrutiny committees. All board members also have incentives to deliver on shared objectives to improve efficiency.

The Parliamentary and Health Service Ombudsman (PHSO)

The PHSO or 'the Ombudsman' is an independent crown servant appointed by the Queen. The Ombudsman's role is to investigate independently complaints that individuals have been treated unfairly or have received poor service from government departments and other public organisations and the NHS in England. Although the service has separate parliamentary and health functions, both come under the same Ombudsman. The Ombudsman can look at complaints about the actions of providers of NHS care, as well as commissioners, and at complaints about the DHSC, NHSE, the CQC and NHSI.

The PHSO is governed by a unitary, decision-making board of executives and non-executives, whose purpose is to lead, provide stewardship and to preserve and build its reputation. PHSO executive directors will be ex-officio executive members of the Board. Executive directors are appointed by the Chair of the

Board, a senior NED and the Managing Director. The Managing Director is appointed by two non-executive directors including the senior non-executive, and the Ombudsman. The Ombudsman is accountable to Parliament through the Public Administration and Constitutional Affairs Committee. The Ombudsman is independent of the NHS.

The Ombudsman had already set out principles that were intended to promote a shared understanding of what is meant by good complaint handling and to help public bodies in the Parliamentary and Health Service Ombudsman's jurisdiction deliver first-class complaint handling to all their customers. The Francis report prompted the Prime Minister and the Secretary of State for Health and Social Care to commission a review of NHS hospital complaints handling, co-chaired by the Rt. Hon. Ann Clwyd and Professor Tricia Hart, which endorsed these principles.

Following the publication of this review, the PHSO suggested that NHS organisations use the option of self-referral for the most serious cases to the PHSO for independent investigation. This allows the PHSO to play its part in delivering justice, discovering what went wrong and ultimately helping the NHS to restore public trust in what is such a key public service.

From April 2016, the Independent Patient Safety Investigation Service (IPSIS) will also offer support and guidance to NHS organisations on investigations into the most serious complaints and carry out some investigations itself.

Healthwatch England and Local Healthwatch

The Healthwatch network consists of two connected levels:

- Healthwatch England works at the national level and supports local Healthwatch organisations. It takes local experiences of health and care and uses them to influence national policy with CQC, NHSE, NHSI and local authorities.
- A local Healthwatch organisation covers every local authority area in England. They take the experiences that people have of local care and use them to help shape local services.

Healthwatch England is the consumer champion for both health and social care and has a role in gathering people's views on their local health and care services. When established, the organisation was hosted by the CQC but reported directly to the DHSC. However, in January 2016, after the departure of its first chief executive, it was announced that a new national director would be appointed who would report to the chief executive of the CQC. Interestingly the national director is still expected to criticise the workings of the CQC where appropriate, despite the conflict created by reporting to the CQC CEO.

Healthwatch's role is to provide national leadership, support and advice to local Healthwatch organisations and to ensure that the collective voice of patients has a direct route into the CQC's decision-making processes operating independently from the CQC. NHSE can escalate concerns about health and social care services raised by local Healthwatch, users of services and members of the public to the CQC. Healthwatch England is also able to provide advice and information (which could include making recommendations and reports) to the Secretary of State, NHSE, NHSI and local authorities. The recipients of Healthwatch England's advice are required in law to respond to Healthwatch England in writing.

The aim of local Healthwatch is to give citizens and communities a stronger voice to influence and challenge how health and social care services are provided within their area. They enable people to share their views and concerns about their local health and social care services to help build a picture of where services are doing well and where they can be improved. Local Healthwatch can also alert Healthwatch England to concerns about specific health and care providers, as well as provide people with information about their choices and what to do when things go wrong – including supporting people who want to complain about NHS services. Local Healthwatch organisations are able to enter and view certain health and social care premises, produce reports and make recommendations that influence the way services are designed and delivered. Local Healthwatch organisations provide information and advice to the public about local services, and pass on views to Healthwatch England. They can also make recommendations to Healthwatch England and the CQC. If a local Healthwatch organisation sends a report or recommendation to a specified provider or commissioner of a local health or social care service, the provider or commissioner is legally obliged to respond to the local Healthwatch organisation in writing.

The Local Government Association (LGA) and the DHSC jointly published a document in 2013 to help local Healthwatch audiences understand the legal requirements that have been set out in regulations. Local Healthwatch Regulations Explained aims to explain and provide clarity in relation to the following issues:

- layperson and volunteer involvement in local Healthwatch; and
- restrictions on activities of a political nature.

Supporting the health and care system

Underpinning the work of primary and secondary care there are a number of special health authorities and national bodies who function it is to take on the national agenda for specific aspects of health and social care delivery.

Special health authorities

Special health authorities are health authorities that provide a health service to the whole of England, not just to a local community. They have been set up to provide a national service to the NHS or the public under section 9 of the NHS Act 1977. They are independent but can be subject to ministerial direction in the same way as other NHS bodies. Examples of special authorities are set out below:

NHS Improvement (NHSI)

From 1 April 2016, NHSI was established, which is the operational name for an organisation that incorporates:

- NHS Trust Development Authority (NHS TDA) (regulator for NHS trusts);
- Monitor (regulator for FTs);
- Patient Safety;
- the National Reporting and Learning System;
- Advancing Change Team; and
- Intensive Support Teams.

NHSI is led by a unitary board consisting of non-executive and executive directors, although it needs to be recognised that both the statutory organisations of NHS TDA and Monitor remain in existence. The NHS TDA was established as a special health authority in June 2012 and Monitor was established as an executive non-departmental public body of the DHSC. This 'merger' was created through a legal workaround; NHS TDA and Monitor now have the same chief executive and chair, while still technically operating with separate boards and producing separate accounts.

NHSI is responsible for overseeing FTs, NHS trusts and independent providers that provide NHS-funded care. It offers the support these providers need to give patients consistently safe, high quality, compassionate care within local health systems that are financially sustainable. By holding providers to account and, where necessary, intervening, it aims to help the NHS to meet its short-term challenges and secure its future. It works closely with NHSE and CQC to ensure alignment and collaboration of support and accountability.

NHSI has set five themes as its strategic objectives. These are in line with Implementing the Forward View. These themes are:

- quality of care;
- finance and use of resources;
- operational performance;
- strategic change; and
- leadership and improvement capability.

More detail on the reporting requirements and assurance role of NHSI can be found in Chapter 18.

NHS Resolution

The NHS Resolution (April 2017) is the operating name that combines the three operating arms of NHS Litigation Authority (NHSLA), the National Clinical Assessment Service and the Family Health Services Appeal Unit to assist the NHS to resolve litigation concerns fairly, as well as share lessons learnt to improve clinical practice and preserve resources for patient care.

The NHSLA was established in 1995 as a special health authority as a not-for-profit part of the NHS. It provides indemnity cover for legal claims against the NHS, assists the NHS with risk management, shares lessons from claims and provides other legal and professional services for its members. As a special health authority, the NHSLA is an arm's-length body of the DHSC. It is an independent body, but can be subject to ministerial direction.

The NHSLA has a unitary board consisting of a non-executive chair, four other non-executive members and four executive members, holding the offices of the CEO and accounting officer (AO), chief finance officer (CFO), and such other executive appointments as required by legislation. The Secretary of State appoints the chair, and other non-executive directors. The DHSC principal accounting officer appoints the chief executive. The chair, chief executive and other non-executive directors are responsible for appointing the executive directors.

The NHS Blood and Transplant Authority (NHSBTA)

The NHS Blood and Transplant Authority is responsible for the supply of blood, organs, plasma and tissues across the NHS. It was established by legislation in 2005. The CQC monitors, inspects and regulates its services to make sure they meet fundamental standards of quality and care.

NHSBT is led by a Board comprised of a non-executive chair, appointed by the SoS for Health and Social Care and not more than eight non-executive members, also appointed by the SoS. One of these members will always include a person with particular experience suited to the interests of Wales. The board also includes a chief executive appointed by the non-executive chair and non-executive members and not more than eight executive board members, including the chief executive, finance director and medical director. The non-executive chair, non-executive members and the chief executive appoint the executive board members.

National bodies

There are a number of other bodies or authorities involved in the provision or organisation of NHS services. They have responsibility for things that are most effectively carried out or coordinated at the national level. Some examples are as follows.

The National Institute for Health and Care Excellence (NICE)

This is the main source of evidence-based guidance and advice for health and social care practitioners, patients, service users and the public on the most effective way to prevent, diagnose and treat disease and ill health. NICE produces quality standards and concise sets of statements that describe what high-quality care looks like for a particular condition or patient group which are used to drive up the quality of health and care services.

It was established in primary legislation in April 2013, becoming an executive non-departmental public body (ENDPB) as set out in HSCA 2012. At this time, it also took on responsibility for developing guidance and quality standards in social care. As an ENDPB, it is accountable to the DHSC, but operationally it is independent of government. The NICE Board sets the strategic priorities and policies, but the day-to-day decision making is the responsibility of the senior management team

The Medicines and Healthcare Products Regulatory Agency
This is responsible for ensuring that medicines and medical devices work and are acceptably safe. It was created by Parliament as an executive agency of the DHSC and is overseen by a unitary board consisting of the MHRA's chairman, nine non-executive directors and two executive members (chief executive and chief operating officer (COO). The non-executive members are appointed by the Secretary of State following open competition.

The Human Fertilisation and Embryology Authority (HFEA)
This is the UK's independent regulator of treatment using eggs and sperm and of treatment and research involving human embryos. They set standards and issue licences to fertility clinics. It is an ENDPB, operating under the provisions in the Human Fertilisation and Embryology Act 1990, as amended. Under the 1990 Act, the HFEA is statutorily independent of government but works in partnership with the DHSC. It is led by a board made up of a non-executive chair appointed by the Secretary of State; a deputy chair and ten authority members, also appointed by the Secretary of State. The board appoints the chief executive, who is not a member of the board.

Education and training

There is a national requirement for appropriately trained staff to ensure the delivery of health and social care. These obligations are also undertaken by a number of special health authorities and national bodies.

Health Education England (HEE)
Originally established as a Special Health Authority in 2012, HEE is a NDPB, as of 1 April 2015, under the provisions of the Care Act 2014. HEE is responsible for promoting high-quality training and education, undertaking national planning and leadership, allocating financial resources, monitoring outcomes and securing the required supply of qualified staff. Long-term national planning is needed because a medical student graduating today will still be providing care in 2050. The DHSC has until recently set HEE's direction and its expectations for the whole education and training system through a document called the Education Outcomes Framework. In October 2018, the DHSC announced HEE would be 'accountable' to and 'report' via NHSI rather than directly to government. The formal arrangements were unclear at the time of publication but it would seem

that whilst HEE will continue to operate as a separate organisation with a board, it will agree its annual plan with NHSI before agreeing the plan with the DHSC. From 1 April 2019, the NHS Leadership Academy moved from HEE to NHSE and NHSI, in order to directly support the leadership and talent management requirements of the NHS Long Term plan. HEE's four regional teams will be restructured to align with the new joint NHSE and NHSI regions.

Clinical senates

Clinical senates are advisory groups of experts from across health and social care. They are non-statutory bodies and do not have a legal duty to commission health services. There are 12 senates covering areas across England providing strategic clinical advice and leadership across a broad geographical area to CCGs, health and wellbeing boards and NHSE. Senates are formed by clinical leaders from across the healthcare system, as well as those from social care and public health. Patients and members of the public will also be involved. They work with strategic clinical networks, academic health science networks, local education and training boards and research networks to develop an alignment of these organisations to support improvements in quality.

Safeguarding patients' interests

Organisations providing NHS services are regulated to ensure they meet essential standards. The boards of organisations providing NHS care have the primary responsibility to ensure the care that they provide is safe and high quality. Regulators exist to ensure providers are fulfilling their obligations to patients and the public. The system of regulation is independent from the government and from the NHS itself. It exists to ensure that the care patients receive is safe and of acceptable quality. The regulators also make sure the bodies or healthcare professionals they regulate are sound and fit for purpose.

The 2013 Francis Report identified a lack of clarity about the roles of NHS regulatory organisations. In response, the government announced that the CQC would focus on assessing the level of quality of care for NHS FTs and NHS trusts whilst Monitor and the NHS TDA would focus on using their powers, where necessary, to intervene to resolve quality failings. There has been further alignment and clarification with the amalgamation of Monitor and the NHS TDA under the umbrella of NHSI. As mentioned previously NHSE and NHSI have announced they will transform the way they work together 'to provide more joined-up, effective and comprehensive system leadership to the NHS'.

Care Quality Commission (CQC)

From April 2009, the safety and quality regulator for all health services has been the CQC, which is also responsible for the regulation of adult social care services. The CQC is responsible for assessing and making judgements as to the level of safety and quality of care provided by providers of health and social care. To make these assessments, CQC can look at information received from the provider itself, its patients, staff and from other organisations; it also conducts its own inspections. Information is published on the CQC website.

Providers of healthcare (including hospitals, care homes, care delivered in the home, dentists, GPs, mental health and other specialist services such as hospices) must register with CQC in order to be able to carry on regulated activities, which include the provision of NHS-funded health services.

The CQC is a NDPB within the DHSC. The CQC board is the senior decision-making structure and it is accountable to the public, Parliament and the Secretary of State for Health and Social Care. The DHSC and CQC agreed a Framework Document in 2010, which set out CQC's purpose, its governance and accountability, management and financial responsibilities and reporting procedures. This was last reviewed in 2014 and is due to be reviewed again to take account of subsequent legislative changes.

The CQC's unitary board is made up of the CQC's chair, NEDs and EDs, including the chief executive and the three chief inspectors (namely, Hospitals, Adult Social Care and General Practice). It also includes the Chair of Healthwatch. All NEDs are public appointees, appointed by the Secretary of State.

The CQC's principal function in relation to healthcare is to:

- register healthcare providers (whether or not they provide services for the NHS);
- monitor compliance with registration requirements and, if necessary, use its enforcement powers to ensure all service providers meet those requirements;
- review and publish comparative information on organisations providing and commissioning healthcare, and undertake reviews or studies of particular types of care; and
- monitor the operation of the Mental Health Act 1983 and Mental Capacity Act 2005.

All healthcare providers are required to be registered with CQC and some of the emerging models of integrated care under STPs and the new vanguards as well as existing large and complex organisations now present challenges for CQC's current approach to registration. The CQC will need to make sure that providers are clear about who has accountability for quality and that, where relevant, CQC adequately reflect the role of head office or board-level leadership when registering these types of organisation. The CQC have set out what good and outstanding care looks like and ensures that services meet fundamental standards below which care must never fall. These are as follows:

- **Person-centred care:** Patients must have care or treatment that is tailored to them and meets their needs and preferences.
- **Dignity and respect:** Patients must be treated with dignity and respect at all times while they are receiving care and treatment.

- **Consent:** Patients (or anybody legally acting on their behalf) must give their consent before any care or treatment is given.
- **Safety:** Patients must not be given unsafe care or treatment or be put at risk of harm that could be avoided. Providers must assess the risks to the patient's health and safety during any care or treatment and make sure their staff have the qualifications, competence, skills and experience to keep patients safe.
- **Safeguarding from abuse:** Patients must not suffer any form of abuse or improper treatment while receiving care (e.g. neglect, degrading treatment, unnecessary or disproportionate restraint or inappropriate limits on their freedom).
- **Food and drink:** Patients must have enough to eat and drink to keep them in good health while they receive care and treatment.
- **Premises and equipment:** The places where patients receive care and treatment and the equipment used in it must be clean, suitable and looked after properly. The equipment used in a patient's care and treatment must also be secure and used properly.
- **Complaints:** Patients must be able to complain about their care and treatment. The provider of a patient's care must have a system in place so they can handle and respond to their complaint. They must investigate it thoroughly and take action if problems are identified.
- **Good governance:** The provider of a patient's care must have plans that ensure they can meet these standards. They must have effective governance and systems to check on the quality and safety of care. These must help the service improve and reduce any risks to the patient's health, safety and welfare.
- **Staffing:** The provider of a patient's care must have enough suitably qualified, competent and experienced staff to make sure they can meet these standards. Their staff must be given the support, training and supervision they need to help them do their job.
- **Fit and proper staff:** The provider of a patient's care must only employ people who can provide care and treatment appropriate to their role. They must have strong recruitment procedures in place and carry out relevant checks such as on applicants' criminal records and work history.
- **Duty of candour:** The provider of a patient's care must be open and transparent with them about your care and treatment. Should something go wrong, they must tell the patient what has happened, provide support and apologise.
- **Display of ratings:** The provider of a patient's care must display their CQC rating in a place where it can be seen. They must also include this information on their website and make the latest CQC report on their service available to them.

Further detail on the role of the Care Quality Commission is set out in Chapter 18.

The Human Tissue Authority

The Human Tissue Authority is an independent watchdog set up in 2005 following events in the 1990s that revealed a culture in hospitals of removing and retaining human organs and tissue without consent. The legislation that established the Authority not only addressed this issue but also updated and brought together other laws that related to human tissue and organs. It protects the public's interest by licensing and inspecting organisations that store and use human tissues and organs for purposes such as research, patient treatment, transplantation, post-mortem examination, teaching and public exhibitions. It was created by Parliament as an executive agency of the DHSC, and is overseen by lay and professional members appointed by the government.

Professional regulators

There are a number of regulatory bodies that are responsible for the regulation of healthcare professionals. An example is the General Medical Council (GMC), which regulates doctors, and the Nursing and Midwifery Council (NMC), which regulates nurses and midwives.

The professional regulators are independent bodies responsible to Parliament that register and regulate the training and practice of health professionals. They safeguard the safety and the quality of the care that patients receive from health professionals. This includes dealing with concerns about misconduct raised by patients, their families or other professionals. Professional regulators certify new practitioners and ensure that they maintain standards and remain fit to practice. Health professionals can be reported to the relevant professional regulator and guidance is available on the website of the Council for Healthcare Regulatory Excellence (CHRE), which provides an oversight role on professional regulation.

Other examples include:

- doctors (GMC);
- nurses and midwives (NMC);
- dental teams (General Dental Council);
- optical professionals (General Optical Council);
- pharmacists (General Pharmaceutical Council);
- chiropractors (General Chiropractic Council);
- osteopaths (General Osteopathic Council); and
- health, psychological and social work professionals (Health and Care Professions Council).

Summary

- This chapter has included a number of figures in an attempt to demonstrate the inter-relationships that exist within the NHS landscape. Every single part of the structure is bound by health service governance guidance – sometimes in a very direct and explicit way, and at other times less so.

- The chapter has also sought to explore the complexity of relationships that exist between the individual part of the NHS as well as setting out the clear accountability models that form each individual part.
- Whilst this chapter has attempted to capture the essence of that landscape, there are further changes planned for the regulatory framework in the light of the 5YFV. As this chapter has tried to highlight, regulators will need to align their approach to oversight of STPs as set out in the recent *Next steps on the NHS five year forward view*, with any framework designed for regulation and oversight.

5
Health Service Governance and the law

Introduction

This chapter considers the extent to which best practice in both health service governance and corporate governance is imposed on organisations by the law. There are two different approaches to establishing a system of best practice in governance. One approach is to establish laws and other regulations for governance that organisations must obey. A second approach is to establish voluntary principles and guidelines and invite (or expect) organisations to comply with them. In practice, many countries combine legal and regulatory requirements with voluntary principles and codes of conduct. This chapter considers the laws and regulations which have been established and their impact on governance.

The chapter identifies both aspects of health service and corporate governance practice that may be regulated by law or regulations. It will demonstrate that laws and regulations on governance vary, so that some sectors and indeed some countries adopt a 'rules-based' approach to governance, while others rely more on a 'principles-based' approach.

Governance and the law

There is no corporate governance law in any country: rather, some aspects of corporate governance are regulated by sections of different laws. Other aspects of governance are not regulated by law at all or are regulated only partially. Even in the US, where there is greater emphasis on regulation of corporate governance, many elements of 'best practice' in corporate governance are voluntary.

Similarly, there is no health service governance law for the NHS. Different aspects of public law and national legislation regulate some aspects of health service governance; there is also a raft of guidance and voluntary codes that have been established for use within the NHS (these are considered in the next chapter).

It is inevitable that some aspects of health service governance practice are regulated by law, and that organisations should be required to comply with 'best practice'. Regulations on health service governance may be found in:

- healthcare law;
- laws on patient and public involvement;

- laws on transparency of information, mental capacity, human rights, bribery, corporate manslaughter, etc.; and
- company law.

Healthcare law

The National Health Service Act 1948 established the NHS in 1948. Since that time, there have been significant amendments and additions to the legislation, which has resulted in a fragmented and piecemeal approach to NHS healthcare law. Rather than list each amendment and addition since 1948, this section sets out the main items of legislation that result in the current form and structure of the NHS.

The NHS Reorganisation Act 1973 provided for lines of authority from NHS providers up to the SoS through the creation of 90 area health authorities (AHAs), which managed both hospitals and community health services. The AHAs were also given joint planning responsibilities with the local authorities. Beneath the AHAs were District Management Teams, which managed hospitals and family practitioner committees (FPCs) that took responsibility for administering contracts for general practitioners (GPs), dentists, pharmacists and opticians. The AHAs were under the supervision of 14 regional health authorities (RHAs), which operated from 1974 to 1996.

The National Health Service Act 1977 set out the obligations of the SoS to promote a comprehensive health service. The SoS's national responsibilities were delegated to special heath authorities such as the National Blood Authority and National Institute for Health and Clinical Excellence (NICE), whilst their local responsibilities were delegated to AHAs. RHAs on behalf of the SoS carried out the management of these functions.

The Health Services Act 1980 abolished the AHAs and District Management Teams and replaced them with district health authorities (DHAs) in 1982.

The National Health Service and Community Care Act 1990 set out how the NHS should assess and provide for patients based on their needs, requirements and circumstances. It established the split between 'purchasers' (health authorities and some family doctors, under the GP fundholding scheme), who were given budgets to commission healthcare; and 'providers' (acute hospitals, organisations providing care for the mentally ill, people with learning disabilities and the elderly, and ambulance services). The Act introduced the concept of the internal market and established the relationship between the purchasers and the providers as a contractual one. The functions of NHS trusts (the 'providers') were partly determined by the 1990 Act and partly through each individual trust's establishment order. The Act also set out key statutory financial obligations such as the obligation to break even, to carry out functions effectively, efficiently and economically, and to hold a public meeting at which the annual report and audited accounts were presented.

The NHS Trusts (Membership and Procedures) Regulations 1990 set out the composition of the board for NHS trusts, the criteria for appointment and tenure of the chair and NEDs. It sets out the rules regarding the meetings and proceedings of NHS trusts and the appointment procedures for EDs. It was updated by regulations in 1998 amending the size and composition of the board and in 2014 allowing existing NHS chairs or non-executive director to hold additional NED positions within other NHS organisations or bodies.

The Health Authorities Act 1995 abolished regional health authorities, district health authorities and family health services authorities and established a single tier of health authorities.

The Health Act 1999 abolished GP fund-holding in England, Wales and Scotland. The Act amended the National Health Service Act 1977 to make provision for the establishment of new statutory bodies in England and Wales, to be known as primary care trusts and provided for NHS trusts in Scotland to take on additional functions.

The Health and Social Care Act 2001 was designed to deliver many of the aspects of the NHS Plan 2000 that required changes to primary legislation. The Act provided for a new form of trust, care trusts, to provide closer integration of health and social services. It outlined a new delivery system for the NHS, which provided for the commissioning of health and social care by care trusts under partnership arrangements. It also strengthened the arrangements for public and patient involvement in the NHS by providing for local authority OSCs, whose role was to scrutinise the NHS and to represent local views on the development of local health services. It also created a duty on NHS organisations to have arrangements for involving patients and the public in decision making about the operation of the NHS. In addition, it legislated for the establishment of the Healthcare Commission as the regulatory body for healthcare and the Health Service Ombudsman to consider complaints about the handling of NHS complaints by any person or NHS body.

The National Health Service Reform and Health Care Professions Act 2002 provided for amendment of the structural framework of the NHS. The Act renamed health authorities as statutory health authorities and conferred most of their functions onto PCTs. Service planning would be undertaken by the PCTs, with the SHAs providing the performance management function for the health services provided within their boundaries. The Act also provided for the creation of an independent 'Patients' Forum', to perform an inspection, monitoring and representation role on behalf of patients and the public. The national Commission for Patient and Public Involvement in Health (CPPIH) was created to oversee this.

The Health and Social Care (Community Health and Standards) Act 2003 provided for the establishment of NHSFTs that have the right to enter into legally enforceable contracts. The Act also established a new regulatory body for healthcare – the Commission for Healthcare Audit and Inspection (CHAI). It also established the duty of each NHS body to put and keep in place arrangements for the purpose of monitoring and improving the quality of health care provided by and for that body. This duty was further reinforced by the principles of the NHS Constitution.

The Directions to NHS bodies on Counter Fraud Measures 2004 set out that each NHS organisation must take all necessary steps to counter fraud in the NHS in accordance with the Directions. Each NHS organisation must require its CEO and director of finance to monitor and ensure compliance with these Directions, and must cooperate with NHS Protect to enable the Counter Fraud and Security Management Service (CFSMS) efficiently and effectively to carry out its counter-fraud functions. Each NHS organisation must also designate a person to undertake specific responsibility for the promotion of counter fraud measures; in the case of an NHS trust this is to be one of the trust's NEDs and in the case of an NHS body other than an NHS trust, it must be one of that organisation's non-officer members.

The National Health Service Act 2006 (NHS Act 2006) redefined the structure of the NHS in England by consolidating much of the existing legislation concerning the health service. The consolidation repealed and re-enacted in its entirety the National Health Service Act 1977, which was itself a consolidation. It also incorporated provisions from:

- the National Health Service and Community Care Act 1990;
- the Health Authorities Act 1995;
- the Primary Care Act 1997;
- the Health Act 1999;
- the Health and Social Care Act 2001;
- the National Health Service Reform and Health Care Professions Act 2002;
- the Health and Social Care (Community Health and Standards) Act 2003; and
- the Health Act 2006.

The Local Government and Public Involvement in Health Act 2007 reformed the existing arrangements (Patients' Forums) for patient and public involvement in the provision of health and social care services with the creation of Local Involvement Networks (LINks).

The Health and Social Care Act 2008 established the CQC as a single, integrated regulator for health and adult social care to replace the Healthcare Commission (health and adult social care regulator in England), the Commission for Social Care Inspection (social care regulator) and the Mental Health Act Commission (monitoring of Mental Health Act 1983).

The Health Act 2009 set out the framework for how the NHS Constitution would operate, including a new legal duty on providers of NHS services in England and other relevant bodies to have regard to the Constitution, and a duty on the SoS to consult on, review and re-publish the NHS Constitution at least every ten years, and to report on its impact. The Act created the obligation to produce

Quality Accounts and gave the SoS powers in relation to their content (including locally agreed elements), format and timing (see Chapter 18). This legislation also amended the NHS Act 2006 to introduce a special administration process. This made provision for the appointment of a Trust Special Administrator (TSA) over an NHS trust, where the SoS considered it in the interests of the health service. The key objective of a TSA appointed to an NHS trust is to develop and consult locally on a draft report and make recommendations to the SoS in a final report about what should happen to the trust and the services it provides to ensure the continued provision of key services (location specific services). The legal framework sets out a maximum period of 120 working days for completion of the process (unless extended by order of the SoS), by which time the SoS must make a final decision on the future of the NHS trust following the TSA's recommendations.

With many hospitals facing significant financial difficulties as a result of a variety of complex factors, it is vital, both politically and socially, that NHS services are maintained. The DHSC assesses NHS trusts according to their performance against a set of financial and quality indicators. If clinical or financial performance is below the required standard and does not improve then the Regime for Unsustainable Providers could be triggered under Chapter 5A of the NHS Act 2006 as the only way in which the DHSC can take decisive action to deal with NHS trusts that are either unsustainable in their current form or significantly failing to make progress towards attaining FT status.

The Health and Social Care Act 2012 (HSCA 2012) extended this regime to include FTs. It enables NHSI to appoint a TSA where the FT is, or is likely to become, unable to pay its debts. The legal framework applicable to FTs is very similar to NHS trusts, although the timetable is longer to enable NHSI to be consulted (a period of 150 days, unless extended). The framework is different from an ordinary administration under general insolvency legislation in that its main objective is to protect patients and staff from failing services and secure the continued provision of patient services. Examples of its use include South London Healthcare NHS Trust and Mid Staffordshire NHS Foundation Trust and Liverpool Community Health NHS Trust.

The HSCA 2012 introduced significant reforms to the structure of the NHS and continued to drive through the implementation of the split of provider/commissioner relationships. It was brought into force by commencement orders. A commencement order is a Statutory Instrument (SI) which is designed to bring into force the whole or part of an Act of Parliament. Different parts of an Act may be brought into force at different times.

The Care Act 2014 (CA 2014) set out a new framework of local authority duties in relation to the arrangement and funding of social care, along with a number of changes to the regulation of social care providers. Whilst primarily aimed at local

HEALTH SERVICE GOVERNANCE AND THE LAW

authorities, the Act has some key implications for NHS organisations due to the growing integration of health and social care, namely:

- a specific duty of candour on health and social care providers registered with the CQC. (The duty of candour itself, along with the fit and proper persons test are set out in the *Health and Social Care Act 2008 (Regulated Activities) Regulations 2014*);
- a clear legal framework for safeguarding adults from abuse or neglect; and
- additional care standards established and made provision for by HEE.

The statutory duty of candour is duty to be open and honest with patients (or 'service users'), or their families, when something goes wrong that appears to have caused or could lead to significant harm in the future. It applies to all health and social care organisations registered with the CQC in England. The key principles are as follows:

- Care organisations have a general duty to act in an open and transparent way in relation to care provided to patients. This means that an open and honest culture must exist throughout an organisation.
- The statutory duty applies to organisations, not individuals, though it is clear from CQC guidance that it is expected that an organisation's staff cooperate with it to ensure the obligation is met.
- As soon as is reasonably practicable after a notifiable patient safety incident occurs, the organisation must tell the patient (or their representative) about it in person.
- The organisation has to give the patient a full explanation of what is known at the time, including what further enquiries will be carried out. Organisations must also provide an apology and keep a written record of the notification to the patient.
- A notifiable patient safety incident has a specific statutory meaning: it applies to incidents where a patient suffered (or could suffer) unintended harm that results in death, severe harm, moderate harm or prolonged psychological harm. Severe and moderate harm definitions are derived from the National Patient Safety Agency (NPSA) Seven Steps to Patient Safety. Prolonged psychological harm means that it must be experienced continuously for 28 days or more.
- There is a statutory duty to provide reasonable support to the patient. Reasonable support could be providing an interpreter to ensure discussions are understood, or giving emotional support to the patient following a notifiable patient safety incident.
- Once the patient has been told in person about the notifiable patient safety incident, the organisation must provide the patient with a written note of the discussion, and copies of correspondence must be kept.

The thresholds for incidents can be confusing, as the threshold is lower for the doctor's ethical duty (any harm or distress caused to the patient) while the thresholds for the contractual and statutory duties are higher and slightly different (with the inclusion of prolonged psychological harm in the statutory duty).

The CA 2014 has also introduced extensions to the special administration timetable to give greater time for the TSA to publish their draft report, extend the consultation period and create an obligation for the TSA to consult:

- other NHS trusts and NHS FTs affected by wider recommendations, their staff and their commissioners;
- any local authority in whose area the trust in administration and other affected trusts are located; and
- any Local Healthwatch organisation in the area of any local authority.

The CQC gained a greater role in dealing with quality and safety failure in FTs by requiring also that NHSI appoint a TSA where the CQC is satisfied that there is a serious failure by an NHS FT to provide services that are of sufficient quality. It also requires NHSI to consult more widely with the CQC in various situations, such as before publishing guidance. In addition, TSAs may not provide draft reports to NHSI without obtaining a statement from the CQC stating that it considers that the recommendations would achieve the sufficient safety and quality of the services.

Laws on patient and public involvement

The HSCA 2012 introduced significant amendments to the NHS Act 2006, especially with regard to how NHS commissioners would function. These amendments included two complementary duties for CCGs with respect to patient and public participation which reflect the public ownership of the NHS enshrined in the NHS Constitution.

The first duty requires CCGs and NHSE to promote the involvement of patients and carers in decisions which relate to their care or treatment. It requires CCGs to ensure that they commission services which promote involvement of patients across the full spectrum of prevention or diagnosis, care planning, treatment and care management.

The second duty places a requirement on CCGs and NHSE to ensure public involvement and consultation in commissioning processes and decisions. A description of these arrangements must be included in a CCG's constitution. It requires the involvement of the public, patients and carers in:

- the planning of commissioning arrangements, which might include consideration of allocation of resources, needs assessment and service specification; and
- any proposed changes to services that may impact on patients.

CCGs must ensure that individuals to whom the services are being or may be provided are involved (whether by being consulted or provided with information or in other ways) in accordance with section 14Z2 of the NHS Act 2006.

There are two other relevant aspects to section 14Z2. Subsection 3 requires all CCGs to include in their constitution a description of their public engagement arrangements and a statement of the principles that they will follow in when implementing them. Subsection 4 empowers NHSE to publish guidance on compliance with this section, which CCGs must have regard to.

Section 13Q of the Act applies to NHSE and contains effectively identical provisions to section 14Z2. Section 242 of the Act contains the same obligations with regard to patient and public involvement for NHS trusts and FTs. Any NHS body considering a change of the services it commissions or provides must be aware of these obligations. The proposals under consideration must have an impact on the manner in which the services are delivered to users of those services or the range of health services available to those users for the sections to apply.

In summary, any significant commissioning decision or reconfiguration of provision will be caught by these statutory requirements. Whilst the statute does not insist on 'consultation', it seeks to make sure that service users are 'involved'. In practice, some form of consultation exercise will be required for any significant proposed change to services to comply with this duty. The biggest area of application and challenge for NHS organisations currently are the requirements and methods of public involvement in the development of STPs.

The most recent NHSE guidance *Patient and public participation in commissioning health and care: statutory guidance for clinical commissioning groups and NHS England* (April 2017) sets out 10 key actions for CCGS and NHSE on how to embed involvement in their work. They should:

1. involve the public in governance;
2. explain public involvement in commissioning plans/business plans;
3. demonstrate public involvement in annual reports;
4. promote and publicise public involvement;
5. assess, plan and take action to involve;
6. feedback and evaluate;
7. implement assurance and improvement systems;
8. advance equalities and reduce health inequalities;
9. provide support for effective involvement; and
10. hold providers to account.

The guidance also explores some of the complexities of commissioning in a changing healthcare landscape, in relation to co-commissioning, devolution and joint arrangements, including accountable care systems (ACSs) (see Figure 5.1).

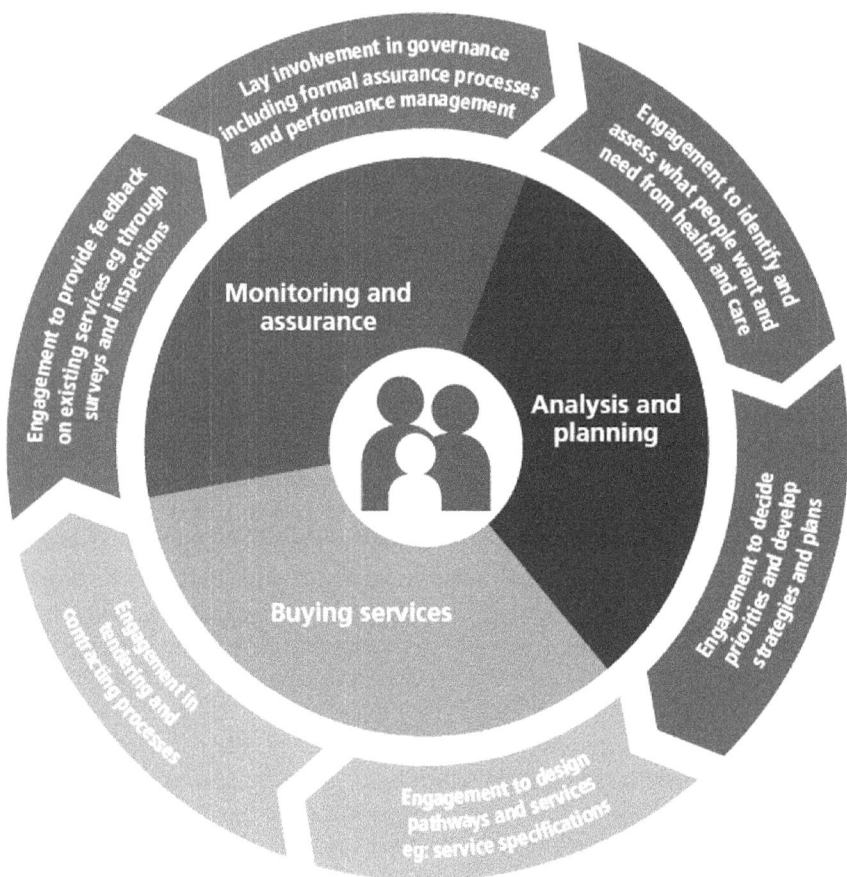

Figure 5.1: How public participation can support the commissioning cycle

Public involvement in commissioning is about enabling people to voice their views, needs and wishes, and to contribute to plans, proposals and decisions about services. The guidance uses the term 'involvement' interchangeably with 'engagement', 'participation', 'consultation' and 'patient or public voice' and there are many different ways to involve patients and the public, as illustrated in the list below. Different approaches will be appropriate, depending on the nature of the commissioning activity and the needs of different groups of people. The guidance sets out an extensive list of ways to involve people:

- Surveys
- Advocate
- Events
- Engage
- World café

- Representation
- Feedback
- Collaborate
- Inform
- Networks
- Facilitation
- Influence
- Community meetings
- Newsletters
- Insight
- Partnership
- Connect
- Consult
- e-Consultation
- Social movement
- You said, we did
- Listen
- Focus groups
- Social media
- Lobby
- Participate
- Co-produce
- Action
- Social
- Power sharing
- Conversation
- Communities of interest
- Citizen panels
- Questionnaires
- Campaign
- Elected Representatives
- Dialogue
- Patient groups.

The guidance goes on to give examples of where the legal duty to involve may arise, such as:
 Changes to commissioning arrangements

- The strategic planning of services:
  - Plans to reconfigure or transform services or improve health.
  - Developing and considering proposals to change commissioning arrangements

Procurement

- Considering or developing proposed models, configurations or specifications for a service.
- Commencing a procurement process.

Contracts

- Entering into a contract with a provider.
- Varying a contract, other than a variation required by law.
- Serving a notice to terminate a contract with a provider.
- Receiving a notice to terminate from a provider.

Overview and scrutiny referral

- Any instance in which a referral has been made to the local overview and scrutiny committee.

Equality

- An equality impact analysis may indicate the need for engagement, for example a lack of evidence relating to certain groups.

The guidance also sets out a three-step process for assessing the benefits of participation and whether the legal duty to involve applies:

- Step 1: Does the activity relate to commissioning responsibilities? If yes, go to step 2,
- Step 2: What type of activity is it? If it is planning, proposals for change and operational decisions, go to step 3,
- Step 3: Would there be an impact on service delivery or the range of services?

An impact on services can arise in two ways:

1. An impact on the way services are delivered to individuals, for example the transfer of a service to another location; and/or
2. The range of health services available to individuals – for example, the decommissioning of a service of limited clinical benefit to fund investment in other services.

In addition, as part of the guidance NHSE developed ten principles of participation based on a review of research, best practice reports and the views of stakeholders.

Reach out to people rather than expecting them to come to you and ask them how they want to be involved, avoiding assumptions.

1. Promote equality and diversity and encourage and respect different beliefs and opinions.
2. Proactively seek participation from people who experience health inequalities and poor health outcomes.

3. Value people's lived experience and use all the strengths and talents that people bring to the table, working towards shared goals and aiming for constructive and productive conversations.
4. Provide clear and easy to understand information and seek to facilitate involvement by all, recognising that everyone has different needs. This includes working with advocacy services and other partners where necessary.
5. Take time to plan and budget for participation and start involving people as early as possible.
6. Be open, honest and transparent in the way you work; tell people about the evidence base for decisions and be clear about resource limitations and other relevant constraints. Where information has to be kept confidential, explain why.
7. Invest in partnerships, have an ongoing dialogue and avoid tokenism; provide information, support, training and the right kind of leadership so everyone can work, learn and improve together.
8. Review experience (positive and negative) and learn from it to continuously improve how people are involved.
9. Recognise, record and celebrate people's contributions and give feedback on the results of involvement; show people how they are valued.

It recommends that STP partners build on the *Six Principles for Engaging People and Communities* (June 2016), in order to work with the knowledge, skills and experience of people in their communities, working in co-production to improve access and outcomes.

The six principles were developed by the People and Communities Board, National Voices, in conjunction with the new models of care 'vanguard' sites, to give practical support to services as they deliver the 'new relationship with people and communities;' set out in the 5YFV (see Chapter 16). These 'six principles' set out the basis of good person-centred, community focused health and care and are set out in Figure 5.2.

Six principles acknowledges that the evidence is increasingly clear that better engagement –which means involvement and co-production – is not a nice to have, it is core business. In fact, there is a growing body of knowledge and practice that demonstrates that engagement is doable and has real impact. However, NHSE recognises that there is a long way to go.

Those who are involved with STPs are also encouraged to use *Engaging local people: a guide for local areas developing sustainability and transformation plans* (September 2016).

As a general rule, the greater the extent of changes and number of people affected, the greater the level of activity that is likely to be necessary to achieve an appropriate and proportionate level of public involvement. However, the nature and extent of public involvement, including the length of consultation required always depends on local circumstances.

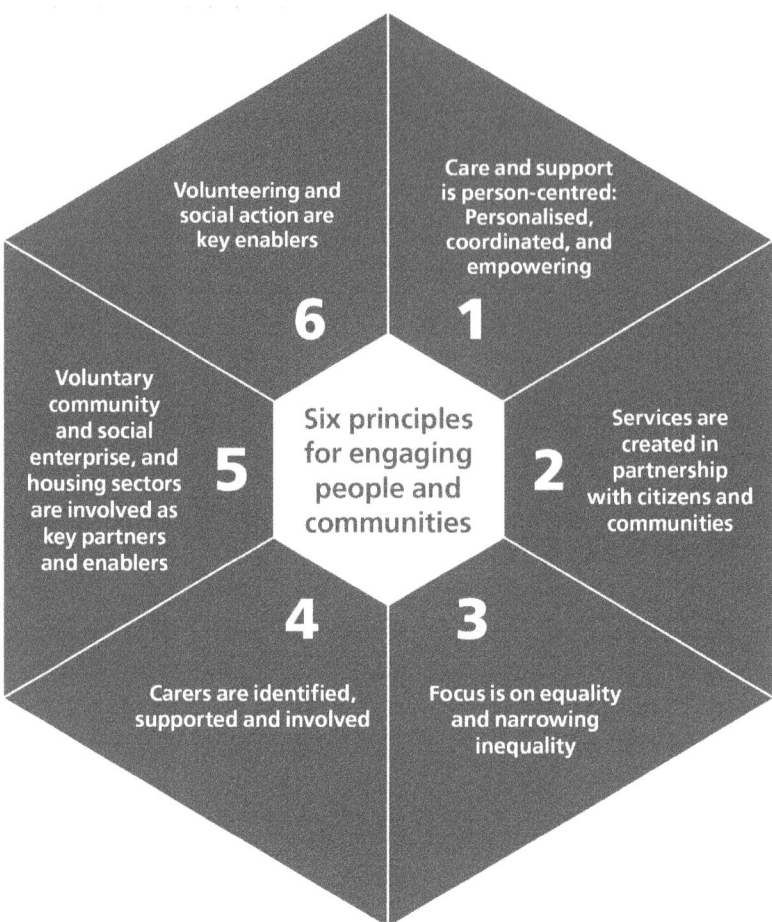

Figure 5.2: Six principles for engaging people and communities: putting them into practice

Whichever methods of involvement are used, it is essential that the approach is documented and agreed through governance structures, and that there is an audit trail of the activity that has taken place, including questions raised and the response to them. This strengthens proposals, highlights likely areas of concern, and provides evidence in the event of subsequent challenge.

Patient and public participation in commissioning health and care: statutory guidance for clinical commissioning groups and NHS England outlines the basic consultation principles as fairness and proportionality. These are set out in the Gunning Principle (resulting from the case *R* v *London Borough of Brent ex parte Gunning* (1985)), providing a helpful overview of what constitutes a fair consultation process:

- Consultation must take place when the proposal is still at a formative stage: consultation cannot take place on a decision that has already been made. Decision makers can consult on a 'preferred option' (of which those being consulted should be informed) and even a 'decision in principle' as long as they are genuinely open to influence.
- Sufficient reasons must be put forward for the proposal to allow for intelligent consideration and response: those being consulted should be made aware of the basis on which a proposal for consultation has been considered and will be considered thereafter, including any criteria to be applied or factors to be considered.
- Adequate time must be given for consideration and response: there is no automatically required time frame within which the consultation must take place unless statutory time requirements are prescribed. A rationale must be set out for any departure from that expected timeframe.
- The product of consultation must be conscientiously taken into account: decision-makers must properly consider the material produced by the consultation.

The Cabinet Office's latest statement of *'Consultation Principles'* (January 2016) echoes many of these issues:

> 'Consultations are also a good way for departments to publicise an issue and demonstrate that they are open to ideas and discussion. Too often though consultations continue to be accused of being too short, not inclusive enough, not publicised, not feeding back and, worst of all, being nothing but a fig leaf for a decision that has already been made.
>
> The same accusations are also made of local consultations as well – those run by schools, the NHS and others. Poor consultation also continues to be an area of successful legal challenge as well. There is a whole set of case law out there where consultations have been challenged and, in many instances, have had to be re-run.'

A public body that fails to involve patients and the public leaves itself open to a challenge by way of judicial review. It may not lawfully be able to take decisions and thus implement the changes until consultation has occurred. The courts may also award legal costs against the NHS body.

Judicial review is a process by which a decision of the SoS or an NHS body can be challenged, on the basis that it is unlawful. This right is derived from administrative law and does not just apply to the failure to involve. It is not a right of appeal and is concerned primarily with how decisions are made, rather than the merits of the decision itself. A decision might be unlawful if:

- the decision-maker does not have power to make the decision, or is using their power improperly;
- the decision is irrational;

- the procedure followed by the decision-maker was unfair or biased;
- the decision was in breach of the Human Rights Act 1998; or
- the decision breaches EU law.

If an application for judicial review is successful, the court has six possible remedies:

1. Quashing orders: the original decision is struck down and the public body has to take the decision again.
2. Prohibiting orders: the public body is forbidden from doing something unlawful in the future.
3. Mandatory orders: the public body is ordered to do something specific which it has a duty to do.
4. A declaration: on the way to interpret the law in future, for example.
5. An injunction: this is usually a temporary remedy until the full application for judicial review is heard.
6. Damages: whilst rare, this may be available for example, where there has been a breach of an individual's rights under the Human Rights Act 1998.

The duty to involve arises whether the changes in health service provision are required in response to financial pressures, clinical requirements or other reasons, or a combination of two or more factors. Changes made to comply with DHSC policy decisions are also subject to the duty to consult. The legal duty to consult both patients and the wider public falls both on the commissioner of health services and on to those providing services. The courts have ruled that, even where a commissioner was simply implementing DHSC policy, the provision of services was still the commissioner's responsibility and therefore it had an obligation to consult.

Finally, *the Local Authority (Public Health, Health and Wellbeing Boards and Health Scrutiny) Regulations 2013* remove the requirement for local authorities to have a Health Overview and Scrutiny Committee as the means by which they discharge their scrutiny function – although most have retained them. Even so, under regulation 23, NHSE, CCGs, and public and independent sector providers of NHS services must consult with the local authority about any proposals for a 'substantial' development or variation of the health service in the authority's area. Whilst substantial is not defined, it would be advisable for an NHS body to tell the local authority when it is proposing to consult. If the local authority ultimately disagrees with the decision of the NHS body, it is entitled to refer the matter up to the SoS for a final decision.

Healthwatch England is a key player for patient and public involvement under HSCA 2012, not least in its role as the independent consumer champion that gathers and represents the views of the public about health and social care services in England. Local Healthwatch organisations were established in April 2013 and have taken over the work previously done by the LINks, but with additional functions (see Chapter 4).

Local Healthwatch has to be representative of its local community as laid out in HSCA 2012. This includes ethnic groups, different users of services and carers.

Other UK law

There are several other specific pieces of UK legislation with a wide remit that are directly applicable to the NHS.

The Employment Rights Act 1996 (ERA 1996) protected employees from detriment if the reason for the employee's action arises from certain cases of whistleblowing – informing on improper practices of employers – where this amounts to a protected disclosure. The whistleblowing legislation is complex. The main principles are as follows:

- a dismissal is automatically unfair if the reason for it is that the employee made a protected disclosure;
- the ERA 1996 sets the parameters of what constitutes a protected disclosure, as well as the manner of the permissible disclosure by the worker; and
- different degrees of protection apply depending upon whether the disclosure was made internally within the employer's organisation, or externally to a third party.

A protected disclosure includes the disclosure of any information by a worker that in their reasonable belief tends to show that:

- a criminal offence has been, is about to be or is likely to be committed;
- a person has failed or is about to fail, to comply with a legal obligation imposed upon them, including an obligation imposed upon them by a contract of employment;
- the health and safety of any person has been or is being or is likely to be endangered;
- a miscarriage of justice has occurred, is occurring or is likely to occur;
- the environment has been or is being or is likely to be damaged; or
- information tending to show that one of the above matters has been, or is likely to be, deliberately concealed.

It is not necessary for the worker to show that the act concerned has or will occur. A reasonable belief is sufficient. It is immaterial whether the act has taken place in the UK or elsewhere. The court determines the state of the employee's disclosure by reference to the date of their dismissal or detriment, not the date on which the disclosure was made.

Where a worker is victimised by the employer as a result of making a protected disclosure, a claim can be brought to an employment tribunal. Dismissals or selection for redundancy for making a protected disclosure are automatically unfair. The worker does not have to have been employed for a minimum period of time to make a claim. There is no limit on the compensation that can be awarded. Employment tribunals can award interim relief in unfair dismissal claims.

The Public Interest Disclosure Act 1998 (PIDA 1998) protects the public by protecting individuals from workplace reprisals for raising a genuine concern, whether a risk to patients or other wrongdoing. The Act's tiered disclosure regime – promoting internal and regulatory disclosures – encourages workplace accountability and self-regulation.

PIDA 1998 protects the public by providing a remedy for individuals who suffer a detriment by any act or any deliberate failure to act by their employer for raising a genuine concern, whether it be a risk to patients, financial malpractice, or other wrongdoing. The Act's tiered disclosure regime promotes internal and regulatory disclosures and encourages workplace accountability and self-regulation.

Under PIDA 1998, workers who act honestly and reasonably are given automatic protection for raising a matter internally. In the NHS, an internal disclosure can go up to the highest level and includes going to the responsible Minister at the DHSC. Protection is also readily available to individuals who make disclosures to prescribed regulators, such as CQC and NHSI.

In certain circumstances, wider disclosures (e.g. to an MP or the media) may also be protected. A number of additional tests apply when going wider, including:

- whether it is an exceptionally serious concern;
- whether the matter has already been raised;
- whether there is good reason to believe that the individual will be subject to a detriment by their employer if the matter were raised internally or with the appropriate regulator; and
- whether disclosure was reasonable given all the circumstances.

The Act covers all workers, including temporary agency staff, persons on training courses and self-employed staff who are working for and supervised by the NHS. It does not cover volunteers. PIDA 1998 also makes it clear that any clause in a contract that purports to gag an individual from raising a concern that would have been protected under the Act is void. Where an individual is subjected to a detriment by their employer for raising a concern or is dismissed in breach of PIDA 1998, they can bring a claim for compensation under PIDA 1998 in an employment tribunal. Awards are uncapped and based on the losses suffered.

The Human Rights Act 1998 came into force in the UK in October 2000. All public bodies (such as courts, police, local governments, hospitals, publicly funded schools, and others) and other bodies carrying out public functions have to comply with the Convention rights. The Act sets out the fundamental rights and freedoms to which individuals in the UK have access.

The Freedom of Information Act 2000 (FOIA 2000) created a public 'right of access' to information held by public authorities. The full provisions of the Act came into force on 1 January 2005. The Act led to the renaming of the Data Protection Commissioner (set up to administer the Data Protection Act 1998 (DPA 1998)), who is now known as the Information Commissioner. The Information Commissioner's Office (ICO) oversees the operation of the Act. It requires public authorities to have an approved publication scheme, which is a means of providing access to information that an authority proactively publishes. The ICO has developed and approved a model publication scheme that all public authorities must adopt.

The scheme:

- sets out the types of information that must be routinely published;
- explains the way the information is provided;
- states what charges can be made for providing information; and
- commits the authority to providing and maintaining a guide to the information provided, how it is provided and any charges.

All public authorities should have adopted the model publication scheme and produced a guide to information using either definition documents or template guides to information provided by the ICO.

The definition documents for the main public sectors give sector-specific guidance on the type of information that authorities are expected to publish and list in their guide to information. The template guides to information are for smaller authorities and are downloadable guides that can be printed off, completed and used without further modification. They have been produced for local councils, schools and NHS practitioners.

The FOIA 2000 means that public authorities must disclose official information when people ask for it (unless there is a good legal reason not to) and they must reply within 20 working days.

This model publication scheme for NHS organisations gives examples of the kinds of information that they are expected to provide to meet their commitments under the model publication scheme. They are required to make the information available unless:

- they do not hold the information;
- the information is exempt under one of the FOI exemptions or Environmental Information Regulations (EIRs) exceptions, or its release is prohibited under another statute;
- the information is archived, out of date or otherwise inaccessible; or
- it would be impractical or resource-intensive to prepare the material for routine release.

FOI requests may be refused if:

- it would cost too much to comply;
- the request is vexatious or repeated; or
- the information is exempt from disclosure under one of the exemptions in the Act.

If any of these criteria apply, the requester must be sent a written refusal notice.

The Act also recognises that there may be valid reasons for withholding information by setting out a number of exemptions from the right to know, some of which are subject to a public interest test. There are 23 exemptions in the FOIA 2000, divided as follows:

- Those that apply to a whole category (or class) of information, for example:
  - information about investigations and proceedings conducted by public authorities;
  - court records; and
  - trade secrets.
- Those that are subject to a 'prejudice' test, where disclosure would, or would be likely to, prejudice, for example:
  - the interests of the UK abroad;
  - the prevention or detection of crime; and
  - the activity or interest described in the exemption.

Information covered by one or more of the exemptions does not have to be disclosed. However, the decision has to be made as to whether the information should nevertheless be released in the public interest. This is called the 'public interest test' and involves considering the circumstances of each case with the exemption that covers the information. The information must be released unless the public interest in maintaining the exemption outweighs the public interest in releasing it.

Under the FOIA 2000, an authority must apply the public interest test separately to each exemption. When the test does apply, these are called qualified exemptions. Those to which the test does not apply are called absolute exemptions.

There are also exemptions for personal information.

- If personal information relates to the applicant, the request must be dealt with as a 'subject access request' made under the DPA 1998.
- If the information requested relates to a third party, a decision on whether to release it must be based on whether releasing it would contravene the DPA 1998.

When refusing a request for information, it is not possible to withhold an entire document because some of the information contained within it is exempt. A redacted version of the document must be provided along with a refusal notice stating why some of the information cannot be released. When refusing a FOI request, the exemption or exemptions applied must be set out, why they have been applied and, where appropriate, the public interest factors for and against disclosure fully explained.

The Mental Capacity Act 2005 (MCA 2005) received Royal Assent in April 2005 and was fully implemented in October 2007. It provides a clear legal framework for people who lack capacity, and their family and carers, to be involved as far as possible in decisions about their care. It sets out five key principles, as well as procedures and safeguards, which are:

- a person must be assumed to have capacity unless it is established that they lack capacity;
- a person is not to be treated as unable to make a decision unless all practicable steps to help them to do so have been taken without success;
- a person is not to be treated as unable to make a decision merely because they make an unwise decision;
- an act done, or decision made, under this Act for or on behalf of a person who lacks capacity must be done, or made, in their best interests; and
- before the act is done, or the decision is made, regard must be had to whether the purpose for which it is needed can be as effectively achieved in a way that is less restrictive of the person's rights and freedom of action.

These principles of the MCA 2005 apply whether the decisions are life-changing or everyday matters. The underlying philosophy is to ensure that individuals are empowered to make decisions where possible and, where this is not possible, that any decision made or action taken is made in their best interests. The MCA Code of Practice also describes the role of the Independent Mental Advocate Service (IMCA) set up under the Act. This service provides support for those particularly vulnerable individuals who lack capacity and have no family or friends so that their views are represented to those working out their best interests.

Deprivation of Liberties Safeguards (DoLS) are an amendment to the MCA 2005. They apply in England and Wales only. The MCA 2005 allows restraint and restrictions to be used – but only if they are in the person's best interests. Extra safeguards are needed if restrictions and restraints used deprive a person of their liberty – these are called DoLS. DoLS can only be used if the person will be deprived of their liberty in a care home or hospital, and then the care home or hospital must ask the local authority if they can deprive the person of their liberty.

The Corporate Manslaughter and Corporate Homicide Act 2007 came into effect on 6 April 2008 and disposed of the need the need to identify a single individual as the 'controlling mind'. This means a trust can be prosecuted as a corporate body.

The Equality Act 2010 legally protects people from discrimination in the workplace and in wider society. It replaced previous anti-discrimination laws with a single Act, making the law easier to understand and strengthening protection in some situations. It sets out the different ways in which it is unlawful to treat someone. The intention of the public sector equality duty is to ensure that a public authority must, in the exercise of its functions, have due regard to three main aims:

1. eliminating discrimination, harassment, victimisation and any other conduct that is prohibited by or under the Equality Act;

2. advancing equality of opportunity between persons who share a relevant protected characteristic and persons who do not share it; and
3. fostering good relations between persons who share a relevant protected characteristic and persons who do not share it.

The Act also prohibits unlawful discrimination in the provision of services on the grounds of 'protected characteristics'. These are:

- age
- disability
- gender reassignment
- marriage and civil partnership
- pregnancy and maternity
- race
- religion or belief
- sex and sexual orientation.

The Bribery Act 2010 came into force in July 2011 and made it a criminal offence for commercial organisations to fail to prevent bribes being paid on their behalf. NHS organisations are included within the definition of 'commercial'. Therefore, if any NHS organisation fails to take appropriate steps to avoid (or at least minimise) the risk of bribery taking place it could face large fines and even the imprisonment of the individuals involved and those who have turned a blind eye to the problem. The Act makes it a criminal offence to give or offer a bribe or to request, offer to receive or accept a bribe, whether in the UK or abroad (the measures cover bribery of a foreign public official), and for a director, manager or officer of a business to allow or turn a blind eye to bribery within the organisation.

The Act also introduces a corporate offence of failure to prevent bribery by persons working on behalf of a commercial organisation. However, organisations will have a defence against prosecution if they can show that they have adequate procedures in place to prevent bribery.

Guidance from the Ministry of Justice describes six guiding principles that set out the approach that organisations should take to prevent bribery occurring in their organisation. These are as follows.

- Proportionate procedures: designed to prevent bribery by anyone associated with the organisation and should be proportionate to the level of bribery risk to the organisation.
- Top-level commitment: senior management teams must show a commitment to preventing bribery, and promote a culture that does not tolerate acts of bribery.
- Risk assessment: an assessment of both internal and external risks of bribery to the organisation should be carried out regularly and documented.

- Due diligence: there must be effective due diligence procedures in place in respect of those involved in the organisation or carrying services out on behalf of the organisation.
- Communication: the organisation's stance on bribery should be clearly communicated to all employees and all those carrying out services on behalf of the organisation. This should include appropriate training.
- Monitoring and review: there should be an ongoing review process that regularly monitors the effectiveness of the procedures in place to prevent bribery.

These principles can be implemented by updating existing documentation, for example:

- updating policies and procedures by adding an anti-bribery statement to the organisation's employee handbook/intranet – this should be adequately communicated to all staff;
- amend whistleblowing policies to make specific reference to bribery, and encourage disclosure of bribery offences;
- training/presentations to make employees aware of the strengthened legislation around 'bribery', particularly in relation to corporate hospitality and the organisation's policy on business conduct (or similar);
- updating/adding a clause on bribery to employment contracts;
- ensuring all employees are under an express obligation to report any potential acts of bribery, including where an employee has personally committed an act of bribery;
- ensuring recruitment checks are robust;
- adding bribery to the matters covered by a disciplinary policy; and
- reviewing remuneration structures so that they comply with the new law where applicable.

The Modern Slavery Act 2015 is designed to tackle slavery in the UK. All businesses with a turnover in excess of £36 million are required to publish an annual statement setting out the steps they have taken to ensure that slavery and human trafficking do not exist in supply chains. The NHS role is twofold: it must review its own supply chains; and it must ensure that its policies, procedures and training in safeguarding are updated to include slavery and human trafficking. In October 2016, the Independent Anti-Slavery Commission published its annual report 2015/16 saying: 'The NHS has a significant role to play in controlling modern slavery and supporting victims. But to do this we need to ensure staff understand that modern slavery exists, and we need to ensure that staff are confident and able to both recognise the signs and symptoms of both victim and perpetrators and know what to do.'

NHS organisations also have statutory responsibilities under the Health and Safety at Work Act 1974, the Management of Health and Safety at Work Regulations 1999, and a number of other health and safety regulations (e.g.

Reporting of Injuries, Diseases and Dangerous Occurrences Regulations 1995, Noise at Work Regulations 1989, Manual Handling Operations Regulations 1992 and the Control of Substances Hazardous to Health Regulations 2002).

There have also been a number of EU Directives that have related to the NHS and time will tell how these are impacted by the Brexit negotiations. For example, the EU Clinical Trials Directive 2001 authorised and regulated the conduct of clinical trials, as trials are often conducted in multiple sites across a number of European countries. A revision of this Directive during 2014 introduced changes to speed up the process for authorising new clinical trials and reducing the administrative burden associated with the conduct of these studies. The new EU Directive takes the form of a Regulation, meaning that it will apply directly in each member state of the EU without the need to be transposed into national law, and thereby will ensure the rules are consistent throughout the EU. The new EU Regulation is expected to apply from 2016.

The EU General Data Protection Regulation 2016 (GDPR 2016) came into force in May 2018 is enshrined in UK Law under the Data Protection Act 2018.

The GDPR will apply to organisations that fall into two broad definitions: 'controllers' and 'processors'. The definitions are similar to those defined in the DPA 1998 in that controllers say how and why personal data is processed, and processors act on the controller's behalf. The GDPR requires organisations to demonstrate compliance by design. This means ensuring there are adequate systems, contractual provisions, documented decisions about processing, and training in place. The GDPR stipulates that any data that can be used to identify an individual is considered to be personal data. It can include things such as genetic, mental, cultural, economic or social information, and IP addresses.

Under the GDPR, organisations must have a valid lawful basis in order to process personal data. There are six lawful bases, as follows:

- **Consent:** the individual has given clear consent for their personal data to be processed for a specific purpose.
- **Contract:** the processing is necessary for a contract with the individual, or because they have asked for specific steps to be taken before entering into a contract.
- **Legal obligation:** the processing is necessary to comply with the law (not including contractual obligations).
- **Vital interests:** the processing is necessary to protect someone's life.
- **Public task:** the processing is necessary to perform a task in the public interest or for official functions, and the task or function has a clear basis in law.
- **Legitimate interests:** the processing is necessary for the organisation's legitimate interests or the legitimate interests of a third party unless there is a good reason to protect the individual's personal data which overrides those legitimate interests. (This does not apply to a public authority processing data to perform their official tasks.)

The GDPR also requires the appointment of a data protection officer (specifically including public bodies), the imposition of privacy impact assessments, adequate systems to manage data breaches, not holding data longer than necessary, not changing the use of the data and compliance with the right to be forgotten.

Company law and other legislation

While the NHS is not governed by UK company legislation, it provides a useful backdrop for understanding health service governance. In the UK, the main item of company legislation is the Companies Act 2006 (CA 2006). This includes regulations relating to:

- the preparation and auditing of annual financial statements, for approval by the shareholders;
- the powers and duties of directors;
- other disclosures to shareholders, such as the requirement for companies to publish an annual business review;
- the disclosure of information about directors' remuneration;
- general meetings of companies, and shareholder rights to call a general meeting; and
- shareholder voting rights at general meetings, including the right to re-elect directors.

The impact of this legislation has been felt in health service governance and is covered throughout this handbook.

A number of EU company law directives also have relevance for the NHS. A proposal for a new or amended EU Directive is initiated by the European Commission in Brussels. Legislation is then agreed by the European Council and the European Parliament in a process known as the 'co-decision procedure'. When a directive has been agreed, its contents must be implemented by all EU member states within a stated timeframe, in either a law or another regulation, if suitable legislation does not already exist. EU Directives on company law have included a requirement for companies to publish an annual business review. Several directives have also been passed affecting companies whose shares are traded on a regulated exchange, including:

- a directive relating to shareholder rights;
- requirements to publish an annual corporate governance statement;
- requirements to have an audit committee; and
- requirements to introduce measures that provide for the independence and ethical conduct of their external auditors.

Companies become insolvent for reasons unconnected with corporate governance. Occasionally, however, the directors of a company may allow it to continue in business when they are aware that it is insolvent and will be unable to pay its creditors or employees. In the UK, the CA 2006 includes provisions that make fraudulent trading a criminal offence; in addition, the Insolvency Act 1986 makes wrongful trading a civil offence.

As discussed earlier, the insolvency framework for NHS organisations is different from an ordinary administration under general insolvency legislation in that its main objective is to protect patients and staff from failing services and secure the continued provision of patient services. The NHS statutory provisions also provide an alternative corporate insolvency procedure for companies to ensure that patients receive uninterrupted services if a provider becomes insolvent.

Money-laundering regulations are also in place to protect the UK financial system. Money laundering is the process of disguising the source of money that has been obtained from serious crime or terrorism, so that it appears to come from a legitimate source. Companies are often used for the purpose of money laundering, which is a criminal offence in most countries, and the owners or directors of the companies concerned are often involved in the money laundering activity themselves. If an organisation is covered by the regulations, it must put in place certain controls to prevent it being used for money laundering by criminals and terrorists. These include:

- appointing a 'nominated officer';
- checking the identity of customers;
- keeping all relevant documents; and
- report any suspicious activity to the Serious Organised Crime Agency.

Whilst NHS organisations are not specifically covered by the regulations, a number of its suppliers will be such as external and internal audit, counter fraud, and law firms.

Summary

- Best practice in both health service governance and corporate governance is found in the combination of legal and regulatory requirements alongside voluntary principles and codes of conduct, which will be considered in the next chapter.
- However, there are some aspects of organisational life where laws are essential to protect the interests of stakeholders such as employees or shareholders. For example, employment laws are needed to give protection to employees against unfair treatment by employers and legal requirements for organisations to prepare annual financial statements and have them audited, and the duties of directors are in place to protect stakeholders.
- In addition, expectations and corporate activity changes and develops, for example, governance has always had some connection with ethical business practice. Some aspects of behaviour may be considered unethical but legal.

- Laws are required to prevent or punish activities that are considered so unethical that they should be illegal. Bribery is an example of behaviour that has been tolerated in the past, but which is now accepted as illegal by most countries.
- Regulation may therefore be needed to address public concerns and maintain public confidence in the governance system. This has been most evident in the US. The Sarbanes-Oxley Act of 2002 was a response to public outrage against the many corporate scandals that emerged after the collapse of Enron. Public fury against the banks following the financial crisis in 2007–09 continues to prompt demands for legislative action that would affect the governance of banks.
- There may be different views about the extent of regulation that is required; however, the need for some regulation seems unquestionable. The key issue at stake here is to prevent the tsunami-like wave of regulations, codes and guidance from obliterating the core principles of good governance.
- This chapter has considered the law and regulations at play for NHS organisations. This establishes a foundation of non-negotiable rules and regulations that have to be followed in order to protect key interests.

6
Voluntary codes of best practice

Introduction

This chapter considers the second approach to establishing a system of best practice in governance, namely, to establish voluntary principles and guidelines and invite (or expect) organisations to comply with them. It will explore the voluntary principles and guidelines that have been established and their impact on health service governance. It will also set out the thinking behind compulsory regulation and/or voluntary best practice as a framework for governance.

As the previous chapter has demonstrated there are aspects of organisational life where laws are essential to protect the interests of stakeholders such as employees or shareholders. In practice, however, many countries combine legal and regulatory requirements with voluntary principles and codes of conduct in order to establish a clear framework for governance.

The chapter will identify both aspects of health service and corporate governance practice that are subject to voluntary codes and guidance; it will also highlight any direct application to the NHS.

Compulsory regulation and voluntary best practice

It is difficult to devise a set of rules that should apply to all organisations in all circumstances. Rules that are appropriate for one organisation might not be appropriate for another whose circumstances are very different. Although a voluntary system of governance (such as the corporate governance system in the UK) places an expectation on organisations to comply with the guidelines, it also allows them to breach the guidelines if it seems appropriate and sensible to do so. As a general rule, governance issues become greater as an organisation gets bigger. A voluntary code of best practice in governance can be targeted at the largest organisations; smaller organisations can then choose whether they want to model their own governance systems on parts of the code for the larger organisations. Governance practices can therefore be adapted to the circumstances of the organisation.

In corporate governance, however, there may be a risk that companies will migrate to those countries where the rules are less onerous if different countries have their own corporate governance regulations. Indeed, governments may compete to offer a corporate governance regime that is more attractive in their country than in other countries in order to attract foreign companies. Excessive regulations may deter companies from becoming a listed company, particularly if the rules for listed companies are stricter than the rules for private companies. In practice, good governance is a combination of regulation and voluntary best practice. In some countries, there is more emphasis on regulation and in others there is greater reliance on voluntary codes of practice for large organisations. However, unless law regulates governance, it is probable that standards of governance will vary substantially between organisations.

Voluntary governance frameworks

A voluntary code of governance is issued by an authoritative national or international body and contains principles or best practice in governance that major companies (listed companies) or organisations are encouraged to adopt and apply.

The principles may consist of main principles with associated supporting principles, and for each principle, there may also be provisions or recommendations about how the principle should be applied in practice. Voluntary codes of corporate governance have been adopted in many countries (e.g. in all the countries of the Commonwealth and all the countries of the EU).

The purpose of a voluntary code is to raise standards of governance. It is principles-based, because there is a recognition that the same set of rules is not necessarily appropriate in every way for all organisations, and that there will be situations where:

- non-compliance with provisions in the code is desirable, given the circumstances that the organisation faces; and
- implementing a principle of best practice is not always best achieved by following the detailed provisions or recommendations in the code, and some flexibility should be allowed.

It is also recognised that a code cannot provide detailed guidelines for every situation and circumstance. The preface to the UK Code in 2010 pointed out:

> 'It seems that there is almost a belief that complying with the Code in itself constitutes good governance. The Code, however, is of necessity limited to being a guide only in general terms to principles, structure and processes. It cannot guarantee effective board behaviour because the range of situations in which it is applicable is much too great for it to attempt to mandate behaviour more specifically than it does.'

'Comply or explain' and 'apply or explain'

There is no statutory requirement for organisations to apply the principles or provisions of a voluntary code. However, a well-established code should attract the support of the significant organisations in that sector, and this develops an expectation that others should adopt the code unless their circumstances are such that non-compliance with some of the code's provisions is a more sensible option. Although voluntary, organisations may be required to adopt the code of governance, or to explain their non-compliance with any aspect of the code and their reasons for non-compliance in their annual report and accounts. For example, NHSE advocates that CCGs adhere to the Good Governance Standard for Public Services 2004. This requirement, common in many countries, is known as 'comply or explain'.

The UK Code (2018) explains:

> 'The effective application of the Principles should be supported by high-quality reporting on the Provisions. These operate on a 'comply or explain' basis and companies should avoid a 'tick-box approach'. An alternative to complying with a Provision may be justified in particular circumstances based on a range of factors, including the size, complexity, history and ownership structure of a company. Explanations should set out the background, provide a clear rationale for the action the company is taking, and explain the impact that the action has had. Where a departure from a Provision is intended to be limited in time, the explanation should indicate when the company expects to conform to the Provision. Explanations are a positive opportunity to communicate, not an onerous obligation.'

The UK Code makes it clear that satisfactory engagement between company boards and investors is crucial to the health of the UK's corporate governance regime. In this way, both companies and shareholders have responsibility for ensuring that 'comply or explain' remains an effective alternative to a rules-based system. It recognises that there are practical and administrative steps to be taken to improve interaction between boards and shareholders, but it also makes it clear that there is scope for an increase in trust, which could generate a virtuous upward spiral in attitudes to the UK Code and in its constructive use.

A similar approach has been taken with some voluntary codes in the NHS. NHSI requires FTs to comply with the FT Code of Governance or to explain any non-compliance. The same is true of the UK Listing Rules, which require listed companies to comply with the UK Code.

The Good Governance Institute in its 2016 version of the Integrated Governance Handbook explains that they are not fans of the traditional Cadbury/Monitor comply or explain approach, preferring the South African King III guidance to apply and explain which for them carries a more thoughtful application of good governance principles. 'You may still have to comply/explain but from a basis of knowing you have sought to do the right thing and you understand why.'

There is also a view that the word 'comply' encourages organisations to follow the provisions of a code in all its details without considering the principles that underpin the code. This may encourage a box-ticking approach, and a view that the detailed provisions must be followed without considering whether the provisions might be appropriate or finding a suitable way of applying the governance principles in the actual circumstances.

For this reason, some countries have adopted governance codes that espouse an 'apply or explain' approach. South Africa in its fourth iteration of King Code, the governance code for South Africa has now moved on to 'apply and explain'. King IV has 17 basic principles,

> '16 of which can be applied by any organisation and all are required to substantiate a claim that good governance is being practised. The required explanation allows stakeholders to make an informed decision as to whether or not the organisation is achieving the four good governance outcomes required by King IV. Explanation also helps to encourage organisations to see corporate governance not as an act of mindless compliance but something that will yield results only if it is approached mindfully with due consideration of the organisation's circumstances.'

'Apply and explain' is a less prescriptive approach but this has been balanced by a greater emphasis on transparency with regard to how the judgement was exercised when considering the recommendations contained in King IV.

- 'Apply' – all principles are phrased as aspirations and ideals that organisations should strive for in their journey towards good governance and realising the governance outcomes. The principles are basic and fundamental to good governance and application is therefore assumed.
- 'Explain' – explanation should be provided in the form of a narrative account, with references to practices that demonstrate application of the principle. The explanation should address which recommended or other practices have been implemented and how these achieve or give effect to the principle.

The detail of information provided in the narrative should be guided by materiality, and should enable stakeholders to make an informed assessment of the quality of an organisation's governance.

The UK Code also recognises the dangers of a 'box-ticking' mentality with 'comply or explain' and stresses that it is not intended to be a set of rules:

> 'The Code is not a rigid set of rules ... It is recognised that [non-compliance with a provision] may be justified in particular circumstances if good governance can be achieved by other means.'

Likewise, the introduction to the FT Code of Governance (2014) (FT Code) makes it clear that some FTs may decide that the provisions are disproportionate or less relevant in their case. Therefore, they should actively consider how to adopt the approach in the code in their particular circumstances.

It should be noted that some principles and recommendations have become legislation (such as with Bribery Act 2010) and the practices required by the legislation then become mandatory.

Codes for health service governance

Governance in the public sector, and specifically in the NHS, is the subject of several reports. Some of the more prominent reports are as follows.

- The Nolan Principles of Public Life (1995): covered in detail the standards of behaviour and principles in public life with particular focus on appointment on merit, with an independent element on all selection panels recommended as the way forward for public bodies (see Chapter 1).
- The Intelligent Board (2006): looked at board level information needs and information flow.
- The Integrated Governance Handbook (2006): looked in detail at the processes and information requirements of sound governance.
- Taking it on Trust (2009): examined how the boards of NHS trusts and FTs in England assure themselves that internal controls are in place and operating effectively.
- The Healthy NHS Board: Principles for good governance (2013): set out the principles of high-quality governance, and is supported by a regularly updated digital compendium, which puts the principles in an operational context.
- The FT Code (2014): set out the governance arrangements for FTs.
- The Integrated Governance Handbook (2016): developing governance between organisations: reviewed the impact of the 2006 Integrated Handbook and explored the growing demands for good governance across organisational boundaries in the light of the developing STPs.
- Developmental Reviews of Leadership and Governance using the Well-Led Framework (2017): intended to support NHS provider organisations in gaining assurance that they are well led.

The intelligent board

This report set out a set of principles and model framework for structuring information to support strategy development and oversight of business delivery and effectiveness. It also suggests practical ways in which boards might use the framework proposed.

The report outlines:

- the information challenge, including discussion of the growing pressure on boards to raise their game and the need to improve the information they receive and how they use it;

- intelligent information for the board, including some key principles that should govern information for the board, together with a proposed framework and minimum data set for reviewing trust performance, supporting decision-making and considering strategy; and
- putting the framework into practice by improving the structure of agendas for the board, developing a 'dashboard' of routine performance indicators and informing the annual cycle of board meetings.

The report was followed by the Intelligent Board series of publications, which includes guidance for mental health trusts, ambulance trusts and clinical commissioners, outlines practical, focused advice for NHS board members on the kind of information they should be using to understand and oversee their organisations' performance.

All the reports in the series are based on the following Intelligent Board principles. All information should:

- cover locally defined priorities as well as national 'must do' requirements;
- focus on outcomes, not systems and processes;
- be available in a timely and understandable format;
- be clearly and simply presented;
- be forward-looking, presenting trends and anticipating future issues;
- allow internal comparison between services and make use of external benchmarks;
- provide interpretation and analysis as well as information; and
- provide a level of detail that is appropriate to the board's governance role.

The Integrated Governance Handbook

The idea of integrated governance was developed by Professor Michael Deighan and Dr Roger Moore with support from Sir William Wells, Professor Sir Ian Kennedy and Bill Moyes. It was first introduced to the NHS in a paper entitled 'Developing Integrated Governance', published by the NHS Confederation in May 2004.

The handbook was published in 2006 by the DH (now DHSC) to ensure that the basic building blocks of integrated governance were in place, with rollout and implementation planned over the following two years. The chief concern that the integrated governance sought to address was the risk of boards governing in silos (e.g. clinical governance, research governance, quality governance, information governance) by moving to an integrated agenda that would enable boards to meet their responsibilities.

Integrated governance is defined as: 'systems, processes and behaviours by which trusts lead, direct and control their functions to achieve organisational objectives, safety and quality of service and in which they relate to patients and carers, the wider community and partner organisations'.

The NHS CEO at the time, Sir Nigel Crisp, said in issue 245 of the Chief Executive Bulletin:

> 'Integrated governance provides the umbrella for all NHS governance approaches. It combines the principles of corporate/financial accountability and it moves towards a single risk sensitivity process which covers all the trust's objectives, supported by a coordinated source of collecting information and subject to coordinated inspection.'

Integrated governance emphasises the critical importance of the board defining, within the overall goals established for the NHS, its own purpose and strategic direction, with clarity of purpose, objective setting and planning of the board's annual cycle of business. The handbook also focused on quality as the driver of change, examined the critical role of clinical governance at the heart of the integrated governance agenda, and covered the legal implications for boards and what they should to do to plan the journey towards good governance.

The key themes were:

- strategic purpose and challenge;
- annual cycle of business;
- strengthened audit committees;
- measuring governance maturity: the matrix;
- board etiquette;
- board secretary role; and
- developing clinical governance and quality.

It was envisaged that the board would take corporate responsibility for all aspects of strategy setting, performance management and quality assurance, as a result of being assured that the appropriate systems were in place to manage the identified risks.

In particular, the handbook suggested a consideration of the 'company secretary' role within health organisations and a development of the role of the audit committee to scrutinise and streamline committee structures and agendas, ensuring all risks (activity, quality and resources) were anticipated, aligned and integrated.

The key task for integration was an examination of the role of the audit committee to ensure that it scrutinised all the sub-committees reporting to the board. At the time, some boards had more than 40 committees (some, of course, were subcommittees) but they reported either through the audit committee or directly to the board. This was unworkable and did not allow NEDs to fulfil their strategic role. The handbook proposed a phased transition to the following structure:

The handbook recommended that boards should be served by the following main standing committees:

- audit
- remuneration and review
- appointments.

Other committees that boards might find useful according to the handbook were:

- risk compliance and assurance
- clinical governance
- health and safety.

More recently, Finance and/or Performance Committees as well as Quality/Assurance Committees have begun to remerge.

This required a change in board meeting reporting structure to ensure that agendas were robust enough to deal adequately with the business from many of the committees that no longer existed. It also relied upon the strengthened audit committee clarifying much of the work prior to it being placed on the board's agenda. The handbook set out a direction of travel for health service governance, which was subsequently updated and revised by a further publication entitled *Integrated Governance: A guide to risk and joining up the NHS reforms* in 2011.

This outlined a governance development programme that clarifies:

- the purpose and behaviours of the board;
- the board structures and systems; and
- the review and improvement process.

Taking it on trust

This report by the Audit Commission was published in April 2009 and examined the rigour with which NHS trust and FT boards operated the processes available to them and obtained the assurance they need.

The report highlighted:

- discrepancies between trust declarations of compliance with Standards for Better Health (now superseded by the CQC) and subsequent Healthcare Commission inspections;
- differences between the Statement on Internal Controls (now known as the annual governance statement (AGS)) and core standards declarations; and
- some major failures in patient care, such as that at Maidstone and Tunbridge Wells NHS Trust and Mid Staffordshire NHS Foundation Trust.

There were significant gaps between the processes on paper and the rigour with which they were applied.

The report stated that the introduction of FTs had reinvigorated governance process and had resulted in the recruitment of NEDs with a greater knowledge of effective risk management and board challenge, drawn from private sector experience. However, the report was critical of assurance processes that had become 'a paper chase' rather than a critical examination of the effectiveness of the trust's internal controls and risk management arrangements.

The report recommended that boards should:

- ensure that their strategic aims and objectives are clearly defined and few in number so they can be widely understood and clearly cascaded throughout the organisation, and that their strategic risks are identified and aligned to their strategic objectives;
- review their risk management arrangements – including the way in which risks are reported to the board and consider how best to promote and demonstrate the value of risk management work to staff;
- ensure they have systems in place to comply with all statutory, regulatory, clinical and contractual requirements;
- consider cascading the Statement of Internal Control (now the AGS) through the organisation by sub-certification by managers, allied with a more effective compliance function, performance information and performance management;
- review how they identify and then evidence assurances on the operation of controls and how these are then evaluated;
- review and increase the assurances they receive from sources other than internal audit, including clinical audit, and in doing so, ensure that their full portfolio of risk is covered;
- maximise the assurance obtained from internal audit by reviewing the scope of internal audit plans and improving its commissioning;
- better align clinical audit programmes to key strategic and operational risks to maximise the assurance provided by the clinical audit function;
- strengthen their compliance mechanisms and distinguish them more clearly from internal audit, which should review the effectiveness of the compliance framework;
- ensure they have robust arrangements for assuring the quality of their data and by developing systematic and formalised review programmes for their data, including checking accuracy back to records; and
- develop policies and guidance on data quality and assurance processes, including defining and allocating responsibility for data quality, to promote consistency and improve awareness of board members.

The Healthy NHS Board: principles for good governance

This 2013 guidance is a refreshed edition of the original guidance, published in 2010. The 2013 guidance was influenced by the Francis Report, and starts from the premise that there is a strong relationship between leadership capability and performance, which is well demonstrated by evidence. It sets out that good leadership leads to a good organisational climate; in turn, good organisational climates lead to sustainable, high-performing organisations via improved staff satisfaction and loyalty.

The report sets out the principles that will allow NHS board members to understand the:

- collective role of the board including effective governance in relation to the wider health and social care system;
- activities and approaches that are most likely to improve board effectiveness; and
- contribution expected of them as individual board members.

The guidance is primarily intended for boards of NHS trusts and FTs, but with some interpretation it is also relevant for organisations operating at a national level. While CCGs, as membership organisations, have developed very specific governance arrangements and are not therefore the primary focus of this guidance, the general principles outlined are relevant to them. It offers a framework that will help them to place reliance on the effective governance of provider organisations.

The guidance sets the three key roles of an effective board as:

- formulating strategy for the organisation;
- ensuring accountability by holding the organisation to account for the delivery of the strategy;
- being accountable for ensuring the organisation operates effectively, with openness, transparency and candour, and by seeking assurance that systems of control are robust and reliable; and
- shaping a positive culture for the board and the organisation.

These are underpinned by three building blocks that allow boards to exercise their role – namely, that boards:

- are informed by the external context within which they must operate;
- are informed by, and shape, the intelligence that provides trend and comparative information on how the organisation is performing together with an understanding of local people's needs, market and stakeholder analyses; and
- prioritise engagement with key stakeholders and opinion formers within and beyond the organisation. The emphasis here is on building a healthy dialogue with, and being accountable to patients, the public, and staff, governors and members, commissioners and regulators.

The three roles of the board and the three building blocks all interconnect and influence one another. The guidance also sets out clear boundaries for the various roles within the board and outlines an established role for a company secretary.

NHS Foundation Trust Code of Governance (FT Code)

The FT Code was first published in 2006 and was revised in 2010. It was updated again in December 2013, following the significant regulatory change as a result of Health and Social Care Act 2012 (HSCA 2012). The FT Code builds on the approach, principles and provisions of the UK Code (and the Combined Codes before it) to bring best practice from the private sector to the NHS.

The legal framework for FTs has been described as being closer to that of a commercial company than that of other trusts. As such, it adopted a much more 'commercial' approach to their regulation. FTs must comply with the NHS provider licence, reporting requirements and the Audit Code used by NHSI. Each FT needs to develop individual standing orders, giving authority to each organisation's standing financial instructions, schemes of delegation and matters reserved for the board.

FTs are created as legal entities as public benefit corporations by the NHS Act 2006. The legislation constitutes FTs with a new governance regime that is fundamentally different from NHS trusts. FT boards of directors have more autonomy to make financial and strategic decisions. They also have a framework of local accountability through members and a council of governors, which was an attempt to move away from central control from the SoS (see Chapter 14).

The provisions of the FT Code, as best practice advice, do not represent mandatory guidance and accordingly non-compliance is not in itself a breach of NHS Foundation Trust Condition 4 of the NHS provider licence (also known as the 'governance condition'). However, FTs should note the relevant statutory requirements that have been highlighted within the FT Code.

The FT Code sets out best practice principles and structures and processes (through its provisions), but also makes clear that only directors and governors can demonstrate and promote the effective board behaviour that is needed to guarantee good corporate governance in practice.

The FT Code explains that satisfactory engagement between the board of directors, the council of governors, members and patients is crucial to the effectiveness of FTs' corporate governance approach. It outlines that both directors and governors have a responsibility for ensuring that 'comply or explain' remains an effective alternative to a rules-based system and a key aspect of this is ensuring improved interaction between directors, governors, members and – crucially – patients, communities and the public.

The FT Code does impose some specific disclosure requirements upon FTs, which are similar to the requirements set out by the UK Listing Authority for listed companies. To meet the requirements of 'comply or explain' each trust must comply with each of the provisions of the FT Code (which in some cases will require a statement or information to be required in the annual report) or, where appropriate, explain in each case why the trust has departed from the FT Code.

In addition, the FT Code also requires a trust, when it opts not to comply with a provision, to explain how its approach still reflects the principles of the FT Code relating to that provision. The form and content of this part of the statement are not prescribed, the intention being that trusts should have a free hand to explain their governance policies in the light of the principles, including any special circumstances applying to them that have led to a particular approach.

Although compliance with the provisions in the FT Code is on a 'comply or explain' basis, it also clearly identifies any relevant statutory requirements that fit closely with the Code. In the first instance, boards, directors and governors should ensure they are meeting the specific governance requirements described in HSCA 2012 (see Chapter 5).

Key aspects of the FT Code are set out in more detail in Chapter 14. In essence, the FT Code adopts a similar structure to the 2016 version of the UK Code, with a series of main principles, supported by a series of supporting principles. It remains to be seen whether the FT Code will be adapted to align with the new 2018 UK Code. The existing main headings are as follows:

Section A: Leadership
A.1   The role of the board of directors
A.2   Division of responsibilities
A.3   The chair
A.4   Non-executive directors
A.5   Governors

Section B: Effectiveness
B.1   The composition of the board
B.2   Appointments to the board
B.3   Commitment
B.4   Development
B.5   Information and support
B.6   Evaluation
B.7   Re-appointment of directors and re-election of governors
B.8   Resignation of directors

Section C. Accountability
C.1   Financial, quality and operational reporting
C.2   Risk management and internal control
C.3   Audit committee and auditors

Section D. Remuneration
D.1   The level and components of remuneration
D.2   Procedure

Section E. Relations with stakeholders
E.1   Dialogue with members, patients and the local community
E.2   Co-operation with third parties with roles in relation to NHS FTs

Developmental Reviews of Leadership and Governance using the Well-Led Framework: Guidance for NHS trusts and NHS foundation trusts

This guidance was published June 2017 following a full consultation on the previous Well-Led Framework (2015). The intention was to create a new Well-Led Framework for all NHS providers, building on the strengths of the earlier version issued by Monitor and the NHS TDA, and to streamline it to cover system governance and leadership, leadership behaviours, promotion of an open and fair culture, and sustainability of high quality, patient-centred care that supports learning and innovation. To support this single Well-Led Framework, the CQC and NHSI worked together to recognise that effective use of resources is also fundamental to enable trusts to deliver and sustain high-quality services for patients.

It is intended that trusts will assure themselves of their leadership and governance through a range of different means, such as external governance reviews (including peer review or consultancy support), advice from professional bodies, and feedback and guidance from regulators; these will be supported by self-reviews, internal audit, CQC inspections and board development programmes. Such developmental reviews reflect the regulators' view of good practice. Developmental well-led reviews will be conducted on a 'comply or explain basis', meaning that trusts should be able to give a robust explanation if they use alternative means to assure themselves. As these reviews are for development purposes, trusts need only feed back that a review has been completed and if it identified any material governance concerns. Trusts' approach to learning from past developmental reviews, and planning for future reviews, would be a source of evidence that would be considered in CQC's regular trust-level well-led assessments.

The depth and breadth of the areas for investigation can be shaped through the trust's self-assessment and/or initial findings of an independent review team at the start of the process. The developmental reviews are intended to complement CQC's trust-level well-led reviews. They will be greater in scope and depth, forward-looking, preventative and focused on improvement. They aim to identify early any factors which may lead to future failings and provide insight into areas for further development.

The Well-Led Framework is based on eight key lines of enquiry (KLOEs), as shown in Figure 6.1.

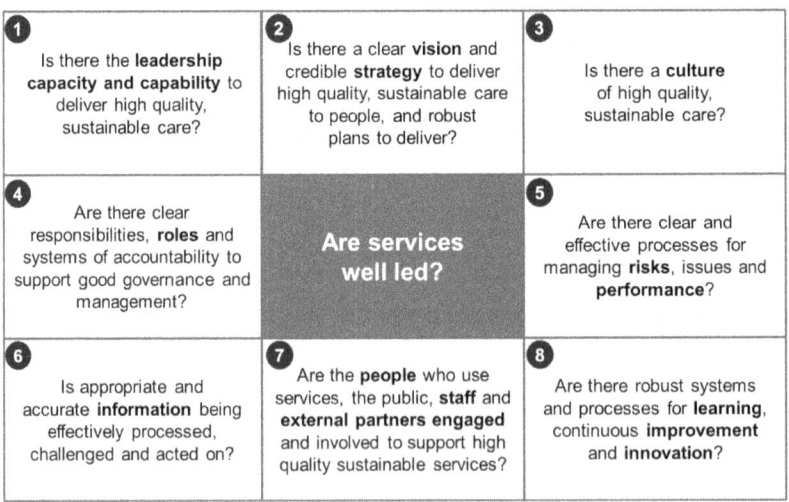

Figure 6.1: The eight KLOEs for the Well-Led Framework

Each of the framework's KLOEs is supplemented by characteristics of good organisations, and detailed descriptions of good practice. The framework sets out the questions that providers and reviewers should ask of themselves under each KLOE. For read-across with the CQC's assessment process, the guidance also includes the prompts that CQC inspection teams use to assess each KLOE. During a developmental review, the self-review should be presented to the external facilitator for comments and further discussion. The reviewer will then agree areas for further scrutiny with the board.

Each of the KLOEs should be rated using a scheme that allows prioritisation of findings and escalation of concerns, informed by the good practice examples in the framework. Each judgement should be backed up by evidence where appropriate. Rating will aid prioritisation and ensure that issues are brought to the attention of the board. Boards should ensure that their approach facilitates continuous improvement rather than a compliance mindset. The reviews should not be about 'meeting a bar', but rather about prioritising improvement actions.

The guidance also contains appendices setting out how to scope a developmental review, commissioning an external facilitator and carrying out a developmental review. The review is likely to include:

- a desktop review of documents;
- board and committee observations;
- a board self-assessment;
- a board skills inventory;
- focus groups with internal and external stakeholders;
- one-to-one interviews with board members, the trust secretary, lead governor, clinical leads and local stakeholders;
- a peer practice assessment; and
- stakeholder surveys.

Choosing an external facilitator is the provider's responsibility. As well as the skills and experience needed to address specific areas of focus arising from self-review, the provider must ensure their supplier can take a holistic view of the organisation, connecting findings from different parts of the review and supporting action-planning, including suggesting appropriate interventions.

Providers should also ensure reviewers are suitably independent of the board. This includes avoiding using reviewers who have done audit or governance related work for the provider in the previous three years, unless there are suitable safeguards against conflict of interest (i.e. information barriers). The UK Code 2018 and the accompanying FRC Board Guidance also offers advice and guidance on how to carry out board evaluation (both internal and external reviews).

Providers are also encouraged to consider involving peer reviewers as part of their external facilitation team, where appropriate, to make use of and enhance leadership and governance capability in the NHS.

Other corporate codes

There are a number of voluntary codes and guidance that have had a significant influence on the development of health service governance, including the following:

- UK Code (2018): a corporate framework of governance that underpins much of health service governance;
- FRC Guidance: numerous documents underpinning health service governance on matters relating to board effectiveness, audit committees and risk management;
- the G20/OECD Corporate Governance Principles; and
- the King IV Code.

The UK Corporate Governance Code

The first version of the UK Corporate Governance Code (the UK Code) was produced in 1992 by the Cadbury Committee. It is a particularly relevant document for FTs, as a significant similarity exists between the FT Code and the UK Code. Chapter 1 outlines the changing emphasis in the UK Code. Even so, the UK Code still contains the classic definition of corporate governance:

> 'Corporate governance is the system by which companies are directed and controlled. Boards of directors are responsible for the governance of their companies. The shareholders' role in governance is to appoint the directors and the auditors and to satisfy themselves that an appropriate governance structure is in place. The responsibilities of the board include setting the company's strategic aims, providing the leadership to put them into effect, supervising the management of the business and reporting to shareholders on their stewardship. The board's actions are subject to laws, regulations and the shareholders in general meeting.'

Corporate governance is, therefore, about what the board of a company does and how it sets the values of the company. It is to be distinguished from the day-to-day operational management of the company by full-time executives. The UK Code has been updated regularly and the most recent version was published in July 2018 and can be found in the Appendix.

The UK Code 2018 contains the broad headings shown below and will be cross-referenced in the later relevant chapters of this handbook:

- board leadership and company purpose;
- division of responsibilities;
- composition, succession and evaluation;
- audit, risk and internal control; and
- remuneration.

The UK Code (2018) is also supported by the FRC Board. This guidance does not set out the 'right way' to apply the UK Code. It is intended to stimulate thinking on how boards can carry out their role most effectively. The FRC Board Guide is designed to help boards with their actions and decisions when reporting on the application of the UK Code's Principles. The board should also consider other guidance by the FRC, as described below.

One of the most significant changes in the UK Code is its emphasis on culture. To this end, it encourages boards to engage effectively with shareholders and key stakeholders, in particular its workforce. More detail can be found this new emphasis on engagement in Chapter 1.

FRC Guidance

The FRC issues guidance and other publications to assist boards and board committees in considering how to apply the UK Corporate Governance Code to their particular circumstances. FRC papers include:

- Guidance on Board Effectiveness (FRC Board Guide);
- Guidance on Risk Management, Internal Control and Related Financial and Business Reporting (FRC Risk Guide);
- Guidance on Audit Committees (FRC Audit Guide);
- Guidance on the Strategic Report;
- Corporate Culture and the Role of Boards; and
- The UK Stewardship Code – sets out good practice for institutional investors on engaging with the companies in which they invest.

In particular, the FRC Board Guide incorporates guidance on the following:

- Board Leadership and Company Purpose
  - An effective board
  - Monitoring culture
  - Decision making
  - Relations with stakeholders
  - Relations with the workforce

- Division of Responsibilities
  - Role of the chair
  - Board committees
  - Role of the senior independent director
  - Role of executive directors
  - Role of non-executive directors
  - Board support and the role of the company secretary

- Composition, Succession and Evaluation
  - Role of the nomination committee
  - Succession planning

- Length of service of the chair and non-executive directors
- Evaluating the performance of the board and directors
- Externally facilitated board evaluations

■ Audit, Risk and Internal Control
- Audit committee
- Viability statements

■ Remuneration
- Role of the remuneration committee
- Remuneration policy

This guidance and the others listed are explored in greater detail in subsequent chapters of the handbook where relevant, as they are key to a good understanding of board and committee's effectiveness.

The G20/OECD Corporate Governance Principles

In 1999, the OECD issued a number of non-binding principles on corporate governance, which were reviewed and amended in 2004. The financial crisis of 2006–08 revealed severe shortcomings in corporate governance. When most needed, existing standards failed to provide the checks and balances that companies need to cultivate sound business practices. The OECD launched an ambitious action plan to develop a set of recommendations for improvements in priority areas such as remuneration, risk management, board practices and the exercise of shareholder rights, which led to revised principles in 2015 in conjunction with the G20 Leaders' Summit.

The G20/OECD Principles are intended to serve as a reference point for countries to use when evaluating their legal, institutional and regulatory provisions for corporate governance. They offer guidance and suggestions for stock exchanges, investors, companies and other bodies involved in developing good corporate governance practices.

The principles deal with six aspects of governance:

■ ensuring the basics for an effective corporate governance framework;
■ the rights of shareholders and key ownership functions;
■ the equitable treatment of shareholders;
■ the role of stakeholders in corporate governance;
■ disclosure and transparency; and
■ the responsibilities of the board.

In the UK, these basics are probably accepted as 'normal' for public companies, but it is a useful reminder that this is not necessarily the case at all times or in all countries.

The King IV Code

The 2016 King IV Code is the corporate governance code for South Africa. It is distinctive because it adopts a 'stakeholder inclusive' approach to corporate governance. In taking this approach, King IV includes some aspects of governance that are not found in other voluntary codes such as the UK Code (e.g. the 'apply and explain' outlined earlier).

> 'Corporate governance for the purposes of King IV is defined as the exercise of ethical and effective leadership by the governing body towards the achievement of the following governance outcomes:
> - Ethical culture
> - Good performance
> - Effective control
> - Legitimacy'.

The objectives of King IV are to:

- promote good governance as integral to running an organisation and delivering governance outcomes;
- broaden the acceptance of the King IV by making it accessible across a variety of sectors;
- reinforce corporate governance as a holistic and interrelated set of arrangements to be understood and implemented in an integrated way;
- encourage transparent and meaningful reporting to stakeholders; and
- present corporate governance as concerned with not only structure and process but also with ethical consciousness and conduct.

Summary

- Having looked at the law and regulation in the previous chapter and voluntary codes in this chapter, it becomes clear how the two approaches work together to provide a framework for governance.
- This is true for both corporate governance and health service governance. In Part 2, this combined approach will be used to explore best practice in a variety of arenas within health service governance (e.g. the role of the chair).
- To paraphrase the UK Code, voluntary frameworks are limited to being a general guide to principles, structure and processes. They cannot guarantee effective board behaviour because the range of situations in which they apply are too great for them to attempt to more specifically mandate behaviour.

7
The board's structure and its committees

Introduction

An efficient and effective board is a key requirement of good governance. The board should have a clear idea of its responsibilities and should fulfil these to the best of its abilities. There should be a suitable balance of skills, experience and power on the board. As a consequence, the role and composition of a board, and the duties and responsibilities of directors and committees, will be important. The ability to identify the characteristics of an effective board, and compare these with the actual practice of boards, is also important.

This chapter concentrates on the structures and processes of the board, while boardroom behaviours and practice will be covered in more detail in Part 3. For the purposes of this chapter, reference to the board should be taken to include a CCG governing body unless expressly set out otherwise.

The board is sometimes referred to as the 'controlling mind' of an organisation or as its 'head'. Though an organisation is not a person in the human sense, it does have characteristics, which support the use of these terms, such as entering into contractually binding arrangements. As the head of the organisation, the board has governance responsibilities to control and lead, while being held to account for delivering the organisation's strategic objectives.

Another way of looking at this is to say that the board acts as the agent for the organisation and exercises powers on its behalf. These powers are delegated to the board under the constitutional documents that establish the organisation, such as statutory instruments, core constitutions or standing orders. Underpinning all of this is the expectation that the board is collectively responsible for its actions, and that the individual members of the board make their decisions in the best interests of the organisation.

Company purpose

The FRC Board Guide (2018) states that:

> 'An effective board defines the company's purpose and then sets a strategy to deliver it, underpinned by the values and behaviours that shape its culture and

the way it conducts its business. It will be able to explain the main trends and factors affecting the long-term success and future viability of the company.'

It is important, therefore, to distinguish between the different NHS organisations as to their purpose as each type of NHS organisation has a different purpose as defined by the relevant law or regulation.

Foundation trusts

According to paragraph 18A of Schedule 7 to the National Health Service Act 2006 (NHS Act 2006) (as inserted by HSCA 2012), the duty of the board, and of each director individually, is to act with a view to promoting the success of the corporation so as to maximise the benefits for the members of the corporation as a whole and for the public. This mirrors the duty as set out in the CA 2006 for companies. This is also set out in the FT Code, which goes on to say that 'every NHS FT should be headed by an effective board of directors. The board is collectively responsible for the performance of the NHS FT'.

Clinical commissioning groups

The duty of the governing body is to ensure that the CCG has made appropriate arrangements for ensuring that the CCG complies with its obligations to exercise its functions effectively, efficiently and economically. It also has a duty to ensure that it complies with relevant generally accepted principles of good governance. Section 14L of NHS Act 2006, as inserted by section 25 of the HSCA 2012, sets out the duties of the governing bodies of CCGs:

- promoting the NHS Constitution in the securing of health services;
- securing continuous improvement in the quality and safety of health services and in the quality of the experience undergone by patients;
- securing continuous improvement in quality of primary medical services;
- reducing inequalities between patients with respect to their ability to access health services, and with respect to the outcomes achieved for them;
- promoting the involvement of patients, their carers and representatives in relation to their health service;
- enabling patients to make choices with respect to aspects of health services provided to them;
- obtaining appropriate professional health service advice to enable it effectively to discharge its functions;
- promoting innovation in the provision of health services;
- promoting research on matters relevant to health services;
- promoting education and training for the persons connected with the provision of health services; and
- securing health services that are provided in an integrated way to improve quality, reduce inequalities of access or outcome.

NHS trust boards

According to the DHSC, NHS trust boards have six key functions. They are held accountable for these by the DHSC on behalf of the SoS. These are to:

- set the strategic direction of the organisation within the overall policies and priorities of the government and the NHS, define its annual and longer-term objectives and agree plans to achieve them;
- oversee the delivery of planned results by monitoring performance against objectives and ensuring corrective action is taken when necessary;
- ensure effective financial stewardship through value for money, financial control and financial planning and strategy;
- ensure that high standards of health service governance and personal behaviour are maintained in the conduct of the business of the whole organisation;
- appoint, appraise and remunerate senior executives; and
- ensure that there is effective dialogue between the organisation and the local community on its plans and performance and that these are responsive to the community's needs.

The Healthy NHS Board (see Chapter 6) states that 'the purpose of NHS boards is to govern effectively and in doing so build patient, public and stakeholder confidence that their health and healthcare is in safe hands'.

It goes on to say that 'in unitary NHS boards, all directors are collectively and corporately accountable for organisational performance'.

Board responsibilities according to the voluntary codes

Alongside each of these prescribed purposes as defined by law or regulation there is also a common understanding around the role of the board and these are set out in the UK Code and the FRC Board Guide.

The UK Code is clear that the board of directors is the key decision-making body in an organisation. Therefore, an organisation should have an effective board of directors dedicated to ensuring that it achieves its objectives. The UK Code states as one of its main principles 'a successful company is led by an effective and entrepreneurial board, whose role is to promote the long-term sustainable success of the company, generating value for shareholders and contributing to wider society'.

The introduction of the phrase 'long-term' into this principle in 2010 recognised that the board should not focus on short-term achievements, if these are inconsistent with longer-term success. The UK Code states that the role of the board should be to:

- establish the company's purpose, values and strategy, and satisfy itself that these and its culture are aligned. All directors must act with integrity, lead by example and promote the desired culture;
- ensure that the necessary resources are in place for the company to meet its objectives and measure performance against them;

THE BOARD'S STRUCTURE AND ITS COMMITTEES

- establish a framework of prudent and effective controls, which enable risk to be assessed and managed;
- ensure effective engagement with, and encourage participation from shareholders and stakeholders; and
- ensure that workforce policies and practices are consistent with the company's values and support its long-term sustainable success. The workforce should be able to raise any matters of concern.

- The preface to the UK Code states:

   'To succeed in the long-term, directors and the companies they lead need to build and maintain successful relationships with a wide range of stakeholders. These relationships will be successful and enduring if they are based on respect, trust and mutual benefit. Accordingly, a company's culture should promote integrity and openness, value diversity and be responsive to the views of shareholders and wider stakeholders.'

The FRC Board Guide states that:

   'A company's purpose is the reason for which it exists. The board is responsible for setting and reconfirming the company's purpose. A well-defined purpose will help companies to articulate their business model, and develop their strategy, operating practices and approach to risk. Companies with a clear purpose often find it easier to engage with their workforce, customers and the wider public.'

One of the new emphases in the UK Code (2018) and supporting FRC Board Guide is that of the value of engagement with stakeholders. The Board Guide defines an effective board as one that 'understands that a company has to engage with its workforce and build and maintain relationships with suppliers, customers and others in order to be successful over the long-term'. It goes on to suggest that the board may wish to refer to *The Stakeholder Voice in Board Decision Making* issued jointly by the ICSA and the Investment Association on how to build stakeholder considerations into board discussions. It builds further on this engagement emphasis with clear recommendations on engaging the workforce. These are set out later in the section on board composition.

The FRC Board Guide also goes on to look at effective decision making in boards, as this is an important board activity. Chapter 6 covers this in more detail.

The South African King IV corporate governance code complements the approach taken by the UK guidance and identifies the distinct roles and responsibilities of the board and management as follows:

   '[The governing body should] steer the organisation and set its strategic direction, on the basis of which management will develop the strategy which is to be approved by the governing body. To give effect to the organisation's strategy, management formulates policy and operational plans, also to be approved by the governing body. Management then, implements and executes strategy in accordance with policy and plans, which are overseen and supervised by the governing body. The governing body finally ensures that there is accountability for organisational performance through, among others, reporting and disclosure. The latter in turn forms the basis for reviewing strategic direction, which starts the business cycle anew.'

King IV goes on to describe the key governance areas of ethics, risk, compliance, remuneration and stakeholder relationship.

Board structures

Unitary boards

Organisations are based around a unitary board structure in many countries. The unitary board consists of both EDs and NEDs under the leadership of the chair. A unitary board makes collective decisions and is accountable to the shareholders or major stakeholders. It is commonly accepted governance practice that the NEDs in a listed organisation should be independent, although this is not a legal requirement.

In the NHS, the concept of a unitary board has not always been well understood or implemented. In 2006, the Integrated Governance Handbook illustrates several dangers of not using a unitary board structure:

> 'To date, NHS boards have performed in a diverse manner by separating out the roles of the various directors, i.e. finance, medical, nursing etc, and the NED/lay individual input. The result of this is that, if the board takes a decision, it is often deemed to be the decision of, say, the finance director or HR director, rather than being a corporate decision. Board corporacy is paramount. Each decision or agreement entered into in the boardroom is a fully accepted corporate decision. If a decision around finance is taken and the information brought to the board clarifies the debate, if there are implications say, one month after the decision, the responsibility is of the corporate whole, rather than just the finance director.'

There is a clear move away from the unitary board structure for the CCGs that were established in 2012. NHSE advocates adherence with the Good Governance Standard as the guidance for best practice in governance; this presupposes a form of leadership not based on the principle of a unitary board. This is in stark contrast to most other NHS organisations (such as FTs) for whom the unitary board is a core principle of governance.

The purpose of the unitary board principle was to ensure that the interests of all stakeholders were properly considered and balanced. As such, CCGs are unlikely to operate in a way that is entirely consistent with the major codes of practice that set out best practice in corporate governance for the NHS – including the UK Code, King IV, the Higgs Report and the FT Code.

The concept of the unitary board is reinforced within the governance structure of the NHS FT, even though there may appear to be a two-tier board structure with a council of governors and a board of directors. The FT Core Constitution and the FT Code make it clear that the concept of the unitary board refers to the fact that NEDs and EDs share the same liability within the board of directors. All directors, ED and NED, have the responsibility to constructively challenge the decisions of the board and help develop proposals on priorities, risk mitigation, values, standards and strategy.

The Healthy NHS Board adds:

> 'A key strength of unitary boards is the opportunity provided for the exchange of views between executives and NEDs, drawing on and pooling their experience and capabilities. Boards are "social systems". The most effective boards invest time and energy in the development of mature relationships and ways of working.'

One of the threats to the principle of the unitary board is the increasing emphasis on the role of the NED. The role of independent scrutiny and constructive challenge undertaken by the NED role can create a tension with their responsibility to provide a strategic oversight and to act collectively alongside the EDs. EDs are not excused from providing scrutiny and challenge, it's just that they cannot be classed as independent.

For example, it has been seen as good practice for NEDs to meet (at least) annually as a group without the chair or EDs present, and also for board committees to be made up solely of NEDs; if not managed correctly, this can divide a unitary board. There is also a further threat, particularly rife in the NHS, which is the increasing requirement for NEDs to be 'champions' for specific areas of management concern (e.g. for whistleblowing or infection control or learning from deaths). This blurs the boundary between governance and management, and between the roles of the NED and the ED.

Interestingly the FRC Board Guide recommends that NEDs do not operate exclusively within the confines of the boardroom but have a good understanding of the business and its relationships with significant stakeholders. Accordingly, it advises them to take opportunities to meet shareholders, key customers and members of the workforce from all levels of the organisation.

Having said all that, the concept of a unitary board is still common practice within the NHS and continues to be the subject of a considerable amount of board development.

Two-tier boards

Some countries, including Germany and Austria, have two-tier boards. A two-tier structure usually consists of a supervisory board and a management board.

The management board is responsible for managing the organisation. It is led by the chair of the management board, normally the CEO, and its members are appointed by the supervisory board. The management board consists entirely of EDs. It develops strategy for the organisation in co-operation with the supervisory board and is responsible for implementing the agreed strategy. It also has responsibility for risk management and for the preparation of the annual financial statements (which are examined by the auditors and the supervisory board). The chair of the management board reports to the supervisory board chair.

The supervisory board is responsible for general oversight of the organisation and of the management board. Members are normally elected by shareholders, except in public companies with more than 500 employees where a minimum proportion of the supervisory board must consist of employee representatives. The supervisory board consists entirely of NEDs. The chair leads the supervisory board, which advises the management board and must be involved in decision-making on all fundamental matters affecting the organisation. These include 'decisions or measures which fundamentally change the asset, financial or earnings situations of the enterprise' (German Corporate Governance Code). The audit committee consists entirely of supervisory board members. In Germany, supervisory board members include:

- representatives of trade unions and/or the organisation's employees;
- representatives of major shareholders; and
- former executives of the organisation.

Supervisory board NEDs are therefore not necessarily independent, particularly employee representatives. It can therefore be difficult to reconcile the differing views of employee representatives and representatives of major shareholders without antagonising the EDs on the management board.

However, if there are a large number of former EDs on the supervisory board, there is a risk that it could take a lenient view of management activities. In addition, some independent supervisory board directors might well be senior managers of other companies, where they are management board members. These individuals might therefore sympathise with the views of the management board.

The success of corporate governance in a two-tier structure depends on a functional relationship between the supervisory board and the management board. The chair of the supervisory board plays a key role. They are responsible for making sure that the two boards work well together. The most powerful individuals in the organisation are the chair of the supervisory board and the CEO. If the relationship between these two works well, the chair will effectively speak for the management at meetings of the supervisory board.

The German Corporate Governance Code states that 'the management board and supervisory board co-operate closely to the benefit of the enterprise' and the management board should discuss the implementation of strategy regularly with the supervisory board.

The main concerns of a two-tier board structure are as follows.

- Supervisory boards are too big, having up to 20 members. German supervisory boards include a large number of employee representatives, and large numbers can result in inefficient meetings.
- It has been common to appoint retired former managers of the organisation to the supervisory board, and these individuals might be tempted to retain some influence over the actions and operational decisions of their successors. This is not the purpose of a supervisory board. However, if former managers are appointed to the supervisory board, it will benefit from their knowledge and experience of the business. In Germany, former managers are now prohibited from 'moving upstairs' to the supervisory board for at least two years, unless the move receives the support of at least 25% of shareholders, because it is thought a former ED will not be sufficiently independent immediately after retiring.
- Companies with more than 500 employees are required to have workers' or trade union representatives on the supervisory board. Companies with more than 2,000 employees are required to have an even greater percentage of employee representatives on the supervisory board. This requirement is an enforcement of the principle of 'co-determination', embodied in German law, that the workers as well as the management and owners should determine the future of their companies. Unfortunately, workers' representatives can lack the competence to consider strategic issues or are not independent from the organisation. In some instances, worker members of a supervisory board opposing planned initiatives by the organisation have been accused of leaking confidential information to the press.
- Concerns about information leaks can damage communications between supervisory and management boards.

The German Corporate Governance Code suggests that the unitary board system and two-tier board system are becoming similar in practice because of intensive interaction between the management and supervisory boards. The German code also suggests that the two types of board structure are equally successful. Developments in some German companies in recent years also suggest that the supervisory boards of large German companies are becoming more responsive to the interests of their shareholders.

The 2009 Walker Report on UK bank corporate governance considered whether unitary boards contributed to the scale of the financial crisis in 2007–09 and whether a two-tier board structure might be more suitable for large banks. Its conclusions were fairly critical of the two-tier structure:

'In practice, two-tier structures do not appear to assure members of the supervisory board of access to the quality and timeliness of management information flow that would generally be regarded as essential for non-executives on a unitary board. Moreover, since, in a two-tier structure, members of the supervisory and executive boards meet separately and do not share the same responsibilities, the two-tier model would not provide opportunity for the interactive exchange of views between executives and NEDs, drawing on and pooling their respective experience and capabilities in the way that takes place in a well-functioning unitary board.'

Matters reserved for the board

Regardless of structure, the board of directors must meet sufficiently regularly to discharge its duties effectively. In addition, the board should have a formal schedule of matters specifically reserved for decision by the board of directors, which will ensure that the main decision-making powers belong to the board of directors. Although the board delegates many of the operational decision-making responsibilities to executive management, it should retain the most significant decisions, and these are recorded in the Matters Reserved for the Board. A key aspect of governance is therefore the nature of the decisions the board reserves for itself (rather than delegating them to executive management).

The FRC Board Guide does not specify which matters should be reserved by the board, but states simply that 'a formal schedule of matters reserved for its decision will assist the board's planning and provide clarity to all over where responsibility for decision-making lies'.

ICSA: The Governance Institute's Guidance Note on matters that should be reserved for the board recommends the following matters be included:

- approval of annual operating and capital expenditure budgets;
- approval of the annual report and accounts;
- approval of formal communications with shareholders;
- approval of major contracts and investments;
- approval of policies on matters such as health and safety, corporate social responsibility (CSR) and the environment approval of strategy;
- changes in corporate or capital structure;
- compliance with legal and regulatory requirements;
- oversight of operations (including accounting, planning and internal control systems); and
- performance review.

The company secretary may be given the task of preparing and maintaining the list of matters to be reserved for the board (for board approval) and reminding the board whenever necessary that certain decisions should not be delegated.

Although this guidance is not specifically aimed at NHS boards, it contains best practice, which NHS boards should actively consider. Though the formal powers of an NHS organisation are vested in its board, the NHS Code of Accountability allows the board to delegate some of its business to board committees and to the EDs.

The board approach to delegation should be consistently set out in:

- its standing orders, which specify how the organisation conducts its business;
- its standing financial instructions, which detail the financial responsibilities, policies and procedures adopted; and
- its scheme of reservation and delegation. This sets out which responsibilities and accountabilities remain at board level and which have been delegated to committees and to the executive, together with the appropriate reporting arrangements that ensure the board has oversight.

The ICSA guidance notes do offer a sample matters reserved for both a FT board of directors and council of governors. A thorough understanding of the matters reserved for the board must underpin a board's approach to delegation. Its schemes of delegation must be subject to regular board review to ensure that the distribution of functions and accountabilities is accurately and appropriately described, and remains appropriate despite changes in the organisation.

Size and composition of the board

The effectiveness of a board of directors depends on its size and composition.

Size

The typical size of a board of directors varies with the size of the organisation and/or the industry or business sector in which it operates. In addition, the average size of boards in listed companies varies between different countries.

A board should not be any larger than it needs to be. Large boards are more difficult to manage, because there are more individuals involved, and board meetings can be very long and time consuming. However, a board should be large enough for its members collectively to have the knowledge, skills and experience to make effective decisions.

The UK Code has previously suggested that the board should be sufficiently large to avoid a situation in which it becomes over-reliant on one or two individuals, for example, as chairmen of board committees (nominations, remuneration, audit and risk committees).

The Walker Review identified that where board membership exceeded 8–12 directors, the risk known as 'group-think' – the phenomenon of a group exhibiting thought processes whereby they seek to minimise conflict and reach consensus without critically testing, analysing and evaluating ideas – increases.

The Healthy NHS Board suggests that:

'NHS boards should not be so large as to be unwieldy, but must be large enough to provide the balance of skills and experience that is appropriate for the organisation. The number of directors is defined in the trust's establishment order, or in a FT's constitution. The composition of the board should achieve a balance between continuity and renewal. Chairs and non-executive directors

(NEDs) of NHS trusts serve a maximum of 10 years in the same NHS post (or two three-year terms for FTs) to ensure this balance. Within this period, any second reappointment must be through open competition. The composition of the board should achieve a balance between continuity and renewal.'

Composition

The composition of a board of directors depends partly on its size. In the UK, the board of a large public company commonly consists of:

- a chair
- possibly a deputy chair
- the CEO
- the senior independent director (SID, who may also be the deputy chair)
- EDs
- NEDs.

Collectively, the members of the board should have sufficient skills and experience to provide effective leadership for the organisation. This suggests that they should have a variety of different backgrounds and expertise.

There should also be a suitable balance of power so that one individual or a small group of individuals is unable to dominate the board and its decision-making. In countries such as the UK, it is considered appropriate to appoint independent NEDs to a board, because they act as a counter-balance to EDs who may give priority to their own interests above those of the shareholders (and other stakeholders). They also have skills and experience that EDs do not have, because they come from a different background and so are able to contribute different ideas and views to board discussions and decision making. As they do not have a strong personal financial interest in the organisation, NEDs are more easily able to represent the interests of the major stakeholders (typically shareholders) and to act (where required) as a restraint on executive management.

These principles relating to board composition are set out in the FRC Guidance on Board Effectiveness as follows:

> 'Appointing directors who are able to make a positive contribution is one of the key elements of board effectiveness. Directors will be more likely to make good decisions and maximise the opportunities for the company's success if the right skillsets and a breadth of perspectives are present in the boardroom. Non-executive directors should possess a range of critical skills of value to the board and relevant to the challenges and opportunities facing the company.'

The UK Code reiterates that

> 'The board should include an appropriate combination of executive and non-executive (and, in particular, independent non-executive) directors, such that no one individual or small group of individuals dominates the board's decision making. There should be a clear division of responsibilities between

the leadership of the board and the executive leadership of the company's business.'

Following on with the emphasis on engagement and in particular the workforce, the FRC Guidance suggests that, one or a combination of the following methods should be used:

- a director appointed from the workforce;
- a formal workforce advisory panel; or
- a designated NED.

If the board has not chosen one or more of these methods, it should explain what alternative arrangements are in place and why it considers that they are effective. Workforce representatives may therefore become an accepted requirement of board composition although there has been considerable criticism of this approach with companies insisting that engagement can be effectively delivered through positive working relationships with their associate trade unions.

The UK Code also sets out different requirements for large listed companies – where at least half of the board, excluding the chair, should be independent NEDs – and for smaller companies (those outside the FTSE 350) should appoint at least two independent NEDs.

Guidelines about the composition of a unitary board differ between countries. The King IV Code, for example, recommends that the majority of directors should be NEDs and the majority of NEDs should be independent, but also adds that there should be at least two EDs on the board – the CEO and chief finance officer (CFO) (finance director).

NHS board composition

The principle that there should be sufficient independent NEDs to create a suitable balance of power is also reflected in the FT Code. However, there is a distinction between NEDs and the role of lay members on a CCG governing body, which is explored in Chapter 15.

In the NHS, the composition of the board is clearly dictated either by:

- the Trust Membership and Procedure Regulations (SI 1998/1975);
- in FTs, by Schedule 7 to the NHS Act 2006; or
- in CCGs by section 14L of the NHS Act 2006 as inserted by section 25 of the HSCA 2012.

There are differences in composition for FTs, CCGs and NHS trusts and whilst the detail or NHS trusts is set out below the details for FTs and CCGs composition is set out in Chapters 14 and 15. The composition for NHS Trusts is as follows:

- The maximum number of directors of an NHS trust shall be 12 excluding the chair and the minimum not less than eight.

- The EDs of an NHS trust shall include the chief officer of the trust; the chief finance officer of the trust; a medical or dental practitioner and a registered nurse or registered midwife.
- There will be a trust chair (appointed by NHS TDA), up to seven NEDs (appointed by the NHS TDA), and up to five EDs (but not exceeding the number of non-officer members) including the CEO and the director of finance.

Board committees

One aspect of best practice in governance is that the board should decide that the EDs be excluded from the decision making or monitoring responsibilities for some issues.

This is achieved by delegating certain responsibilities to committees of the board. A board committee might consist entirely or mostly of NEDs and have the responsibility for dealing with particular issues and making recommendations to the full board. The full board is then usually expected to accept and endorse the recommendations of the relevant board committee. Despite this, the committees only have delegated authority from the board; they do not have the capacity to act independently.

According to the Walker Review, the optimum size for a sub-committee is between five and nine members. It states 'at five a group becomes more of a team, at seven thinking is optimised; above nine the ability of the cognitive limit of the group is exceeded'.

Three standing committees are recommended by the UK Code:

- an audit committee
- a nomination committee
- a remuneration committee.

Some boards might establish other committees. For example, an organisation might have an environment committee if its business activities are likely to have important consequences for the environment – especially if it involves an exposure to government regulation, the law and public opinion. The Walker Review recommended that all banks and life assurance companies establish a risk committee with responsibility for 'oversight and advice to the board on the current risk exposures to the entity and future risk strategy'. In recognition of the emphasis on workforce engagement in the UK Code, the FRC Board Guide suggests that a board can delegate responsibility for reviewing non-pay-related workforce policies to a board committee with relevant responsibilities where one exists, for example, a people committee, a sustainability committee or a corporate responsibility committee.

Guidance for the NHS can be found in the DH (now DHSC) publication the Intelligent Board, which recommended that all NHS trusts should have an audit committee, a nomination committee and a remuneration (and terms of service)

THE BOARD'S STRUCTURE AND ITS COMMITTEES

committee as part of their governance arrangements. All report to the board of directors.

Nowadays, the model standing orders for NHS Trusts requires an audit committee as well as a remuneration and terms of service committee. In line with its role as a corporate trustee, the board should also establish a charitable funds committee. This enables it to administer any funds held in trust either as charitable or non-charitable funds, in accordance with any statutory/legal requirements or best practice required by the Charity Commission.

The FT core constitution for FTs requires the board to establish:

- a committee consisting of the trust chair, the CEO and the other NEDs to appoint or remove the other EDs (nomination committee); and
- a committee of NEDs to decide the remuneration and allowances, and the other terms and conditions of office, of the CEO and other EDs (remuneration committee).

According to the FT Code, FTs may choose to have two nomination committees, one dealing with NEDs and one with EDs. Where an NHS FT has two nomination committees, the nomination committee responsible for the appointment of NEDs should consist of a majority of governors. If only one nomination committee exists, when nominations for NEDs are being discussed – including the appointment of a chair or a deputy chair – there should be a majority of governors on the committee, and a majority of governors on the interview panel. The core constitution also requires the FT to establish a NED committee as an audit committee to perform monitoring, reviewing and other functions. It also requires the council of governors to approve the appointment of all NEDs, including the trust chair.

CCGs are required by statute to appoint an audit committee and a remuneration committee (see section 14M(1) of the NHS Act 2006, as inserted by section 25 of HSCA 2012). The NHS England guidance *Towards Establishment: Creating responsive and accountable clinical commissioning groups* also recommends that CCGs consider the establishment of a quality committee to:

- provide assurance on the quality of services commissioned; and
- promote a culture of continuous improvement and innovation with respect to safety of services, clinical effectiveness and patient experience.

In practice, most NHS organisations also have a board committee that covers quality assurance, governance and/or risk.

Boards should ensure that they delegate authority to committees in line with their constitutional documents, set out clear terms of reference for them – including the composition and quoracy requirements – and provide a clear statement of the remit of the committee. These committees do not absolve the board of its responsibility in their respective areas of scrutiny: rather, they should support the board in carrying out its responsibilities of strategic leadership and holding to account.

The three main committees (audit, nomination and remuneration) are set out in detail in later chapters. Here is a brief summary of their functions.

The audit committee

The FRC Audit Guide states that the 'audit committee has a particular role, acting independently from the executive, to ensure that the interests of shareholders are properly protected in relation to financial reporting and internal control'. The guidance contains recommendations about the conduct of the audit committee's relationship with the board, with the executive management and with internal and external auditors:

> 'The essential features of these interactions are a frank, open working relationship and a high level of mutual respect. The audit committee must be prepared to take a robust stand, and all parties must be prepared to make information freely available to the committee, to listen to their views and to talk through the issues openly.'

At times, it may be necessary for the committee to challenge the position of the external auditors or other professional advisers. The committee should comprise a minimum of three independent NEDs and have clear terms of reference. The chair of the board may only be a member of the committee in smaller companies, and even then, may not chair the committee.

These principles are reflected in the NHS Audit Committee Handbook, published by the Healthcare Financial Management Association (HFMA). The HFMA handbook says the audit committee plays a key role by:

> 'critically reviewing and reporting on the relevance and robustness of the governance structures and assurance processes on which the board places reliance. In particular, this requires the committee to understand and scrutinise the organisations overarching framework of governance, risk and control'.

The HFMA handbook stipulates that the chair of the board should not chair the audit committee nor be a member of the committee. It also specifies that at least one member of the committee should have 'recent and relevant financial experience' (in line with the FRC Audit Guide mentioned above).

The audit committee should summarise its work during the year, submitting an annual report to the board promptly after the year-end but before it considers the organisation's annual report and statutory declarations. The UK Code also provides that a separate section of the annual report should describe the work of the committee. This deliberately puts the spotlight on the audit committee and gives it an authority that it might otherwise lack.

The UK Code (2018) sets out the role of the audit committee more fully and this is set out in more detail in Chapter 6.

The nomination committee

This committee gained a higher profile after the publication of the Higgs Report, which resulted in the UK Code recommending that all listed companies should establish a nomination committee. Its remit covers the review of the structure, size and composition of the board, including:

- the oversight of the board's succession planning requirements for EDs, NEDs, the company secretary and other senior management positions);
- the identification and assessment of potential board candidates; and
- making nominations to the board for its approval as appropriate.

The FRC Board Guide states that 'the nomination committee is responsible for board recruitment and will conduct a continuous and proactive process of planning and assessment, taking into account the company's strategic priorities and the main trends and factors affecting the long-term success and future viability of the company'.

In particular, the FRC Board Guide emphasises the importance of diversity of background and of personal attributes. It recommends that the nomination committee, by working with human resources, must take an active role in setting and meeting diversity objectives and strategies for the company as a whole, and in monitoring the impact of diversity initiatives. Examples of the type of actions the nomination committee could consider encouraging include:

- a commitment to increasing the diversity of the board by setting stretching targets;
- dedicated initiatives with clear objectives and targets; for example, in areas of the business that lack diversity;
- a focus on middle management;
- mentoring and sponsorship schemes;
- a commitment to more diverse shortlists and interview panels; and
- positive action to encourage more movement of women into non-traditional roles.

The committee membership is appointed by the board and should comprise the chair, CEO and NEDs. The majority of its members must be independent NEDs. The chair of the board should chair the committee, except when it is dealing with the appointment of a successor chair: the SID should chair the committee in this instance. The Committee is usually made up of at least three members who are free of any conflict of interest. Members conflicted on any aspect of an agenda presented to the committee are required to declare their conflict and withdraw from discussions.

These guidelines are largely followed by NHS organisations in their standing orders or constitutional documents.

Further details on the main duties of the nomination committee can be found in Chapter 9.

The remuneration committee

This committee received an increased profile following the publication of the Kay Review and the stirrings of the 'Shareholder Spring' in 2012 when investors refused to back multi-million pound bonuses for EDs when coupled with extremely poor corporate performance.

There has been a greater emphasis on public disclosure of executive remuneration, and a culture change of shareholders refusing to accept severance pay arrangements. Changes in 2013 to the CA 2006 saw increased levels of reporting on remuneration in the annual report and greater voting powers for shareholders. More recently, the consultation on employee representation on boards may also impact remuneration levels for senior managers and directors. See the section on board composition above.

The Enterprise and Regulatory Reform Act 2013 underlines the importance of boards and investors engaging on directors' remuneration. The UK Code recommends that the committee determines an appropriate balance between fixed and performance-related, and immediate and deferred remuneration; that performance conditions should be relevant, stretching and designed to promote the long-term success of the company; and that incentives should be compatible with risk policies and systems. The committee should also consider whether the directors should be eligible for annual bonuses and/or benefits under long-term incentive schemes.

The UK Code states that the committee should comprise at least three independent NEDs (although two is permissible for smaller companies). In addition to the independent NEDs, the chair of the board may also be a member of the committee if they were considered independent on appointment as chair, but may not chair the committee. Before appointment as chair of the remuneration committee, the appointee should have served on a remuneration committee for at least 12 months. The ICSA's model terms of reference for the remuneration committee states that it is good practice for the company secretary to act as secretary to the committee, although this is not a provision in the UK Code.

The FRC Board Guide defines the role of the remuneration committee as having delegated responsibility for designing and determining remuneration for the chair, EDs and the next level of senior management and that it is vital that the committee recognises and manages potential conflicts of interest in this process.

The remuneration committee is also tasked with reviewing workforce remuneration and related policies. The purpose of this review is to:

- ensure the reward, incentives and conditions available to the company's workforce are taken into account when deciding the pay of EDs and senior management;
- enable the remuneration committee to explain to the workforce each year how decisions on executive pay reflect wider company pay policy; and

THE BOARD'S STRUCTURE AND ITS COMMITTEES

- enable the remuneration committee to feed back to the board on workforce reward, incentives and conditions, and support the latter's monitoring of whether company policies and practices support culture and strategy.

The review should include matters such as any pay principles applied across the company, base pay, benefits, and all incentives and aspects of financial and non-financial reward that drive behaviour – for example, sales compensation – regardless of where this is managed in the business.

Under the UK Code, there should be a description of the work of the remuneration committee in the annual report, including:

- an explanation of the strategic rationale for EDs remuneration policies, structures and any performance metrics;
- reasons why the remuneration is appropriate using internal and external measures, including pay ratios and pay gaps;
- a description, with examples, of how the remuneration committee has addressed the factors in Provision 40 which established guidelines for executive director remuneration policy and practices;
- whether the remuneration policy operated as intended in terms of company performance and quantum, and, if not, what changes are necessary;
- what engagement has taken place with shareholders and the impact this has had on remuneration policy and outcomes;
- what engagement with the workforce has taken place to explain how executive remuneration aligns with wider company pay policy; and
- to what extent discretion has been applied to remuneration outcomes and the reasons why.

HM Treasury also requires NHS organisations to provide a remuneration report in a prescribed format within their annual report and accounts.

The principal duties of the remuneration committee

A list of duties of the remuneration committee were at one time included as an annex to the UK Code, and they are now set out in ICSA's guidance note on the terms of reference for a remuneration committee (see Table 7.1). Typically, the duties of a remuneration committee in the corporate sector are as follows.

- The committee should determine and agree with the main board the remuneration policy for the CEO, the chair of the board and any other designated executive managers. This policy should provide for executive managers to be given appropriate incentives for enhanced performance.
- To maintain and assure their independence, the committee should also decide the remuneration of the company secretary.
- The committee should decide the targets for performance for any performance-related pay schemes operated by the organisation.
- It should decide the policy for and scope of pension arrangements for each ED.

- It should ensure that the contractual terms for severance payments on termination of office are fair to both the individual and the organisation, that failure is not rewarded and that the director's duty to mitigate losses is fully recognised.
- Within the framework of the agreed remuneration policy, it should determine the remuneration package of each individual ED, including any bonuses, incentive payments and share options.
- It should be aware of and advise on any major changes in employee benefit structures throughout the organisation or group.
- It should agree the policy for authorising expense claims from the chair and CEO.
- It should ensure compliance by the organisation with the requirements for disclosure of directors' remuneration in the annual report and accounts.
- It should be responsible for appointing any remuneration consultants to advise the committee.
- In the annual report, it should report the frequency of committee meetings and the attendance by members.
- It should make available to the public its terms of reference, setting out the committee's delegated responsibilities. Where necessary these should be reviewed and updated each year.

NHS remuneration committees are also required to declare the relationship between the remuneration of the highest-paid director in their organisation and the median remuneration of the organisation's workforce in its annual report in line with the Hutton Fair Pay Review (see Chapter 15).

Protecting the independence and effectiveness of board committees

As a way of protecting the independence and improving the effectiveness of board committees, the UK Code recommends that consideration should be given to the benefits of ensuring that committee membership is refreshed when deciding the chairship and membership of board committees (membership rotation). It adds that undue reliance should not be placed on particular individuals.

In addition, the only individuals who are entitled to attend meetings of the nomination, remuneration and audit committees are the chair and members of the committee, although other individuals may attend at the invitation of the committee.

The UK Code recommends that the effectiveness of the board committees be reviewed annually and included within the overall annual review of board effectiveness.

Nominations committee	Audit committee	Remuneration committee
Chair should be the chair of the board	Chair should be an independent NED	Chair should be an independent NED with at least 12 months' experience of the committee
Majority of members should be independent NEDs	All independent NEDs – in large companies, at least three, in smaller companies two	All independent NEDs – in large companies, at least three, in smaller companies two
If the board chair is the committee chair, s/he should not act as chair when the committee is considering their successor	In smaller companies, the chair of the board may also be a member of the audit committee (but not chair of the committee), in addition to the independent NEDs – but only if they were independent on appointment to the chair	The chair of the board may be a member of the committee if they were considered independent on appointment as chair, but may not chair the committee
	At least one member of the committee should have recent and relevant financial experience	

Table 7.1: Summary of the UK Code's recommendations regarding membership of board committees

Governance checklist

- Does the board act as the controlling mind of the organisation?
- Does it provide strategic and entrepreneurial leadership?
- Are there prudent and effective controls to manage the principal risks faced by the organisation?
- Do EDs and NEDs fulfil their roles individually and collectively within a unitary board structure?
- Are the statutory board committees properly constituted?
- Do they provide effective oversight in their respective areas?
- How does assurance flow from committee to board and between committees?
- Are the board committees properly constituted with delegated powers and clear terms of reference?

- Does the board make the appropriate public disclosures about its work and the work of its committees?

Summary

- The unitary nature of the board is a key issue in understanding the governance arrangements for the board.
- The board acts as the 'controlling mind' or head of the organisation: checks and balances need to be in place to make sure that it is held fully to account by stakeholders for the decisions that it takes.
- There is a distinct difference for governing bodies of CCGs, which are not established as unitary boards.
- On all boards, however, the distinct roles for EDs and NEDs (lay members in CCGs) must be recognised, while at the same time maintaining collective responsibility.

8
Directors' duties and liabilities

Introduction

It is an accepted governance tenet that boards have a collective responsibility for the way they act and make decisions. However, the individual directors who make up the board also have key duties and responsibilities as a consequence of their roles – and they will be liable for certain outcomes that result from the actions and decisions of the board. There is extensive legal precedent on this subject, which cannot be covered in detail in this handbook. However, the information collected here will form the basis of a good understanding for those individuals who take on a director role within an NHS organisation.

As set out in Chapter 7, the directors act as agents of the organisation, binding the organisation in its relationships with a number of third parties. They can do this with 'actual authority' or 'apparent authority' (the directors represented to the third party that they had the authority to act on behalf of the organisation).

This power to act is constrained by the duties that are expected of those directors. These duties stem from two sources – common law and statute. The duties enshrined in common law should be considered for directors of NHS organisations. As far as the legislation is concerned, a 'company' means a company formed and registered under the companies' legislation. NHS organisations that are organisations created by statutory instrument – not registered companies – are not bound by this legislation. Even so, it is good practice to have an understanding of the general principles of the companies' legislation and the nature of the original common law duties.

A distinction should be made between the powers and duties of EDs as board members and their responsibilities as managers of the organisation. Managers have neither powers nor duties to bind the organisation. The relationship they have with the organisation (including their authority and responsibilities) is established by their contract of employment and by the law of agency.

Who can be a director?

Anyone can become a director under companies legislation, with a few exceptions. The following cannot be a company director:

- someone who is disqualified by the company's own articles of association (the rules relating to the running of the company);
- an undischarged bankrupt;
- someone disqualified by a court order; or
- the company's auditor.

If someone effectively acts as a director, even without the title, they may still legally be seen as a director. The law on a director's duties and liabilities also specifically includes a person who is classed as a 'shadow director'; this is anyone who, despite not officially being a 'director', regularly attends board and strategy meetings and upon whose advice the directors are accustomed to act. This could apply to a lawyer or accountant (or a FT governor acting outside of their role) who advises a company's directors and whose guidance the directors usually take.

NHS directors

The 'fit and proper persons' test for NHS directors was introduced under the Health and Social Care Act 2008 (Regulated Activities) Regulations 2014. This means the CQC will assess whether directors are:

- of good character;
- have the necessary qualifications, skills and experience;
- are able to perform the work that they are employed for; and
- can supply information, such as certain checks and a full employment history.

The 'fit and proper person' requirement for directors will have a wider impact, in both the scope of its application and the nature of the test. It makes it clear that individuals who have authority in organisations that deliver care are responsible for the overall quality and safety of that care and, as such, can be held accountable if standards of care do not meet legal requirements. The test applies to people who have director level responsibility for the quality and safety of care. This includes any executive and non-executive, permanent, interim and associate positions, irrespective of their voting rights.

It will apply to all directors and 'equivalents'. This will include executive directors (EDs) and non-executive directors (NEDs) of NHS trusts and FTs and members of clinical commissioning group (CCG) governing bodies. It will be the responsibility of the healthcare provider and, in the case of FTs and CCGs, the chair, to ensure that all directors meet the fitness test and do not meet any of the 'unfit' criteria. For NHS trusts, NHS Improvement (NHSI) is responsible for ensuring NEDs meet the criteria.

In addition to the usual requirements of good character, health, qualifications, skills and experience, the regulation bars individuals who are prevented from holding the office of director (e.g. under a directors' disqualification order). It also excludes from office people who:

'have been responsible for, been privy to, contributed to or facilitated any serious misconduct or mismanagement (whether unlawful or not) in the course of carrying on a regulated activity, or discharging any functions relating to any office or employment with a service provider.'

In addition, a director will fail the 'fit and proper person' test if they:

- are an undischarged bankrupt;
- are the subject of a bankruptcy order or an interim bankruptcy order; or
- have an undischarged arrangement with creditors.

The CQC will require the chair of the board or NHSI to confirm that the fitness of all new directors has been assessed in line with the regulations and to declare to the CQC in writing that they are satisfied that they are fit and proper individuals for that role. NHSI have also made explicit that health and social care providers have to undertake an enhanced DBS check for directors to check whether they are on the children's and/or safeguarding barred list where they meet an eligibility criteria.

The standing orders of an NHS organisation may also include grounds upon which a person is disqualified from office. These include:

- people who have received a prison sentence or suspended sentence of three months or more in the last five years;
- people who are the subject of a bankruptcy restriction order or interim order;
- anyone who has been dismissed (except by redundancy) by any NHS body;
- in certain circumstances, those who have had an earlier term of appointment terminated;
- anyone who is under a disqualification order under the Company Directors' Disqualification Act 1986;
- anyone who has been removed from trusteeship of a charity;
- in most circumstances, civil servants within the DHSC, or members/employees of the CQC;
- a member of the council of governors or a chair or member of the governing body of a CCG – or an employee of such group or a member of the local authority's OCS;
- a person who is the spouse, partner, parent or child of a member of the board of directors (including the chair) of the trust;
- a person whose tenure of office as a chair or as an officer or director of a health service body has been terminated on the grounds that their appointment is not in the interests of the health service, for non-attendance at meetings, or for non-disclosure of a pecuniary interest;
- a person who has had their name removed or been suspended from any list prepared under the National Health Service Act 2006 (NHS Act 2006) who has otherwise been suspended or disqualified from any healthcare profession, and has not had the suspension lifted or qualification reinstated; and

- anyone who has previously been or is currently subject to a sex offender order and/or required to register under the Sexual Offences Act 2003, or has committed a sexual offence prior to the requirement to register under current legislation.

The fit and proper persons test has been the subject of a detailed review by Tom Kark QC and Jane Russell (Barrister) (February 2019), and further developments in this area are expected.

The powers of directors

The powers of the board of directors are set out in an organisation's constitution. In UK companies, formed under the CA 2006, this means the articles of association. These are similar to, for example, a CCG's or FT's constitution or NHS trust's standing orders. Article 3 of the model articles of association states:

> 'Subject to the articles, the directors are responsible for the management of the company's business, for which purpose they may exercise all the powers of the company.'

In health service governance, the powers of the board of directors are set out in their governing document. For example, FTs have a written constitution, which has to be approved by both the FT board and council of governors and in some circumstances by the FT members at the AGM. This is then further defined by:

- the schedule of matters reserved for the board;
- the scheme of delegation;
- standing orders; and
- standing financial instructions.

These will be covered in more detail later in this chapter.

The duties of directors to their organisation

Directors act as agents of their organisation. They have certain duties, which are to the organisation itself – not to its shareholders, its employees or any person external to the organisation, such as the general public. Although an organisation is a legal person in law, it is not human. Since the relationship between directors and the organisation is by its very nature impersonal, it might be wondered just what 'duty' means.

The concept of duty is not easy to understand, and it is helpful to make a comparison with the duties owed by other individuals or groups.

Examples of individuals owing a duty to something inanimate are uncommon, although personnel in the armed forces have a duty to their country. It is more usual to show loyalty to something inanimate than to have a duty. For example, individuals might be expected to show loyalty to their country and they might voluntarily show loyalty to their sports team, group of friends or work colleagues. Arguably, solicitors have a duty to their profession to act ethically, although the solicitors' practice rules in the UK specify that solicitors owe a duty of care to their clients. Similarly, doctors have a duty to act ethically, but their duty is to their patients. Duty is normally owed to individuals or a group of people. It might therefore be supposed that directors should owe a duty to their shareholders and possibly to the organisation's employees, but this is not the case.

- Accountability and responsibility should not be confused with duty.
- Directors have a responsibility to use their powers in ways that seem best for the organisation and its shareholders or major stakeholders.
- They should be accountable to the 'owners' of the organisation, for the ways in which they have exercised their powers and/or the performance of the organisation.
- They have duties to the organisation.

If a person is guilty of a breach of duty, there should be a process for calling them to account. There might be an established disciplinary procedure, for example, in a court or before a judicial panel, with a recognised set of punishments for misbehaviour.

The common law duties of directors

Until the CA 2006 came into force, the main legal duties of directors to their organisation were duties in common law – a fiduciary duty and duty of skill and care to the organisation.

The CA 2006 has now written the common law duties of directors into statute law. It states that these general duties 'are based on certain common law rules and equitable principles as they apply to directors and have effect in place of those rules and principles as regards the duties owed to an organisation by a director' (CA 2006, s. 170). The Act goes on to state that the statutory general duties should be interpreted in the same way as the common law rules and equitable principles.

Fiduciary duty of directors

'Fiduciary' means given in trust, and the concept of a trustee (as established in US and UK law) is applicable. The directors hold a position of trust because they make contracts on behalf of the organisation, and control its property. Since this is similar to being a trustee of the organisation, a director has a fiduciary duty to the organisation (not its shareholders).

If a director were to act in breach of their fiduciary duty, legal action could be brought against them by the organisation. In such a situation, 'the organisation' might be represented by a majority of the board of directors, a majority of the shareholders or a single controlling shareholder.

A director would be in breach of their fiduciary duty in carrying out a particular transaction or series of transactions in any of the following circumstances:

- The transaction is not in any way incidental to the business of the organisation. For example, the CEO of a building construction organisation might decide to trade in diamonds and lose large amounts of money in these diamond-trading transactions.
- The transaction is not carried out bona fide (in good faith) with honesty and sincerity.
- The transaction has not been made for the benefit of the organisation but for the personal benefit of the director or an associate. A director has a fiduciary duty to avoid a conflict of interest between themselves personally and the organisation and must not obtain any personal benefit or profit from a transaction without the consent of the organisation. In other words, it would be a breach of fiduciary duty for a director to make a secret profit from a transaction by the organisation in which they have a personal interest.

Director's duty of skill and care

Directors are also subject to a duty of skill and care to the organisation. A director should not act negligently in carrying out their duties and could be personally liable for losses suffered by the organisation due to such negligence.

The standard of skill and care expected of a director is the higher of the skill that they have or the skill that would objectively be expected of a director of the particular organisation. In the case Re D'Jan of London [1993], the judge ruled that the common law duty of care was the equivalent to the statutory test applied by section 214 of the Insolvency Act 1986. This statutory test refers to what would be expected of 'a reasonably diligent person' having both:

- the general knowledge, skill and experience that may reasonably be expected of a person carrying out the same functions as are carried out by that director in relation to the organisation; and
- the general knowledge, skill and experience that that director has.

A director is expected to show the technical skills that would reasonably be expected from someone of their experience and expertise. If the finance director of a scientific research organisation is a qualified accountant, they would not be expected to possess the technical skills of a scientist but would be expected to possess some technical skill as an accountant.

However, the duty of skill and care does not extend to spending time in the organisation. A director should attend board meetings if possible, but at other times is not required to be concerned with the affairs of the organisation. This requirement is best understood with NEDs, who might visit the organisation only for board or committee meetings. The duties of a director are intermittent in nature and only arise from time to time, such as when the board meets. If a director holds an executive position in the organisation, a different situation

DIRECTORS' DUTIES AND LIABILITIES

arises, because he is an employee of the organisation with a contract of service. This contract might call for full-time attendance at the organisation or on its business. However, this requirement arises out of their job as a manager, not out of their position as a director.

It is also not a part of the duty of skill and care to watch closely over the activities of the organisation's management. Unless there are particular grounds for suspecting dishonesty or incompetence, a director is entitled to leave the routine conduct of the organisation's affairs to the management. If the management appears honest, the directors may rely on the information they provide. It is not part of their duty of skill and care to question whether the information is reliable, or whether important information is being withheld.

A board of directors might make a decision that appears ill-judged or careless. However, the courts in the UK are generally reluctant to condemn business decisions made by the board that appear, in hindsight, to show errors of judgement. Directors can exercise reasonable skill and care, but still make bad decisions.

For a legal action against a director to succeed, an organisation would have to prove that serious negligence had occurred. It would not be enough to demonstrate that some loss could have been avoided if the director had been a bit more careful.

Wrongful trading and the standard of duty and care

The standard of duty and care required from a director has been partly defined in a number of UK legal cases relating to wrongful trading. Under the Insolvency Act 1986, directors may be liable for wrongful trading by the organisation when they allowed the organisation to continue trading but knew (or should have known) that it would be unable to avoid an insolvent liquidation. When such a situation arises, and an organisation goes into liquidation, the liquidator can apply to the court for the director to be held personally liable for negligence.

When there is a question about the extent of the director's duties and responsibilities, a significant factor could be the level of reward that the director was entitled to receive from the company. Prima facie, the higher the rewards, the greater the responsibilities should be expected.

The statutory duties of directors

NHS organisations are not registered companies but organisations created by statutory instrument. As such, they are not bound by the CA 2006. Good practice, however, would require an understanding of the general principles of the Act, which are set out here.

The duties of directors were introduced into UK statute law by the CA 2006 (ss. 171–177). These consist of a duty to:

- act within powers;
- promote the success of the organisation;
- exercise independent judgement;

- exercise reasonable care, skill and diligence;
- avoid conflicts of interest;
- not accept benefits from third parties; and
- declare any interest in a proposed transaction or arrangement.

Duty to act within powers

A director must act within their powers in accordance with the organisation's constitution and should only exercise these powers for the purpose for which they were granted. If a director acts outside their powers to make a contractual agreement with a third party, the organisation is still liable for any obligation to the third party, provided that the third party has acted in good faith.

Directors should also ensure that they comply with the organisation's constitution. For example, when a group of directors meets, it must be clear whether the meeting is a full board meeting, a meeting of a board committee or an unofficial meeting of directors. Unless the meeting is a formal board meeting, the directors would be acting outside their powers if they took a decision on a matter that is reserved for decision making by the board.

Duty to promote the success of the organisation

A director must act, in good faith, in the way that they consider would be most likely to 'promote the success of the organisation for the benefit of its members as a whole'. The Act does not define 'success', but the term is likely to be interpreted as meaning 'increasing value for shareholders'. However, in so doing, a director must also have regard, among other matters, to the:

- likely long-term consequences of any decision;
- interests of the organisation's employees;
- need to foster the organisation's relationships with its customers, suppliers and others;
- impact of the organisation's operations on the community and the environment;
- desirability of the organisation maintaining its reputation for high standards of business conduct; and
- need to act fairly as between members of the organisation.

The Act does not create a duty of directors to any stakeholders other than the shareholders (members), but it requires directors to consider the interests of other stakeholders in reaching their decisions. The Act specifically mentions employees, customers, suppliers and the community.

FT directors now have the same responsibility to promote the success of the corporation so this particular duty is directly applicable to FTs.

Duty to exercise independent judgement

A director must exercise independent judgement. However, this requirement does not prevent a director from acting in a way authorised by the organisation's constitution (such as accepting resolutions passed by the shareholders in general meeting) or from acting in accordance with an agreement already entered into by the organisation that prevents the director from using discretion. The requirement for independent judgement does not prevent a director from taking advice and acting on it.

The ICSA Guidance on Directors' General Duties (2015) comments as follows on this duty.

- A director should ensure that they do not allow personal interests, for example in a particular contract, to affect their independent judgement in the interest of the company. A director should ideally excuse themselves from any meeting at which a decision is to be taken in respect of their own property or interest.
- Importantly, where someone is an ED, they must not promote a collective executive line, but should give the board the benefit of their own independent judgement, including their appreciation of the risks involved in a particular course of action.
- This duty does not prevent a director from exercising their power to delegate, but they must still exercise their own judgement in deciding whether to follow the action suggested by that person(s).
- Similarly, a director would not be prevented by this duty from seeking legal or other professional advice but, ultimately, the director's final judgement would need to be independent.
- A director associated with a major shareholder should set any 'representative' function aside and make decisions on their own merits. This is of particular importance in joint venture situations where there may be constraints imposed by joint venture agreements. However, the Act states that this duty is not infringed by a director acting in accordance with an agreement duly entered into by the company that restricts the future exercise of discretion by its directors, or in a way authorised by the company's constitution.
- Likewise, a director who is a family representative in the business may consult their family but must understand that they will make the final decision.
- A director of a subsidiary would need to take into account the interests of the parent company and the other subsidiaries, but not insofar as this would prejudice the solvency of the subsidiary itself. This might apply, for instance, in relation to a transfer of assets within a group.

Duty to exercise reasonable care, skill and diligence

This is similar to the common law duty of care. For example, if a NED had an accounting qualification, they would be expected to exercise more active scrutiny of the accounts (such as on the appropriateness of accounting policies) than a director without such a qualification.

Duty to avoid conflicts of interest

A director has a duty to avoid conflicts of interest with the interests of the organisation. However, this duty is not breached if the director declares to the board their interest in a transaction and the interest is authorised/approved by the board. In the commercial world, it is inevitable that many directors will have a potential conflict of interest with their organisation (whether direct or indirect). For example, one organisation might be planning to trade with another organisation in which one of its directors is a shareholder. In such a situation, the director concerned is required to declare their interest in the proposed contract and must not make a secret profit.

A director or a connected person might have a material interest in a transaction undertaken by the organisation. For example, the organisation might award a contract to a firm of building contractors to rebuild or develop a property owned by the organisation, and the director or their spouse might own the building organisation.

A director might also have a direct or indirect interest in a contract (or proposed contract) with the organisation. For example, the director might be a member of another organisation with which the organisation is planning to sign a business contract. Such a contract is not illegal, although the organisation can choose to rescind it, should it wish to do so.

If a director has an interest in a contract with the organisation and has failed to disclose it, and has received a payment under the contract, they will be regarded as holding the money in the capacity of constructive trustee for the organisation (and so is bound to repay the money).

The CA 2006 recognises three situations in which an actual or potential conflict of interests may arise.

- A conflict of interest may arise in a situation where the organisation is not a party to an arrangement or transaction, but where the director might be able to gain personally from 'the exploitation of any property, information or opportunity'. For example, a director might pursue an opportunity for their personal benefit that the organisation might have pursued itself.
- A conflict of interest may arise about a proposed transaction or arrangement to which the organisation will be a party. If a director has a direct or indirect personal interest in any such transaction or arrangement, they must disclose their interest to the board of directors before it is entered into by the organisation. An example would be a proposal to acquire a target company in which a director owns shares.
- A third type of conflict of interest arises with existing transactions or arrangements in which the organisation is already a party. It can be a criminal offence for a director not to make or update their declaration of interest in an arrangement or transaction to which the organisation is a party.

DIRECTORS' DUTIES AND LIABILITIES

This is key principle for NHS directors. There are specific guidelines for NHS directors to follow with regard to conflicts of interest, in line with the Nolan Principles, which are set out in the NHS Code of Conduct and Accountability and in the NHSE Guidance on Managing Conflicts of Interest (covered later in this chapter).

Duty not to accept benefits from third parties

A director must not accept benefits from a third party unless they have been authorised by the shareholders or cannot reasonably be regarded as creating a potential conflict of their interest. Clearly, accepting a bribe from a supplier in return for awarding a supply contract would be a breach of this duty. It would also be illegal to accept lunch or dinner from the same supplier or customer every week, accepting an all-expenses-paid holiday or accepting frequent invitations to 'hospitality' events. However, it should be within the law to accept an invitation to a day out to tennis at Wimbledon or an invitation to dinner to celebrate the successful completion of a project.

Many listed companies already have strict policies on the acceptance of gifts and corporate hospitality, especially from other companies that are or might be about to tender for business with the organisation. A policy might include a requirement for a director to obtain clearance from another director before accepting any such benefits, and for all instances of gifts or hospitality to be recorded in a register.

The Bribery Act 2010 sets out that an organisation may be liable for failing to prevent a person from bribing on its behalf, but only if that person performs business services for it. It contains a full defence for an organisation that shows it had adequate procedures in place to prevent bribery. It is important to note that guidance on the Act specifically sets out that while hospitality is not prohibited by the Act, facilitation payments are classed as bribes.

The Bribery Act is applicable to NHS organisations, and there are a number of steps that they can consider. These include:

- carrying out a bribery and corruption risk assessment;
- putting in place anti-bribery procedures that are proportionate to the identified risks;
- ensuring that when proportionate anti-bribery procedures are put in place, the principles outlined in the guidance are taken into account (top-level commitment, due diligence, communication and training, and monitoring and review);
- being clear that NHS organisations and their employees, contractors and agents are covered by corporate liability for bribery;
- taking steps to make their trust employees and contractors aware of the standards of conduct expected of them, particularly in known risk areas such as procurement; and

- recording any steps taken, as they provide the defence against corporate liability under the Act.

Duty to declare interests in proposed transactions with the organisation

This duty is linked to the duty relating to conflicts of interest. A director must declare the nature and extent of their interest to the other directors, who may then authorise it. The NHS Code of Conduct and Accountability also covers this for NHS directors.

A director may have a personal interest in a proposed transaction with the organisation. For example, a director may own a building that the organisation wants to buy or rent; or a director may be a major shareholder in another organisation that is hoping to become a supplier or customer. Proposed transactions do not necessarily create a conflict of interest, but they must, nevertheless, be declared and subject to approval by the rest of the board. If a conflict of interest would arise from the proposed transaction, the director must take measures to ensure that the conflict is avoided.

Other statutory duties

Directors' responsibilities to third parties

Although the duty of directors is to their organisation, a breach of that duty could also affect outsiders. When the directors make a contract with an outsider, the contract is binding on the organisation when it is made according to its constitutional documents. However, the directors might exceed their powers in making the contract – for example, because they should have obtained stakeholder approval first, but failed to do so. Contracts entered into without proper authority are known as 'irregular contracts' and might seem to be void.

The main provision of UK company law is that an irregular contract is binding on an organisation when an outsider, acting in good faith, enters into the contract and the board of directors has approved the contract. The directors will be liable to the organisation for any loss suffered. This rule means that irregular contracts do not affect third parties (outsiders). Instead, when they occur, they would be a corporate governance problem.

Related party transactions and the UK Disclosure and Transparency Rules for listed companies

In listed companies, the requirements of UK law are reinforced by the UK Disclosure and Transparency Rules, which include a section on related party transactions. In broad terms, a related party means a substantial shareholder of the organisation, a director of the organisation, a member of a director's family or an organisation in which a director or family member holds 30% or more of the shares. A related party transaction is a transaction between an organisation and a related party, other than in the normal course of business and results in a disclosure being made to the stock market and the shareholders. The effect of the rules should be to prevent directors or major shareholders of UK listed companies from obtaining a personal benefit from any non-business transaction with their organisation, unless the shareholders have given their approval.

The NHS Code of Conduct and Accountability covers this for directors and stakeholders of NHS organisations.

Borrowing powers of directors

In the UK, there is no restriction in law on how much the directors can borrow on behalf of their organisation unless the constitutional documents include a specific restriction. As far as the law is concerned, the borrowing powers of companies are limited only by what lenders are prepared to make available to them. Conceivably, the directors could therefore put the investment of their shareholders at risk by borrowing more than the organisation can safely afford.

FTs are also free to borrow from banks and other private sector lenders to improve the facilities and equipment available to patients. They are, however, subject to statutory controls – unlike voluntary or private providers of healthcare – which give NHSI powers to set limits on the amount they can borrow.

Duty to break even

Although the break-even duty is a statutory requirement solely for NHS trusts, all NHS bodies including FTs are expected to operate a balanced budget ensuring that total expenditure does not exceed total income.

Paragraph 2(1) of Schedule 5 to the NHS Act 2006 states: 'Each NHS trust must ensure that its revenue is not less than sufficient, taking one financial year with another, to meet outgoings properly chargeable to revenue account.' This is known as the 'breakeven duty'. NHS trusts and CCGs should normally plan to meet this duty by achieving a balanced position on their income and expenditure accounts each and every year. The breakeven duty includes the phrase 'taking one financial year with another'. This provides some flexibility on the time-scale for matching income with those costs whose incidence is uneven and when managing the recovery of an NHS trust with serious financial difficulties.

An agreement was reached in 1997 with the Treasury and the Audit Commission that the duty will be assumed to have been met if expenditure is covered by income over a rolling three-year period. Exceptionally, the breakeven duty is assumed to be met if the cumulative deficit being recovered is covered by subsequent surpluses over a four or five-year period.

NHSI issued guidance in April 2018 *Statutory Breakeven Duty: A guide for NHS trusts* which stated that since 2009/10 was the first year of International Financial Reporting Standards (IFRS) implementation then this was a suitable point from which the breakeven duty should now be assessed.

In 2017/18, 44% of all provider trusts (acute, ambulance, community, mental health and specialist providers) ended the year in deficit and these were largely in the acute sector (i.e. 66% of acute trusts). In 2016/17, the provider sector deficit was reduced to £791 million from the record position of a £2.45 billion deficit in 2015/16; however, the sustainability and transformation fund of £1.8 billion was required to support providers during this period.

Where an NHS trust or CCG is recovering a cumulative deficit position, the organisation would be required to produce and agree a robust recovery plan with either the NHSI or NHSE (see the section on financial special measures in Chapter 18).

Duty to improve quality

The Health Act 1999 (and 2003) introduced a statutory 'duty of quality' for services commissioned and provided by all NHS trusts, for which trust CEOs are accountable. The DHSC expected this duty of quality to be discharged, at trust level, through the implementation of clinical governance. The relevant section was repealed by the Health and Social Care (Community Health and Standards) Act 2003 but was restated as:

> 'It is the duty of each NHS body to put and keep in place arrangements for the purpose of monitoring and improving the quality of health care provided by and for that body.'

This duty was further reinforced by the principles of the NHS Constitution.

Liability of directors

The starting point for considering the liabilities of individual directors is to understand the role of the board and the corporate nature of the specific NHS organisation (NHS trust, CCG or FT). Any such organisation will be a corporate entity in its own right and will take decisions as such. As noted earlier, this has implications for the role of directors, who are collectively responsible for all decisions.

The corporate nature of the organisation will mean that, in most instances, even if a decision is open to criticism, individual directors will not be legally liable. There are also specific statutory protections where they are acting in good faith (see Public Health Act 1875, s. 265). This section covers the circumstances where such personal liability can arise.

Criminal liability

An individual who, in the course of their activities as a director, commits a criminal offence will carry personal responsibility and liability. Perhaps more significantly, a director can be held to have committed a criminal offence where the offence arises under statute that includes explicit provision to hold a director liable. Examples are the Health and Safety at Work Act, the Environmental Protection Act and the Data Protection Act.

Prior to the Corporate Manslaughter Act 2007 coming into force, it was possible for a corporate entity, such as a company, to be prosecuted for a wide range of criminal offences, including the common law offence of gross negligence manslaughter. However, in order for the corporate entity to be guilty of the offence, it was also necessary for a senior individual who could be said to embody the company (also known as a 'controlling mind') to be guilty of the offence. The new law was wider, meaning a corporate entity can be convicted if it can be proven that there was a gross breach of duty of care by senior management, instead of just one individual.

Civil liability to third parties

Civil liability, which generally relates to the payment of compensation, can arise in either contract or tort. Liability in contract will only occur if the contract is entered into in the personal name of the director rather than that of the trust or where a contract entered into by the trust is found to be ultra vires and the director has given a personal warranty or representation that the trust has appropriate powers. Directors therefore need to be careful about what assurances they give about the powers of the organisation.

The more usual risks are for the individual to have a claim in tort made against them, most commonly in relation to either negligence or defamation. A tort can be defined as a wrongful act resulting in injury to another's person, property or reputation, for which the injured party is entitled to seek compensation where there has been no contractual relationship. Negligence arises where an individual acts without due care towards a person to whom they owe a duty of care, and causes foreseeable loss. Usually, as with clinical negligence claims, the claim is pursued against the trust, not the individual and NHS Resolution will provide cover. Indeed, the Liabilities to Third Parties Scheme includes cover for directors similar to that available in the commercial market by way of directors' and officers' liability insurance.

Defamation is a potential risk, and while some degree of protection is afforded where public officers are acting honestly and in the course of their business, there are risks if they step outside the strict parameters of the role.

A potential threat is misfeasance in public office. In practice, this is very rare and requires the establishment of deliberate malice, targeting the individual or a limited class of people who has/have suffered loss.

Claims by the NHS organisation

A final area of risk is that of claims by the NHS organisation itself. All directors owe a duty of care and skill to the NHS organisation, and breaches could give rise to claims. There is a material difference in this matter between the position of EDs and NEDs (or lay members). The latter are protected by the terms of the standard HM Treasury indemnity, unless they have been reckless. However, EDs could in theory be the subject of claims, even if they have only been negligent.

Although there are some high-profile corporate cases, such as Equitable Life, in practice claims against the directors for negligently carrying out their duties are rare. It does, however, underline the need for directors to use care and skills in carrying out their role. Where a matter is outside their competence, they may want to consider whether they need independent advice.

A further area of claim by an NHS organisation would be for breach of fiduciary duty or for repayment of benefits improperly received. This can arise in two main ways. The first is where a director abuses their position to make private gain. This could occur where a director arranged for a contract with a company in which they had an interest, without declaring the relevant interest. In such circumstances, the trust can call for an account of the proceeds.

Secondly, and perhaps more commonly, situations may arise where the auditors call into question officers' severance or retirement packages. Irrespective of the propriety of the individual's conduct, if the award of the package was outside the powers of the NHS organisation or decided upon improperly, it can be clawed back.

Indemnity

As indicated above, directors have a degree of protection against claims. Non-executives will typically have the benefit of the Treasury approved wording (HSG 1999/104):

> 'A chair or non-executive member or director who has acted honestly and in good faith will not have to meet out of his or her own personal resources any personal civil liability that is incurred in the execution or purported execution of his or her board function. Save where the person has acted recklessly.'

This indemnity may be extended to members of those committees that have delegated powers to make decisions or take actions on behalf of NHS boards. This covers the director for acts carried out in good faith in the execution or purported execution of the functions of the trust, short of recklessness. It does not cover criminal liability, and no indemnity could do so.

There is some doubt about the position where the director is in fact acting outside the powers of the organisation, particularly where to enforce the indemnity would be to allow a collateral enforcement of an ultra vires obligation against the trust.

EDs will generally be indemnified in relation to claims against them arising from third parties, but difficult issues can arise when staff make allegations of harassment, and trusts will need to tread carefully in such cases.

DIRECTORS' DUTIES AND LIABILITIES

NHS Code of Conduct and Accountability

It is a long-established principle that public sector bodies, which include the NHS, must be impartial and honest in the conduct of their business, and that their employees and officers should remain beyond suspicion. It is also an offence under the Bribery Act for a person to offer, promise or give a financial or other advantage to another person where the intention is either:

- to bring about the improper performance by another person of a relevant function or activity or to reward such improper performance; or
- that the acceptance of the advantage offered, promised or given in itself constitutes the improper performance of a relevant function or activity.

Given the scale and magnitude of the procurement of contracts and services within the NHS, there is clearly a significant need to regulate the behaviour of both the board and NHS staff in regard to managing conflicts of interests.

The Code of Conduct: Code of Accountability (Second revision 2004) is quite clear in that NHS staff should act in a way that protects the interest of the NHS in the way they undertake their business.

- Accountability: Everything done by those who work in the NHS must be able to stand the test of parliamentary scrutiny, public judgements on propriety and professional codes of conduct.
- Probity: There should be an absolute standard of honesty in dealing with the assets of the NHS: integrity should be the hallmark of all personal conduct in decisions affecting patients, staff and suppliers, and in the use of information acquired in the course of NHS duties.
- Openness: There should be sufficient transparency about NHS activities to promote confidence between the NHS organisation and its staff, patients and the public.
- Public service values matter in the NHS. The Code of Conduct makes it clear that chairs and board directors should act impartially, and should not be influenced by social or business relationships. Where there is a potential for private interests to be material and relevant to NHS business, the relevant interests should be declared and recorded in the board minutes, and entered into a register, which is available to the public. When a conflict of interest is established, the board director should withdraw and play no part in the relevant discussion or decision.

It is vital that NHS board directors should set an example to their organisation in the use of public funds and the need for good value in incurring public expenditure. The use of NHS monies for hospitality and entertainment, including hospitality at conferences or seminars, should be carefully considered. All expenditure on these items should be capable of justification as reasonable in the light of the general practice in the public sector. NHS boards should be aware that expenditure on hospitality or entertainment is the responsibility of management and is open to be challenged by the internal and external auditors and that ill-considered actions can damage respect for the NHS in the eyes of the community. NHS boards should also have an explicit procedure for the declaration of hospitality and sponsorship offered by, for example, suppliers. Their authorisation should be carefully considered and the decision should be recorded. NHS boards should be aware of the risks in incurring obligations to suppliers at any stage of a contracting relationship.

NHS boards should ensure that staff have a proper and widely publicised procedure for voicing complaints or concerns about maladministration, malpractice, breaches of this code and other concerns of an ethical nature. This has been developed further in whistleblowing procedures, which are set out in more detail in Chapter 19.

Conflicts of interest

The NHSE guidance Managing Conflicts of Interest in the NHS came into force in June 2017. This guidance:

- introduces common principles and rules for managing conflicts of interest;
- provides simple advice to staff and organisations about what to do in common situations; and
- supports good judgement about how interests should be approached and managed.

The guidance is applicable via the statutory guidance to CCGs issued by NHSE (see Chapter 15), to NHS trusts and FTs and NHSE itself. Organisations may adopt their own policy, but it must meet the standards in the guidance as a minimum. Such policies must also be consistent with and should be read in conjunction with the following NHS publications as appropriate on this matter:

- Standards of Business Conduct for NHS Staff (October 2018) – NHSE.
- NHS Trusts Example Standing Orders – Section 8 Standards of Business Conduct.
- Commercial Sponsorship – Ethical Standards for the NHS (November 2000) – DH (now DHSC).
- Nolan Principles of Public Life – HMSO.
- Good Medical Practice (2014) – General Medicine Council.
- The Code (2018) – Nursing and Midwifery Council.
- Code of Conduct Payment by Results (2013) – DH (now DHSC).

Underpinning this guidance there is of course the statutory duty described earlier for directors to act in the best interests of that organisation, in accordance with the governing document, and to avoid situations where there may be a potential conflict of interest. The Bribery Act 2010 also sets out legal obligations for organisations to take steps to prevent bribes being paid on their behalf.

For NHS FTs, there is also a requirement for the board of directors to adopt appropriate standards of conduct and to be open and transparent in their decision making and the manner in which conflicts of interest are managed. This was clarified further in section 152 of HSCA 2012 as follows:

> 'The duties that a director of a public benefit corporation has by virtue of being a director include in particular
> a) a duty to avoid a situation in which the director has (or can have) a direct or indirect interest that conflicts (or possibly may conflict) with the interests of the corporation;
> b) a duty not to accept a benefit from a third party by reason of being a director or doing (or not doing) anything in that capacity.
>
> This duty is not infringed if the situation cannot reasonably be regarded as likely to give rise to a conflict of interest, or the matter has been authorised in accordance with the constitution, or if acceptance of the benefit cannot reasonably be regarded as likely to give rise to a conflict of interest.
>
> If a director of a public benefit corporation has in any way a direct or indirect interest in a proposed transaction or arrangement with the corporation, the director must declare the nature and extent of that interest to the other directors. And if a declaration under this section proves to be, or becomes, inaccurate or incomplete, a further declaration must be made. Any declaration required by this section must be made before the corporation enters into the transaction or arrangement. The section did not require a declaration of an interest of which the director was not aware or where the director was not aware of the transaction or arrangement in question.'

Conflicts of interest are a major governance issue for CCGs. NHSE provided guidance for CCGs in Managing Conflicts of Interest in the NHS: revised statutory guidance for CCGs (June 2017). This will be covered in more detail in Chapter 15. However, the core of the issue is neatly summarised in the quote below from the September 2011 briefing paper on managing conflicts of interest by the Royal College of General Practitioners (RCGP) and NHS Confederation.

> 'If conflicts of interest are not managed effectively by CCGs, confidence in the probity of commissioning decisions and the integrity of clinicians involved could be seriously undermined. However, with good planning and governance, CCGs should be able to avoid these risks.'

CCGs need to provide clear guidance to their members and employees on what might constitute a conflict of interest, providing examples that are likely to arise. They should also highlight the following points to members and employees:

- a perception of wrongdoing, impaired judgement or undue influence can be as detrimental as any of them actually occurring;
- if in doubt, it is better to assume a conflict of interest and manage it appropriately rather than ignore it; and
- financial gain is not necessary for a conflict to exist.

The Healthy NHS Board reinforces the importance of NHS boards acting – and being seen to act – with integrity and in the best interests of the organisation:

> 'Probity requires that the board maintains an up-to-date register of board members' interests. Board agendas should include an opportunity for board members to declare conflicts of interests that may relate to specific agenda items so that they can be managed appropriately.'

It is, therefore, essential that there are clear and robust systems in place for identifying and managing real and potential conflicts of interest of board members to protect the reputation and tangible assets of the NHS organisation, as well as the reputation of individual board members.

What are conflicts of interest?

The CA 2006 defines a conflict of interest as arising when the interests of directors, or 'connected persons', are incompatible or in competition with the interests of the organisation. Such situations present a risk that directors may make decisions based on these external influences, rather than the best interests of the organisation. The Act goes on to define 'connected persons' (s. 252(2) of CA 2006) as:

> 'a) members of the directors' family
> (section 253 defines these as spouse or civil partner; any other person with whom the director lives as a partner in an enduring family relationship, the directors' children or step-children, a partners' children or step-children under 18 years of age; and the directors' parents);
> b) a body corporate with which the director is connected;
> c) a person acting in their capacity as a trustee of a trust –
>   (i) the beneficiaries of which include the director or a person who by virtue of (a) or (b) is connected with them, or
>   (ii) the terms of which confer a power on the trustees that may be exercised for the benefit of the director or any such person, other than a trust for the purposes of an employees' share scheme or pension scheme;
> d) a person acting in their capacity as a partner –
>   (i) of the director, or
>   (ii) of a person who by virtue of (a) to (c) is connected with that director;
> e) a firm that is a legal person under the law by which it is governed and in which –
>   (i) the director is a partner,
>   (ii) a partner is a person who by virtue of (a) to (c) is connected with the director, or
>   (iii) a partner is a firm in which the director is a partner or in which there is a partner who by virtue of (a), (b) or (c) is connected with the director.'

The NHSE guidance (2017) defines a conflict of interest as:

> 'A set of circumstances by which a reasonable person would consider that an individual's ability to apply judgement or act, in the context of delivering, commissioning, or assuring taxpayer funded health and care services is, or could be, impaired or influenced by another interest they hold.'

It follows the CA 2006 in its definition of 'connected persons'.

A conflict of interest may be actual where there is a material conflict between one or more interests, or potential where there is the possibility of a material conflict between one or more interests in the future. The guidance recommends caution as staff may hold interests in which they cannot see potential conflict, but others may see it differently. It will be important, therefore, for them to exercise judgement and to declare such interests, as there is a risk of implied improper conduct. Interests can arise in a number of different contexts. A material interest is one, which a reasonable person would take into account when making a decision regarding the use of taxpayers' money because the interest has relevance to that decision. Such interests fall into the following categories:

- **Financial interests:** where an individual may get direct financial benefit (over and above the agreed remuneration and terms of their service package) from the consequences of a decision they are involved in making. This is the most easily recognisable form of conflict of interest. Examples include the award of a contract to a company or other business with which a director is involved, and the sale of assets at below market value to a director.
- **Indirect interests:** where an individual has a close association with another individual who has a financial interest, a non-financial professional interest or a non-financial personal interest who would stand to benefit from a decision they are involved in making. An example is when a close relative of a director benefits from the decision. Directors will also benefit indirectly if their financial affairs are bound with those of the relative in question through the legal concept of 'joint purse', as would be the case if the relative were the spouse, partner, dependent child of the director, or directly connected in some other way
- **Non-financial professional interests:** where an individual may obtain a nonfinancial professional benefit from the consequences of a decision, they are involved in making, such as increasing their professional reputation or promoting their professional career. For instance, to gain some other intangible benefit or kudos, or awarding contracts to friends or personal business contacts.
- **Non-financial personal interests:** where an individual may benefit personally in ways which are not directly linked to their professional career and do not give rise to a direct financial benefit, because of decisions they are involved in making in their professional career. For example, directors may have competing loyalties between the trust to which they owe a primary duty and

some other person or entity which could inhibit free discussion resulting in decisions or actions that are not in the interests of the trust.

The guidance provides additional examples for each of these types of interests. It recognises that a benefit may arise from the making of gain or avoiding a loss and explains that associations may arise through relationships with close family members and relatives, close friends and associates, and business partners and that a common-sense approach should be applied to these terms.

It would be unrealistic to expect staff to know of all the interests that people in these classes of association might hold. However, if staff do know of material interests (or could be reasonably expected to know about them), these should be declared. The guidance also distinguishes between staff generally and those who are more likely than others to have a decision-making influence on the use of public monies because of their role. Board and governing body members are clearly decision-making staff for the purposes of the guidance, as are:

- members of advisory groups which contribute to direct or delegated decision making on the commissioning or provision of taxpayer-funded services;
- those at Agenda for Change band 8d and above;
- administrative and clinical staff who have the power to enter into contracts on behalf of their organisation; and
- administrative and clinical staff involved in decision making concerning the commissioning of services, purchasing of good, medicines, medical devices or equipment, and formulary decisions.

The NHSE guidance is comparable to the companies legislation requirements.

Decisions made under a conflict of interest may be legally challenged and could result in personal liability for the director. The aim of a conflict of interest policy, therefore, is to protect both the organisation and the individuals involved from any appearance of impropriety.

Declaration of interests

Having interests is not in itself negative, but not declaring them or managing them is. Consequently, where there is potential for an interest to be material and relevant to NHS business, then the relevant interest should be declared and recorded in a register of interests. The company secretary must maintain the Register of Directors' Interests and ensure that arrangements have been made for staff interest to be recorded within the organisation as appropriate.

Once recorded, then appropriate action needs to be taken and the NHSE guidance includes the following possibilities:

- deciding that no action is warranted;
- restricting an individual's involvement in discussions and excluding them from decision making;
- removing an individual from the whole decision-making process;

- removing an individual's responsibility for an entire area of work;
- removing an individual from their role altogether if the conflict is so significant that they are unable to operate effectively in the role; and
- keeping an audit trail of the actions taken.

The guidance outlines situations with associated principles and rules, which may give rise to a possible conflict of interest. These are:

- gifts;
- hospitality;
- outside employment;
- shareholdings and other ownership interests;
- patents;
- loyalty interests;
- donations;
- sponsored events;
- sponsored research;
- sponsored posts; and
- clinical private practice.

Hospitality & gifts policy and associated registers

A hospitality & gifts policy is intended to assist all employees of an NHS organisation (and this includes all board members) in following the NHS guidance and relevant legislation on the giving and receipt of hospitality or gifts. This covers both the receipt and delivery of hospitality and gifts. Any hospitality, gifts or benefits accepted should be entered on the hospitality & gifts register by means of a standardised form. Each employee has a personal responsibility to declare hospitality and gifts in accordance with the policy.

Under the Prevention of Corruption Acts 1906 and 1916, it is an offence for employees corruptly to accept any gifts or consideration as an inducement or reward for; doing, or refraining from doing, anything in their official capacity; or showing favour or disfavour to any person in their official capacity. Under the 1916 Act, any money, gift or consideration received by an employee in public service from a person or organisation holding or seeking to obtain a contract will be deemed to have been received corruptly unless the employee proves to the contrary.

Under NHS Standing Orders and European Commission Directives on Public Purchasing for Works and Supplies, there is a requirement for fair and open competition between prospective contractors or suppliers.

Circular HSG (93) 5, 'Standards of Business Conduct for NHS Staff' (January 1993), provides guidelines for NHS employers and employees. This sets out that NHS employers are responsible for ensuring the guidelines are brought to the attention of all employees, and that machinery is put in place to ensure they are effectively implemented. A hospitality policy is intended to fulfil these requirements by providing clear guidance to employees and by establishing a hospitality register.

The NHSE guidance (2017) also sets out that it is the responsibility of staff to ensure that they are not placed in a position which risks, or appears to risk, conflict between their private interests and their NHS duties. This applies to both staff who commit resources directly (ordering of goods or services) or indirectly (by policy development).

Examples of hospitality, gifts or benefits where a declaration may be necessary include:

- meals and drinks;
- crates and bottles of wine or spirits;
- tickets for sporting events/theatre, etc.;
- events where the cost of accommodation is paid for by a research company;
- national and international seminars where the placement has been paid for by the company organising the seminar;
- sponsored golf events;
- lecture trips (national and international);
- site visits to prospective suppliers of goods and services where hospitality, gifts or benefit is provided or loaned; and
- gifts of equipment by drug companies.

The above list is not exhaustive, but it will give an indication of the types of items that may need to be declared. The NHSE guidance (2017) stipulates that low-cost branded promotional items from suppliers valued at more than £6 in total must be declared. Gifts of cash or vouchers to individuals from patients or families should always be declined and gifts of over £50 can only be accepted on behalf of the organisation (e.g. to the organisations' charitable funds). Modest gifts under a value of £50 do not, however, need to be declared, but multiple gifts over a 12-month period should be declared if the total value exceeds £50.

Hospitality (meals, refreshments, accommodation, tickets etc.) may only be accepted where there is a legitimate business reason and it is proportional to the event itself. If the value is under £25 then it does not need to be declared, however if the meal and/or refreshments are valued at more than £75 then it should be refused unless senior approval is given. All other hospitality must be declared and recorded. However, the recipient should not allow themselves to reach a position whereby they might be deemed by others to have been influenced in making a business decision as a consequence of accepting such hospitality.

Where it is not easy to decide whether the hospitality or gift should be accepted or not, advice should be sought from the line manager.

Outside employment

The NHS relies on staff with good skills, broad knowledge and diverse experience. Many staff bring expertise from sectors outside the NHS, such as industry, business, education, government and beyond. The involvement of staff in these outside roles alongside their NHS role can therefore be of benefit, but their existence should be well known so that conflicts can be either managed or avoided. Staff should declare any existing outside employment on appointment, and any new outside employment when it arises.

Shareholding and other ownership interests

Staff should declare, as a minimum, any shareholdings and other ownership interests in any publicly listed, private or not-for-profit company, business, partnership or consultancy that is doing, or might be reasonably expected to do, business with their organisation. There is no need to declare shares or securities held in collective investment or pension funds or units of authorised unit trusts.

Clinical private practice

Service delivery in the NHS is done by a mix of public, private and not-for-profit organisations. The expertise of clinicians in the NHS is in high demand across all sectors and the NHS relies on the flexibility that the public, private and not-for-profit sectors can provide. It is therefore not uncommon for clinical staff to provide NHS-funded care and undertake private practice work either for an external company, or through a corporate vehicle established by themselves.

Existing provisions in contractual arrangements make allowances for this to happen and professional conduct rules apply. However, these arrangements do create the possibility for conflicts of interest arising. Therefore, these provisions are designed to ensure the existence of private practice is known so that potential conflicts of interest can be managed.

Clinical staff should declare all private practice on appointment, and/or any new private practice when it arises including:

- where they practise (name of private facility);
- what they practise (specialty, major procedures); and
- when they practise (identified sessions/time commitment).

In situations where a conflict of interest arises, NHS commitments must take precedence over the private work.

Managing conflicts of interest

Interests must be declared as soon as they become apparent and any change in interests should be declared as soon as it is recognised.

The register of interests (directors) is maintained by the company secretary who formally records the declarations of interests made by members of the board. These details must be kept up-to-date by means of at least an annual review of the register in which any changes to interests declared during the preceding months will be incorporated. The register is available to the public and to the trust's internal and external auditors; it should be published on the trust's website, to ensure compliance with ICO Publication Scheme. The details of the interests of board members must be published in the trust's annual report.

If a board member has an actual or potential interest, the chair should consider the following approaches and ensure that the reason for the chosen action is documented in minutes or records:

- Require the member not to attend the meeting.
- Ensure that the member does not receive meeting papers relating to the nature of their interest.
- Require the member not to attend all or part of the discussion and decision on the related matter.
- Note the nature and extent of the interest, but judge it appropriate to allow the member to remain and participate.
- Remove the member from the group or process altogether.
- Any interest that arises during the course of a meeting should be declared immediately and should be recorded in the relevant minutes. When a conflict of interest is established, the person should withdraw and play no part in the relevant discussion or decision.

The default response should not always be to exclude members with interests, as this may have a detrimental effect on the quality of the decision being made. An example is the need for clinical involvement, when clinicians may hold and represent a diversity of interests. Good judgement is required to ensure proportionate management of risk. The composition of groups should be kept under review to ensure effective participation.

An interest should remain on the register(s) for a minimum of six months after the interest has expired. Organisations should retain a private record of historic interests for a minimum of six years after the date on which it expired. Sanctions for the failure to declare a conflict of interests could include:

- disciplinary sanctions – verbal, written or dismissal;
- professional regulatory sanctions – fitness to practice;
- civil sanctions misfeasance in public office; and
- criminal sanctions – fraud, bribery and corruption.

Governance checklist

- Are the directors aware of the extent of their authority and powers and the purposes for which they have been granted?
- Are directors aware of the boundaries set out in the matters reserved for the board and in the standing orders/standing financial instructions?
- Are directors aware of the implications of the common law and statutory duties that could be the benchmark their actions are judged against?

- Are board members provided with sufficient and accurate information and advice for them to exercise reasonable care, skill and diligence?
- Does that information enable them to make decisions that will fulfil their function – for example, promoting the success of the corporation in a FT?
- Are the directors confident in identifying potential conflicts of interest, how to declare them and how to manage them?
- When was the register of interests last updated?

Summary

- Individual directors who compose the board have key duties and responsibilities as a consequence of the role.
- Consequently, they will be liable for certain outcomes that result from the actions and decisions of the board.
- Directors need to have a clear understanding of these duties and liabilities: this should form a key part of their induction and ongoing development as board members.
- Conflicts of interest are a key governance issue for NHS organisations.

9
Maintaining an effective board

Introduction

This chapter deals with governance issues relating to the effectiveness of the board (and again this should be taken to include the governing body of a CCG). Board performance and operation has been highlighted in a number of NHS publications, but the key guidance can be found in The Healthy NHS Board (2013) and the Well-Led Framework (2017), which are intended to support NHS boards in gaining assurance on their effectiveness in carrying out their role of setting strategy, leading the organisation and overseeing operations, and being accountable to stakeholders in an open and effective manner.

Though such guidance is helpful in setting out clear processes and procedures, it is important to recognise the vital interplay of the different roles, personalities and relationships around the board table. Defining an effective board merely in terms of its processes and procedures, without recognising that behaviours and culture are the essential ingredients, is a recipe for poor governance and failing organisations.

In the corporate sector a similar realisation is dawning – the global financial crisis and other governance failings of large organisations (e.g. BHS, Volkswagen, Tesco) have demonstrated that, as the old saying goes, 'culture eats strategy for breakfast'. This had also been apparent during the failed corporate mergers and restructures of the 1980s and 1990s and yet the lesson had failed to be learned.

The FRC study Corporate Culture and the Role of Boards (2016) explores the relationship between corporate culture and long-term business success in the UK. Sir Winfried Bischoff, Chairman of the FRC, writes:

> 'There needs to be a concerted effort to improve trust in the motivations and integrity of business. Rules and sanctions clearly have their place but will not on their own deliver productive behaviours over the long-term. This report looks at the increasing importance which corporate culture plays in delivering long-term business and economic success.
>
> A healthy corporate culture is a valuable asset, a source of competitive advantage and vital to the creation and protection of long-term value. It is the board's role to determine the purpose of the company and ensure that the company's values, strategy and business model are aligned to it. Directors should not wait for a crisis before they focus on company culture.'

It is now accepted that stakeholders and society in general have a vested interest in healthy corporate values, attitudes and behaviours that lead to sustainable growth and long-term economic success. The study also asks stakeholders and investors to consider their behaviours too, so that they 'engage constructively to build respect and trust, and work with companies to achieve long term value'.

Consequently, the FRC Board Guide encourages boards to think more deeply both about culture and about how engaging with stakeholders will help the boards to be more effective in their role.

The board and culture

Boardroom practice describes the way in which a board conducts its procedures and reaches its decisions. The board's practice is an essential part of establishing the corporate culture and sets the tone for the rest of the organisation.

The FRC Board Guide states:

> 'The board sets the framework of values within which the desired corporate culture can evolve and thrive. Ownership of the values will be stronger if a collaborative approach is taken and both the leadership and the workforce are involved in a two-way process to define the company's values.
>
> It is important for trust that companies avoid giving contradictory messages through their decisions, strategies or conduct. Directors can reinforce values through their own behaviour and decisions. To do this effectively, EDs and NEDs may need to increase their visibility.'

The guidance continues to say:

> 'The boardroom should be a place for robust debate where challenge, support, diversity of thought and teamwork are essential features. Diversity of skills, background and personal strengths is an important driver of a board's effectiveness, creating different perspectives among directors, and breaking down a tendency towards "group think".'

The common attributes of a healthy culture are defined by the FRC Board Guide as:

- honesty;
- openness;
- respect;
- adaptability;
- reliability;
- recognition;
- acceptance of challenge;
- accountability; and
- a sense of shared purpose.

The guidance recommends some questions for boards to consider:

- How have the values and expected behaviours been reinforced in the recruitment, promotion, reward, performance management and other policies, processes and practices?
- Do reward structures produce appropriate incentives that encourage desired behaviours and responsible risk-taking?
- What steps has management taken to communicate values and expected behaviours widely and clearly across the company?
- What assurance is there that the code of conduct and ethics training programmes are up to date, adequately communicated and understood by the workforce?
- What steps has management taken to ensure that suppliers meet expected standards of behaviour?
- Has management identified appropriate KPIs that are properly aligned to desired outcomes and behaviours?

The guidance also suggests some sources of culture insights that boards could adopt for its monitoring of culture. These include:

- turnover and absenteeism rates;
- training data;
- recruitment, reward and promotion decisions;
- use of non-disclosure agreements;
- whistleblowing, grievance and 'speak-up' data;
- employee surveys;
- board interaction with senior management and workforce;
- health and safety data, including near misses;
- promptness of payments to suppliers;
- attitudes to regulators, internal audit and employees; and
- exit interviews.

The guidance offers further questions that boards might want to consider in monitoring culture:

- What does the workforce say about 'the tone from the top' and the 'tone from the middle'?
- What evidence is there that the CEO is willing to listen, take criticism and let others make decisions?
- What do examples of communications from leadership and middle management tell the board about the commitment to values, openness and accountability?
- What action does the board take against leaders or top performers who do not uphold the company's values?
- How are key promotions decided?

- Is management using root cause analysis where cultural issues are found, examining not just what went wrong but why?
- How can the board use technology to analyse, interpret and present information?
- Does the board need to invest in human resources or internal audit, develop skills and capabilities or encourage the use of multi-disciplinary teams?
- How does the company deal with breaches of company rules or codes of conduct?
- Does internal audit have the degree of independence needed and a clear mandate to look at culture?
- How will the board address any negative trends or misalignment between values and behaviours?

Interestingly this line of approach, which is also adopted in the King IV Code, is also beginning to have more profile in health service governance. The Well-Led Framework (2017) clearly sets out capacity and culture as a domain for evaluation in a board's self-effectiveness.

Culture and constructive challenge

There is a general consensus among recently published reports and reviews in both corporate and health service sectors that the quality of governance depends ultimately on the culture and behaviour of individuals, and consequently the ability of procedures and regulation to provide good governance is limited.

The Walker Report argued that both character and culture of the board members are important for an effective board. It commented that:

> 'Board conformity with laid-down procedures ... will not alone provide better corporate governance overall if the chair is weak, if the composition and dynamic of the board is inadequate and if there is unsatisfactory ... engagement with its owners.'

The report went on to argue that the main weaknesses in the boards of banks had been caused by behavioural factors and a failure to challenge.

> 'The sequence in board discussion on major issues should be: presentation by the executive, a disciplined process of challenge, decision on the policy or strategy to be adopted and then full empowerment of the executive to implement. The essential "challenge" step in the sequence appears to have been missed in many board situations and needs to be ... clearly recognised and embedded for the future.'

Back in 2004, the NHS Confederation published *Effective Boards in the NHS*, which identified the behaviour and culture of a board as key determinants of the board's performance. From the interviews, the research identified four characteristics of effective boards:

- a focus on strategic decision making;
- board members who trust each other and act cohesively/behave corporately;
- constructive challenge by board members of each other; and
- effective chairs who ensure meetings have clear and effective processes.

Some boards appear to be too trusting, with little constructive challenge or debate about strategic issues. Reasons for this lack of challenge include the desire to present a united public face in public meetings. Perceived differences between NEDs and EDs roles needed to be addressed, as challenge should not be seen as the preserve of NEDs scrutinising the executive team. This will create a culture that enables board business to be conducted in a sharp and focused, making clear what decisions are required of the board and what action will follow as a result of the decisions.

Deffenbaugh (2015) describes the behaviour of board members as 'the how' of the challenge function:

> 'I have worked with boards where challenge has been inappropriate. I have seen executives suit up with armour in advance of a board meeting because their expectation is that they will be challenged in a manner that borders on the unprofessional. I have observed instances where a robust challenge may have been merited due to performance issues, but was carried out in a way that became counterproductive.'
>
> ('Effective Challenge on a Unitary Board', *British Journal of Healthcare Management* 2015 Vol 21 No 11)

Building on this analysis, The Healthy NHS Board identified boards as 'social systems'. It summarised the techniques and practices that support and hinder the effectiveness of these social systems (see Table 9.1).

In 2009, ICSA: The Governance Institute submitted a report, entitled *Boardroom Behaviours*, to Sir David Walker, who was reviewing the corporate governance issues that contributed to the 2007–09 banking crisis in the UK. The report suggested that best practice in boardroom behaviour is characterised by:

- a clear understanding of the role of the board;
- the appropriate deployment of knowledge, skills, experience and judgement;
- independent thinking;
- the questioning of assumptions and established orthodoxy;
- challenge, which is constructive, confident, principled and proportionate;
- rigorous debate;
- a supportive decision-making environment;
- a common vision; and
- the achievement of closure on individual items of board business.

The report also provided an outline of the guidance that might be useful to directors about boardroom behaviours:

Ways of working that support good social processes	Ways of working that obstruct good social processes
Building a crystal clear understanding of the roles of the board and individual board members	Board members behaving in a way that suggests a 'master–servant' relationship between non-executive and executive
Actively working to develop and protect a climate of trust and candour	Executive directors only contributing in their functional leadership area rather than actively participating across the breadth of the board agenda
Building cohesion by taking steps to know and understand each other's backgrounds, skills and perspectives	Demonstrating an unwillingness to consider points of view that are different from individual directors' starting positions
Encouraging all board members to offer constructive challenges	Challenge primarily coming from non-executive directors, rather than all directors feeling empowered to challenge one another in board meetings
Sharing corporate responsibility and collective decision making	Challenging in a way that is unnecessarily antagonistic and not appropriately balanced with appreciation, encouragement and support
Ensuring that neither chair nor chief executive power and dominance act to stifle appropriate participation in board debate	Working in ways that do not demonstrate overall confidence in the executive and that feed individual anxiety and insecurity about capability

Table 9.1: Techniques and practices that support and hinder boards

- All directors, including EDs, need to improve their performance in these important areas of boardroom behaviours. The process of achieving this for NEDs can be made more effective by giving them greater exposure to the organisation's operations.
- A knowledgeable board is a function of board balance and there may be insufficient balance if the board is shrunk to just two EDs (CEO and finance director) in order to achieve a majority of NEDs without making the board too big.
- Diversity of board membership is necessary to provide sufficient independent challenge.
- High standards of performance evaluation are needed to increase the effectiveness of a board.

- At the moment, the remuneration of EDs appears to focus on maximising short-term 'value' rather than pursuing the goal of a sustainable business. Remuneration arrangements should give more emphasis to the behaviours of directors in the boardroom, working in the long-term interests of the organisation.
- In terms of developing a wider perspective of the business, directors should look 'forward and out, as well as backwards and in'.
- The board should lead by example, 'evidenced by high levels of visibility and integrity, strong communications, and demanding expectations'.
- Practical issues, such as the timely circulation of board papers, 'can have a disproportionate effect on the quality of decision-making'.

The NHS Leadership Model from the NHS Leadership Academy is also helpful in that it describes nine behaviours that together contribute towards strong and effective NHS leaders. NHSI expects board members to demonstrate this range of behaviours and the highest standards of conduct required to contribute effectively in this board level role. The behaviours are:

- inspiring shared purpose;
- leading with care;
- evaluating information;
- connecting our service;
- sharing vision;
- engaging the team;
- holding to account;
- developing capability; and
- influencing for results.

In the report *Responses to Francis: changes in board leadership and governance in acute hospitals in England since 2013* (January 2018), five main roles were identified as relevant for effective healthcare boards in the wake of Francis:

- the board as conscience – guardian of its values, and the custodian and monitor of its culture;
- the board as sensor – being able to sense problems, rather than seek comfort from internal and external data;
- the board as diplomat – being curious about and attending to the diverse range of stakeholder interests and perspectives;
- the board as coach – instilling a restless urge for the achievement of higher ambitions; and
- the board as shock absorber – distilling the attention and challenge of multiple national regulators and arm's length bodies into clear organisational messages.

It is interesting to see that these relate closely to the main board roles from the literature on board governance in relation to agency, stewardship, stakeholder, resource dependency and power, but the report develops them specifically to relate to the context and the pressures of the NHS in England since the Francis Report.

Constructive challenge and effective decision making

If the culture and tone set by the board establishes a culture of constructive challenge then the next issue for boards to consider is how to develop and support well-informed and high-quality decision making. This does not happen by accident. Boards can minimise the risk of poor decisions by investing time in the design of their decision-making policies and processes, including the contribution of committees and obtaining input from key stakeholders and expert opinions when necessary.

The FRC Board Guide describes the following as risk factors for poor decision making:

- a dominant personality or group of directors on the board, inhibiting contribution from others;
- insufficient diversity of perspective on the board, which can contribute to 'group think';
- excess focus on risk mitigation or insufficient attention to risk;
- a compliance mindset and failure to treat risk as part of the decision-making process;
- insufficient knowledge and ability to test underlying assumptions;
- failure to listen to and act upon concerns that are raised;
- failure to recognise the consequences of running the business on the basis of self-interest and other poor ethical standards;
- a lack of openness by management, a reluctance to involve NEDs, or a tendency to bring matters to the board for sign-off rather than debate;
- complacent or intransigent attitudes;
- inability to challenge effectively;
- inadequate information or analysis;
- poor quality papers;
- lack of time for debate and truncated debate;
- undue focus on short-term time horizons; and
- insufficient notice of meetings and supply of papers.

The guidance goes on to suggest the following questions for boards to consider:

- Have relevant members of the executive team been invited to explain the issues at the earlier stages, enabling all directors to share concerns or challenge assumptions well before the point of decision?
- Does the board have a clear idea of the success criteria related to a particular decision?
- What are the board doing to test key decisions for alignment with values? Can the board give examples and explain how this was considered?

- What are the risks that the decision could encourage undesirable behaviours or send the wrong message?
- Can the board explain how the impact on key stakeholders has been taken into account?

The guidance sets out that the board should have clear policies about what matters need a board decision or approval, and the processes required for each type of decision. Good decision making can be improved by giving directors sufficient time to prepare for meetings, allowing sufficient time for issues to be discussed at board meetings, and making clear to EDs what action they must take to implement board decisions.

The guidance goes on to say that 'most complex decisions depend on judgement, but the decisions of well-intentioned and experienced leaders can, in certain circumstances, be distorted. Factors known to distort judgement are conflicts of interest, emotional attachments, unconscious bias and inappropriate reliance on previous experience and decisions.'

For significant decisions, therefore, a board may wish to consider extra steps, for example:

- Describing in board papers the process that has been used to arrive at and challenge the proposal prior to presenting it to the board, thereby allowing directors not involved in the project to assess the appropriateness of the process as a precursor to assessing the merits of the project itself.
- Where appropriate, putting in place additional safeguards to reduce the risk of distorted judgements by, for example, commissioning an independent report, seeking advice from an expert, introducing a devil's advocate to provide challenge, establishing a sole purpose sub-committee, or convening additional meetings. Some chairs favour separate discussions for important decisions (e.g. concept, proposal for discussion, proposal for decision). This gives EDs more opportunity to put the case at the earlier stages, and all directors the opportunity to share concerns or challenge assumptions well in advance of the point of decision.
- Boards can benefit from reviewing past decisions, particularly those with poor outcomes. A review should not focus just on the merits of the decision itself but also on the decision-making process.
- As well as receiving relevant and timely information, directors should be given access to independent professional advice, at the organisation's expense, when they consider this necessary in order to fulfil their duties as director. For example, a director might ask to consult a lawyer for advice on a matter where the legal position is not clear.
- NEDs and possibly EDs may also need administrative support or advice on routine matters. Board committees should be provided with sufficient resources to carry out their duties, and all directors should have access to the advice and assistance of the company secretary.

The FRC Board Guide also notes that some boards favour separate discussions for important decisions; for example, separating discussions about concepts, proposals for discussion and proposals for decision. This gives EDs more opportunity to put their case at the earlier stages, and all directors the opportunity to share concerns or challenge assumptions well in advance of the point of decision.

Effective decision making and stakeholder engagement

The recent updates to the UK Code have really been to focus on culture and engagement with stakeholders as a means to greater effectiveness for boards. As the FRC Board Guide states, an 'effective board will appreciate the importance of dialogue with shareholders, the workforce and other key stakeholders, be proactive in ensuring that such dialogue takes place and that the feedback is taken into account in the board's decision making. How the board approaches this will provide useful insight into the company's culture'.

The guidance goes on to make recommendations about relations with shareholders, other key stakeholders and in particular the workforce. It sets out clear recommendations for gathering the views of the workforce and gives examples of workforce engagement activities such as:

- hosting talent breakfast/lunches, town halls and open-door days;
- listening groups for frontline workers and supervisors;
- focus or consultative groups;
- meeting groups of elected workforce representatives;
- meeting future leaders without senior management present;
- inviting colleagues from different business functions to board meetings;
- involvement in training and development activities;
- surveys;
- digital sharing platforms; and
- establishing mentoring between NEDs and middle managers.

It also recommends that NEDs and, in particular, the chair should consider ways of reaching out to increase their visibility with the workforce and gain insights into the culture and concerns at different levels of the business.

The legislation requirements and best practice for stakeholder engagement for the NHS have been set out in Chapter 1, but it is interesting to see the direction of travel for the corporate sector in order to address some of the failings of corporate governance in recent times.

Other factors affecting board effectiveness

The role of the chair

The Association of British Insurers (ABI) Report on Board Effectiveness (2012) makes it quite clear that the chair has a key role to play in the effective board.

While the report found no 'one size fits all' approach to the role, with different chairs having different approaches based on what is best for the individual company and board, it did find a significant amount of consensus about the role and responsibilities of the chair.

The report emphasised a number of aspects to the role of the chair on the following five themes:

- creating the right board dynamic and having the right people around the boardroom table;
- helping to set the board agenda, ensuring the board has the right information and is debating the right issues;
- managing the board's relationship with the EDs and in particular the CEO;
- being an ambassador for the company; and
- being fully engaged in the business and understanding what is happening on the ground.

The role of the chair is covered in more detail in Chapter 10.

Board meetings

A basic requirement of an effective board is that there should be regular board meetings. The UK Code states simply that the board should meet sufficiently regularly to discharge its duties effectively and there should be a formal schedule of matters reserved for the board.

The agenda for board meetings is a governance issue in the sense that the chair decides what the board will discuss when they set the agenda. Although directors can raise matters as 'any other business', most of the time at board meetings is spent in discussion of the items listed on the agenda. It is therefore important that the agenda should include all matters reserved for board decision, whenever they arise. The company secretary can assist the chair by providing advice and reminders.

To contribute effectively to board discussions, directors must be provided with relevant information. They should receive relevant documents in advance of a board meeting, so that they have time to read them and think about the issues they deal with. The UK Code states that 'the board should be supplied in a timely manner with information in a form and of a quality sufficient to enable it to discharge its duties'.

The chair has the responsibility for ensuring that directors receive the information that they need in sufficient time. The UK Code states that management has an obligation to provide the required information, but that the directors should ask for clarification or additional information if required.

The Intelligent Board report states that 'every member of the board needs sufficient information at a high enough level to be confident that the organisation is well run, but not so much information that it becomes difficult to tell what is important' and that 'good governance is underpinned by intelligent information'.

Such information enables the board to:

- set an appropriately challenging, but achievable, strategic direction;
- identify the strategic issues that require discussion or decision, and distinguish these issues from operational detail;
- provide constructive challenge;
- ensure taxpayers are receiving value for money (VFM);
- identify trends in performance;
- enable comparisons with the performance of similar organisations;
- understand the needs, views and experiences of users and non-users from all backgrounds and communities;
- ensure users are receiving a high-quality service;
- anticipate the potential impact of key policy, technological and socioeconomic developments; and
- assure themselves that the organisation is complying with standards and other regulatory requirements.

All information should:

- be presented clearly and simply, including graphic overviews as well as brief commentary;
- be updated in a timely manner;
- direct the board's attention to significant risks, issues and exceptions; and
- provide a level of detail appropriate to the board's role.

Information flows should be both formal and informal. Information is provided formally in documents or files, but this is supplemented by informal communication by e-mail, telephone or face-to-face conversation. Whether providing information formally or informally, the company secretary should ensure that there are good information flows between the board and its committees, between committees and between EDs and NEDs.

Managing conflicts of interest

Whilst much of the detail on conflicts of interest is dealt with in Chapter 8, it is important to take such conflicts into account when considering how to maintain the effectiveness of the board. Failing to declare and manage conflicts of interest will essentially jeopardise the ability of the board to act in the best interests of that organisation.

Appointments to the board

The appointment of the chair and NEDs for NHS trusts is overseen by NHSI. The SoS has the power to make these appointments but has delegated this to the NHS TDA, which is now under the umbrella of NHSI.

Foundation trust (FT) chairs and NEDs are appointed by the council of governors and will be covered in Chapter 14. The appointment processes for CCGs will be covered in Chapter 15, as they are quite distinct to the procedures illustrated here.

The main functions of the NHSI in this regard are to:

- appoint, re-appoint and, where necessary, terminate the appointment of chairs and NEDs of NHS trusts;
- ensure chairs and NEDs receive relevant and appropriate training;
- ensure through annual performance review that chairs and NEDs are supported and developed in their role and feel valued;
- ensure chairs and NEDs receive all necessary support through mentoring programmes; and
- ensure that overall NHS boards add value to the NHS locally and more widely.

NHSI follows The Government's Governance Code (December 2016), which sets out the regulatory framework for public appointments processes within the Commissioner's remit. NHSI must comply with the following principles of the Code:

- **Selflessness:** Ministers, when making appointments, should act solely in terms of the public interest.
- **Integrity:** Ministers, when making appointments, must avoid placing themselves under any obligation to people or organisations that might try inappropriately to influence them in their work. They should not act or take decisions in order to gain financial or other material benefits for themselves, their family or their friends. They must declare and resolve any interests and relationships.
- **Merit:** All public appointments should be governed by the principle of appointment on merit. This means providing ministers with a choice of high-quality candidates, drawn from a strong, diverse field, whose skills, experiences and qualities have been judged to meet the needs of the public body or statutory office in question.
- **Openness:** Processes for making public appointments should be open and transparent.
- **Diversity:** Public appointments should reflect the diversity of the society in which we live, and appointments should be made taking account of the need to appoint boards that include a balance of skills and backgrounds. Public appointment competitions that are open and/or have not completed on the day notified should continue to run to completion under the previous Code of Practice published by the Commissioner for Public Appointments.
- **Assurance:** There should be established assurance processes with appropriate checks and balances. The Commissioner for Public Appointments has an important role in providing independent assurance that public appointments are made in accordance with these Principles and this Governance Code.

- **Fairness:** Selection processes should be fair and impartial and each candidate must be assessed against the same criteria for the role in question.

NEDs hold a statutory office under the National Health Service Act 2006, and their appointment does not create any contract of service or contract for services between the individual and the NHS trust. Chairs and NEDs are not employees. HMRC has determined that the nature of the appointment means that the status of chairs and NEDs is 'employment-like' and their remuneration is taxable under Schedule E and subject to Class 1 NI contributions but it is not pensionable. NEDs are also eligible to claim allowance for travel and subsistence costs incurred necessarily on NHS business in line with rates set centrally within the DHSC. The legislation governing the payment of chairs and NEDs of boards means that they can only be paid remuneration at the levels determined by the SoS. This includes any work on any of the organisation's committees.

At present, NHSI engages and supports NHS trusts throughout the entire recruitment and selection process. It works with the trust's nomination committee (covered later in this chapter) to conduct a full recruitment campaign, including developing a job description and person specification, advertising the post and supporting the interview process. The NHSI's Appointments Committee makes the final appointment decision based on the recommendation of the selection panel that assesses the merit of each application received.

NHSI rules state that, in most circumstances, civil servants within the DHSC, members/employees of the CQC, chairs and members of the governing body of a CCG, and employees of such a group are ineligible as a NED of an NHS trust. The National Health Service Trusts (Membership and Procedure) Amendment Regulations 2014 removed the disqualification that prevents a person being appointed as chair or NED of an NHS trust where they are:

(a) a chair, NED or member of certain health service bodies;
(b) providers or performers of primary health services; or
(c) an employee of such health service bodies or of such performers or providers.

NHSI has a duty to ensure that the chairs and NEDs it appoints meet the requirements of the 'fit and proper persons' regulations. Consequently, a number of checks may be undertaken to ensure that these requirements are met. They include:

- Disclosure and Barring Scheme (DBS) checks;
- Occupational Health Assessment (OHA);
- photographic proof of ID;
- proof of qualifications, where appropriate;
- search of insolvency and bankruptcy register;
- search of disqualified directors register; and
- check with relevant regulators, where appropriate.

The 'fit and proper person' text is being reviewed, and recommendations for change were issued in February 2019 by Tom Kark QC and Jane Russell (Barrister).

Suspension or removal from office

The NHSI has principles and processes that it will use to establish whether and how a chair or NED of an NHS trust should be suspended or removed from office. The policy incorporates three separate but interconnected pathways:

- seeking resignation;
- suspending the office holder; and
- terminating the appointment.

Where there is clear evidence supporting the removal of a NED from office, the individual may choose to resign or a resignation may be actively sought. This is the preferred course of action in most cases. As these posts are public appointments, information about those appointed and removed is in the public domain. Resignation enables the person to be removed from office with dignity and in a managed way that normally meets the needs of both the individual and the organisation. However, there are circumstances when this would not be appropriate or in the public interest.

If the circumstances associated with an appointee's removal from office are actually or potentially so damaging that it would not be in the public interest for them to be able to take up another NED role in the NHS, it might be more appropriate to pursue the suspension and/or termination of appointment procedures.

If the office holder submits their resignation during the course of a suspension or termination procedure, the NHSI reserves the right to continue with the procedure. This includes completing any investigation until a conclusion is reached, which may then form part of the person's formal appointment record.

When an appointment to an NHS trust is terminated, an automatic disqualification period lasting two years applies. The NHSI may specify a longer period, such as potentially indefinitely in serious cases. The appointee may apply to the NHSI to reduce the period of disqualification.

Regulation 9 of the NHS Trusts (Membership and Procedure) Regulations 1990 sets out the grounds on which a NED appointment may be terminated with immediate effect. They are:

(i). If they are, or become, disqualified for appointment.
(ii). If it is considered that it is not in the interests of the health service that they should continue to hold office.
(iii). If they do not attend a meeting of the trust for a period of three months.
(iv). If they do not properly comply with the requirements of the regulations with regard to pecuniary interests in matters under discussion at meetings of the trust (e.g. a failure to disclose such an interest).
(v). If they fail to disclose a non-pecuniary conflict of interest.

(vi). If they are appointed following a nomination from a university or local authority and they cease to hold a post with the nominating body.

The following list also provides examples of matters which may indicate that it is no longer considered to be in the interests of the health service that a NED continues in office. It is not intended to be exhaustive or definitive; NHSI will consider each case on its merits, taking account of all relevant factors.

- If they are found to be an unfit person as set out in the Health and Social Care Act 2008 (Regulated Activities) Regulations 2014.
- If an annual appraisal or a sequence of appraisals is unsatisfactory.
- If they no longer enjoy the confidence of their chair, other board members, the public or local community or NHSI in a substantial way.
- If (as chair) they fail to ensure that the board monitors the performance of the trust in an effective way.
- If they fail to meet agreed objectives.
- If there is a breakdown in essential relationships (e.g. between them and the chair, them and the CEO, them and NHSI, or between them and other members of the board).
- If they fail to apply the Nolan Principles of Public Life.
- If they fail to comply with the letter and/or principle of the trust's internal policies and procedures, as applicable.
- If an investigation into allegations of wrong doing results in a finding against them.
- If a capability or other board effectiveness review indicates that they are not making a full contribution to the board.
- If a chair has reviewed the contribution of the trust's NEDs directors and identified performance issues and/or skills gaps.

If a NED is disqualified from continuing as a chair or NED on any of the grounds set out above, they should immediately give notice in writing to NHSI. They are also required to declare immediately if they have ever been arrested, have any pending prosecutions or convictions (including driving offences) or if they have accepted any police cautions.

Appointments in the corporate sector

Corporate governance is less prescriptive than health service governance when it comes to appointments, although it is an accepted principle of good corporate governance that the power over board appointments should rest with the whole board. Under UK corporate governance, new appointments can be made to the board at any time during the year, but each newly appointed director must offer themselves for re-election at the next annual general meeting (AGM). The company chair and the board committees' chairs are appointed by the board. These appointments are not subject to shareholder approval at the next AGM.

Recommendations about new appointments should not belong exclusively to the chair and/or the CEO. Appointments should be made on merit and against objective criteria; however, in practice, criticism has been expressed about the way in which most appointments are made, particularly appointments of NEDs. This criticism centres on the fact that most NED appointments come from a relatively small circle of successful businesspeople, many of whom know each other, whereas the net should be cast much wider and individuals from more diverse backgrounds should be chosen.

The UK Code states that there should be 'a formal, rigorous and transparent procedure for the appointment of new directors to the board'. The procedure of identifying candidates for a directorship should be rigorous, and candidates should be investigated thoroughly before the directorship is offered. It goes on to say that appointments should be made on 'merit' and 'against objective criteria'. However, it does not specify what these 'objective criteria' should be.

The procedure should be transparent so that shareholders and other stakeholders are able to see what is happening (what type of person the company is looking for and why a particular individual has been appointed). A formal procedure involves the nomination committee.

The Davies Report

Perhaps somewhat controversially, the UK Code also states that appointments to the board should be made 'with due regard to the benefits of diversity on the board, including gender'. This reflects the widely expressed concern that the boards of major UK companies are dominated by middle-aged to older white males with a commercial or financial background and that there are not enough directors with different attributes, talents and experience to provide boards with an appropriate balance. The relative shortage of female board directors has been well-publicised in the Davies Report, Women on Boards (February 2011).

The report made a strong case for greater diversity on boards, recommending in particular that there should be a greater proportion of women on the boards of FTSE 350 companies. Its general argument in favour of greater diversity was that diverse and balanced boards 'are more likely to be effective boards, better able to understand their customers and stakeholders, and to benefit fresh perspectives, vigorous challenge and broad experience. These in turn lead to better decision making.'

The report rejected the view, for example, that directors (and particularly NEDs) should have had experience of financial responsibilities before their appointment: 'although there is a real need for financial literacy, financial responsibility … can be taught and should not be a pre-requisite for appointments.'

The report recommended a voluntary business-led strategy to bring about a culture change at the heart of business. Chapter 1 sets out the reviews in 2013 and 2015. NHSI has declared that it is committed to achieving the goal of 50/50 gender balance on all NHS boards by 2020.

Roger Kline's paper, 'The "Snowy White Peaks" of the NHS' (2014), explores the links between good diversity management and improved service delivery. Kline stated that 'the case for an inclusive and diverse leadership at trust board level – and indeed across the NHS – is now a convincing one'. In London, the proportion of trust board members from a BME (black and minority ethnic) background was 8%, which had declined from 9.6% almost a decade earlier – in a city where 41% of staff and 45% of the population were from a BME background. Kline also reported that the proportion of women in London on trust boards was 40%, which was well below that of the NHS workforce (77%) or the population as a whole (51%) – women were especially under-represented at chair and CEO level.

Ruth Sealy of Cranfield University in The Female FTSE Board Report (2015) has also reported on the better governance resulting from more gender diverse boards such as enhanced independence, better induction, more accountability, better self-evaluation, more awkward questions, improved innovation and decision-making processes, and improved stakeholder relations. All of which affect organisation performance.

Nomination committee

The role of the nomination committee in FTs and CCGs will be covered in Chapters 14 and 15 (respectively), as they are quite distinct to the procedures that follow here. However, best practice as to composition and process should be used as a useful benchmark as far as possible. Chapter 7 has already set out the background for the nomination committee, along with its basic role and composition.

It is important to note that a nomination committee does not have the authority to make new appointments; it simply carries out the search and makes the recommendation. Appointing new directors is a matter for the board, therefore the whole board should make decisions.

It is also important to note that the need for a new board appointment, or a replacement for an existing board member (succession planning), is not necessarily decided by the nomination committee. The chair has responsibility for ensuring that the composition of the board is appropriate. The need for a new NED may also emerge from the annual review of board performance, if an existing NED has not been performing as well as expected or if a gap is identified in the range of skills and experience that the board needs. The chair is also responsible for ensuring that there is succession planning for board positions and may therefore ask the nomination committee to identify potential successors.

The existence of a majority of NEDs should ensure that the chair and CEO do not dominate the appointments process. The committee should consider new appointments to the board and make recommendations to the full board. The full board should then reach a decision about offering a position to the individual concerned so that final responsibility for board appointments remains with the board as a whole.

The main duties of the nomination committee

For NHS trusts, the work of the nomination committee in the appointment of NEDs is supported and underpinned by NHSI. In general, however, the main role of the nomination committee is to:

- regularly review the structure, size and composition (including the skills, knowledge and experience) required of the board compared to its current position, and make recommendations to the board with regard to any changes;
- give full consideration to succession planning for all board members in the course of its work, taking into account the challenges and opportunities facing the trust, and what skills and expertise are therefore needed on the board of directors in the future;
- before any appointment is made by the board of directors, evaluate the balance of skills, knowledge and experience on the board, and, in the light of this evaluation, prepare a description of the role and capabilities required for a particular appointment. In identifying suitable candidates the committee shall:
  - use open advertising or the services of external advisers to facilitate the search
  - consider candidates from a wide range of backgrounds
  - consider candidates on merit and against objective criteria, taking care that appointees have enough time available to devote to the position;
- review the job descriptions of the director role as required;
- keep under review the leadership needs of the organisation, with a view to ensuring the continued ability of the organisation to deliver services effectively;
- keep up-to-date and fully informed about strategic issues and commercial changes affecting the trust and the environment in which it operates; and
- review annually the performance evaluation process for EDs ensuring it is fit for purpose.

The committee shall also make recommendations to the board of directors concerning:

- formulating plans for succession for EDs;
- membership of the audit and remuneration committees, in consultation with the chairs of those committees; and
- any matters relating to the continuation in office of any ED at any time including the suspension or termination of service.

The committee also ensures that the full range of eligibility checks have been performed and references taken and found to be satisfactory.

This is based on the principal duties of the nomination committee, which were summarised in the suggestions for good practice in the Higgs Report. These have been adopted in the NHS; a further useful document is the ICSA guidance note NHS Foundation Trust – Non-Executive Directors Nomination Committee.

The UK Code requires that a separate section of the annual report should describe the work of the nomination committee, including the process it used in relation to appointments that were made during the year. An explanation should be given if neither the services of an external search consultancy ('headhunters') nor advertising were used in making the appointment of chair or NED. If the vacancy was not advertised nor a headhunter used, this would suggest that the appointment was made of a person that the nomination committee already knew or who was recommended privately: this would be contrary to the requirement for a formal, rigorous and transparent appointment procedure. Executive directors may be appointed from within the organisation, so the requirement applies only to the appointment of a chair or NED.

The UK Code includes several provisions about criteria for appointment to the board that are reflected in health service governance for NHS organisations.

- The search for board candidates should be conducted, and appointments made on merit, against objective criteria and with due regard for the benefits of diversity on the board, including gender.
- The nomination committee should evaluate the balance of skills, experience, independence and knowledge on the board and, in the light of this evaluation, prepare a description of the role and capabilities required for a particular appointment.
- On initial appointment, the chair should meet the criteria for independence.
- For the appointment of a chair, the nomination committee should prepare a job specification, including an assessment of the time required and recognising the need for the chair's availability in times of crisis.
- The departing chair should not chair the nomination committee when it is meeting to consider the appointment of the successor to the role of chair.
- A proposed new chair's other significant commitments should be disclosed to the board before an appointment is made and included in the annual report (subsequent changes should also be disclosed and reported).

In the NHS, the requirement to advertise all NED appointments openly under the auspices of NHSI has gone some way to addressing issues of ethnicity and gender. The Equality Act 2010 also imposes a duty on public bodies to achieve equal opportunities in the workplace and in wider society. The Act is supported by specific duties, which require public bodies to publish relevant, proportionate information demonstrating their compliance with the equality duty and to set themselves specific, measurable equality objectives. NHS trusts must set objectives that eliminate unlawful discrimination, harassment and victimisation, advance equality of opportunity and foster good relations.

Succession planning and refreshing board membership

The key positions on the board of directors are the chair of the board and the CEO. The individuals holding these positions will retire or resign at some time, perhaps because the individual has reached retirement age or has come to the end of a fixed-term contract.

The board of directors should try to ensure a smooth succession, with a replacement lined up to take the place of the departing individual. In the case of a departing CEO, the successor might be an existing executive manager who has been groomed for the role. In the case of a departing chair, the successor might be an external appointment. A smooth succession is desirable to avoid disruptions to the organisation's decision-making processes or changes in policy or direction. The succession can also be planned well in advance, so that the newly appointed individuals will have an opportunity to learn about their new role before the actual succession occurs.

The FRC Board Guide states that EDS may be recruited externally, but that companies should also develop internal talent and capability. Initiatives to encourage this could include middle management development programmes, facilitating engagement between middle management and NEDs, as well as partnering and mentoring schemes.

The positions of chair and CEO (and director of finance or CFO) are important. It is undesirable to have vacancies in these positions for more than a short period. Ideally, the successor should be in place for immediate appointment. This is why succession planning should be carried out in advance and should be delegated to the nomination committee.

Succession planning should be delegated to the nomination committee. If the board of a listed company intends to breach the governance code by appointing the current CEO as the next chair, it would be advisable for a suitable representative of the board (such as the chair of the nomination committee or the SID) to discuss the reasons for their choice with major shareholders and representative bodies of the institutional shareholders. These discussions should take place well in advance of any final decision about the appointment.

There should also be succession planning for NEDs to allow for compliance with the FRC Board Guide on lengths of terms of service (more details can be found in Chapter 7).

The FT Code and the UK Code state that there should be 'progressive refreshing of the board'. Succession planning as outlined above, in terms of horizon scanning for the right skills and experience to manage the future challenges the board will face, is one way of refreshing the board. However, the nomination committee should also be aware of when a vacancy is expected to arise and should plan in advance to appoint the type of person it considers would improve the balance of skills and experience on the board. In addition, there has been increasing pressure for board appointments to be regularly reviewed under a process of annual re-election.

The financial crisis in banking between 2007 and 2009 led to a re-assessment of the UK Code, when it was argued that some or all of the board should be subject to annual re-election. Annual re-election increases the accountability of the directors to the shareholders and gives more power to the shareholders, who are able to threaten to vote against a director at the next AGM (instead of possibly having to wait up to three years before having the opportunity).

After extensive consultation, the UK Code now requires:

- annual re-election of directors of FTSE 350 companies;
- annual re-election of all NEDs who have served longer than nine years on the board; and
- the same recommendations as before for directors of other companies subject to the UK Code: all other directors to be subject to re-election at the first AGM following their appointment and re-election subsequently at intervals of no more than three years.

The UK Code also requires that, when the board proposes a NED for election at an AGM, they should present reasons why the directors believe that the individual should be appointed. When a director is proposed for re-election, the chair should confirm to the shareholders that following a formal performance evaluation of the individual, they have concluded that the individual's performance continues to be effective and the individual remains committed to the role.

The requirement for the board to ensure planned and progressive refreshing means that re-election of current directors, particularly NEDs, should not be an automatic process. As indicated earlier, plans to refresh the board with new NEDs should be a part of succession planning.

Induction and training of directors

Induction of new directors

The induction of directors is a process by which new directors familiarise themselves with the business, its services and how it operates. New directors need induction in order to become effective contributors to the board decision-making process. The need for induction is more important for NEDs than for EDs, particularly internally appointed EDs, who should be familiar with much of the business before their appointment to the board. However, newly appointed EDs may not be familiar with all the responsibilities and duties of being a director; they may also need induction to make them more aware of what will be expected of them in their new role.

In the NHS, NHS Providers offers structured inductions for new chairs, NEDs, EDs and CCG lay members around key issues. It includes:

- an introduction to NHS board roles;
- sessions on structures, roles, patient safety and individual liabilities; and
- an introduction to their governance responsibilities; including risk assurance, financial obligations and the board role in delivering a safe and high-quality service.

The UK Code states that all directors should receive an induction on joining the board and that 'to function effectively, all directors need appropriate knowledge of the organisation and access to its operations and staff'.

The chair is responsible for ensuring that new directors receive 'full, formal and tailored' induction. Although there is no specific reference to the company secretary, the chair will probably ask the company secretary to arrange for each director to receive a personalised induction programme. The aim should be to make the director an effective member of the board quickly. An induction programme may therefore focus initially on providing essential information and familiarity with the organisation, such as visits to key sites, meetings with senior management and staff and providing copies of previous board meetings and copies of any current strategy documents. Over time, further induction may then be provided.

Reading is an effective way for an individual to absorb new information quickly, and the company secretary might therefore wish to give a new director a selection of documents as an induction pack.

Training and professional development

Directors should keep their knowledge and skills up to date so they can continue to perform effectively. The organisation should ensure this is provided. The appropriate training and personal development for each individual director will depend on the director's personal situation. All directors may need training or updating when there is a change in an important aspect of the law or when new regulations are introduced that affect the organisation's operations or its governance. Members of board committees may need to be updated or may need to acquire greater in-depth knowledge of matters affecting the work of their committee. Directors may need to be informed about an important new service or product or an important new acquisition for the organisation.

Reflecting as it does the UK Code, the FT Code states that:

> 'The chair should ensure that the directors continually update their skills and the knowledge and familiarity with the organisation required to fulfil their role both on the board and board committees. The organisation should provide the necessary resources for developing and updating its directors' knowledge and capabilities.'

The chair, as part of their annual appraisal, should assess the particular training and development needs for each individual director. Each director should also be able to make suggestions about the type of training or development that might be suitable for them personally. The UK Code includes a provision that the chair should agree a personalised approach to training and development with each director. This should be reviewed regularly. The obvious time to do this is during the annual performance review of the director.

Performance evaluation of the board, its committees and individual directors

Requirement for annual evaluation

A possibly contentious issue in both corporate and health service governance is the extent to which the performance of directors should be monitored and assessed, and what form such assessments should take.

In the UK, a requirement for company directors to undergo formal performance appraisals each year was introduced into the UK Code in 2003. Both the FT Code and the UK Code state as a main principle that the board should undertake a 'formal and rigorous annual evaluation of its own performance and that of its committees and individual directors'. The evaluation should consider the 'balance of skills, experience, independence and knowledge of the organisation on the board, its diversity, including gender, how the board works together as a unit, and other factors relevant to its effectiveness'.

Evaluation of individual directors should aim to show whether each director continues to contribute effectively and demonstrates commitment to the role (such as in terms of time spent carrying out director's duties, attendance at board and committee meetings, and on other duties). The evaluation of performance is particularly important for NEDs. Executive directors commit all or most of their time to the organisation and should be fully familiar with the business and the organisation's operations. In contrast, NEDs spend only a part of their time with the organisation, even though they make up the membership of key committees of the board – the audit and remuneration committees in particular. There is a possibility that NEDs will lose some of their enthusiasm for the organisation and may get into a habit of missing meetings and spending less time with the organisation than expected. In some cases, a director may fail to keep up to date with an important area of his supposed expertise. The respective chapters for the chair, EDs and NEDS set out the performance evaluation process for each role, respectively. In addition, the processes for these roles in FTs and CCGs are set out in Chapters 14 and 15, respectively.

The FRC Board Guide states that 'evaluation should be bespoke in its formulation and delivery' and provides a non-exhaustive list of areas that might be considered, such as:

- the mix of skills, experience and knowledge on the board, in the context of developing and delivering the strategy, the challenges and opportunities, and the principal risks facing the company;
- clarity of, and leadership given to, the purpose, direction and values of the company;
- succession and development plans;
- how the board works together as a unit, and the tone set by the chair and the CEO;

- key board relationships, particularly chair/CEO, chair/senior independent director, chair/company secretary and EDs/NEDs;
- effectiveness of individual directors;
- clarity of the senior independent director's role;
- effectiveness of board committees, and how they are connected with the main board;
- quality of the general information provided on the company and its performance;
- quality and timing of papers and presentations to the board;
- quality of discussions around individual proposals and time allowed;
- process the chair uses to ensure sufficient debate for major decisions or contentious issues;
- effectiveness of the company secretary/secretariat;
- clarity of the decision-making processes and authorities, possibly drawing on key decisions made over the year;
- processes for identifying and reviewing risks; and
- how the board communicates with, and listens and responds to, shareholders and other key stakeholders.

According to the FRC Board Guide, the chair has overall responsibility for the process, and should select an effective approach, involving the senior independent director as appropriate. The senior independent director should lead the process that evaluates the performance of the chair and, in certain circumstances, may lead the entire evaluation process. The chair should consider ways in which to obtain feedback from the workforce and other stakeholders (for example, the auditors) on the performance of the board and individual directors. Chairs of board committees should be responsible for the evaluation of their committees.

The outcomes from the board evaluation should be shared with and discussed by the board. They should be fed back into the board's work on composition, the design of induction and development programmes, and other relevant areas. It may be useful for a company to review how effective the board evaluation process has been and how well the outcomes have been acted upon. The chair is encouraged to give a summary of the outcomes and actions of the board evaluation process in their statement in the annual report.

The FT Code and the UK Code both require that the board should state in the organisation's annual report how the performance evaluation of the board, its committees and individual directors has been carried out. In addition, the FT Code requires the outcomes of the evaluation of the EDs to be reported to the board of directors, and for the CEO to take the lead on the evaluation of the EDs.

Board evaluation – what does it mean to be well-led?

In the UK, the potential value of external consultants has been recognised, and the 2018 Corporate Governance Code states that for the evaluation of the board as a whole, the evaluation of the board of FTSE 350 companies should be 'externally facilitated' at least every three years. In other words, the company should use specialist external consultants at least once every three years, and where the company uses external consultants, it should identify them in the annual report and make a statement of whether the consultants have any other connection with the company. The FRC Guide on Board Effectiveness sets out clear guidance for corporate organisations in how to select and brief an external evaluation.

Much of this is echoed in the FT Code and was formalised in the Well-Led Framework (2017). The 2017 framework aligns the view of a well-led organisation with CQC's assessments and ratings and with NHSI expectations under the Single Oversight Framework. The Framework replaced Monitor's Quality Governance Framework (QGF) and the Board Governance Assurance Framework (BGAF), which were effectively incorporated within this framework.

In-depth, regular and externally facilitated developmental reviews of leadership and governance are good practice across all industries and such reviews should identify the areas of leadership and governance of organisations that would benefit from further targeted development work to secure and sustain future performance, rather than assessing current performance. The external input is vital to safeguard against the optimism bias and group think to which even the best organisations may be susceptible. The Well-Led Framework recommends that all providers carry out externally facilitated, developmental reviews of their leadership and governance using the Well-Led Framework every three to five years, according to their circumstances.

The structure of the framework (key lines of enquiry (KLOEs) and their characteristics) is wholly shared with the CQC and underpins CQC's regular regulatory assessments of their well-led assessment. This means that information prepared for regulation can also be used for development, and vice versa. The main elements of the framework are also reflected in NHSE IAF.

However, while CQC's regulatory assessments are primarily for assurance, developmental reviews are primarily for providers themselves to facilitate continuous improvement.

The Well-Led Framework is a move in the right direction as previously the assessment of board effectiveness was largely determined using national access and quality targets to produce a governance risk rating. Recognising that a board's leadership and performance must also be assessed for its contribution to strategy and culture and as well as holding the EDs to account for the day-to-day performance of the organisation aligns health service governance with the similar movement in corporate governance (e.g. UK Code 2018 and FRC study in corporate culture).

Whilst the specific detail of the 2017 framework has already been set out in Chapter 6, essentially the aligned framework sets out a clear expectation of what 'good' looks like for any well-led NHS organisation.

It is encouraging to see that the guidance has moved away from a checklist approach: recognising that a mechanical 'ticking off' of each item is unlikely to lead to better performance. Much more important to the development of leadership and good governance is the attitude of organisational leaders to the review process, the connections they draw between the framework's different areas, and their judgements about what needs to be done to improve continually. Consequently, providers are encouraged to engage with the review processes openly and honestly, selecting an external facilitator to provide tailored support and prioritise actions arising from reviews. Providers are also encouraged to make more use of peer review, to utilise and enhance skills within the NHS, draw on learning from others and share learning back with the system. This is how providers, individually and together, will gain the greatest benefit from these reviews. To assess the performance of the board, a comparison should be made between what the board should be expected to achieve, and what it has actually achieved. One way of doing this may be to provide answers to a set of questions about performance, possibly through discussions at a special board meeting.

Questions that may provide a useful basis for assessment of board performance are set out below:

- Does the board have any specific performance objectives (e.g. in terms of business performance or quality measures)? How well has the board performed against any such targets?
- What has the board contributed to the development of strategy and what has it done to oversee the implementation of strategy and achievement of strategy targets?
- What has the board contributed to ensuring that the organisation has a robust and effective risk management system?
- Is the board concerning itself with the appropriate issues? Is the list of matters reserved for the board suitable or should it be amended?
- Is the board an appropriate size and is the mix of members suitable (in terms of spread of experience, knowledge, skills and/or background)? Are changes needed?
- How well does the board communicate with patients, the public, management, employees and other stakeholders?

Questions may also be asked about the effectiveness of boardroom practice:

- Do board members receive relevant and clear information in good time for board meetings and decision making? Is the amount and quality of this information adequate?
- Have there been sufficient board meetings in the past year?
- Are the board meetings too short to be effective or too long?

Evaluation of board committees

Board committees should be evaluated in a similar way to the board as a whole. For each committee, there should be a comparison between what the committee is responsible for doing and what it has actually done. For example:

- Has the nomination committee been successful in identifying suitable individuals for board appointments?
- Have any individuals been appointed to the board who, in retrospect, were not as good as originally thought?
- Has the nomination committee done any succession planning, and if so, how good have its plans been?
- Has the committee made clear recommendations to the board, and has the board acted on its recommendations?
- Is the committee an appropriate size and is the mix of members suitable? Are changes needed?
- Have there been enough committee meetings during the past year?

Similar questions can be asked about the remuneration and audit committees as well as any other committees established by the board.

Using the results of a performance review

To obtain practical value from an annual evaluation of the board, its committees and its individual directors, the board should be prepared to act on its findings whenever performance is not considered to be as good as it should be. The chair has the responsibility for acting to deal with poor performance.

According to the FRC Board Guide, the chair is responsible for making sure the board gets the most from an externally facilitated board evaluation and should ensure it is not approached as a compliance exercise. The chair is likely to find the board evaluation process more valuable if:

- its recommendations are constructive, meaningful and forward-looking;
- there is a clear set of recommendations and actions, and a time-period for review of progress against agreed outcomes by the evaluator with the board;
- it includes views from beyond the boardroom (e.g. shareholders, senior executives who regularly interact with the board, auditors and other advisors, and the workforce);
- it includes peer reviews of directors and the chair plus feedback on each director;
- good practice observed in other companies is shared;
- the evaluator observes the interaction between directors and between the CEO and chair;
- there is a robust analysis of the quality of information provided to the board;
- feedback is provided to each individual board member; and
- the board is challenged on composition, diversity, skills gaps, refreshment and succession.

The chair may also consider the need for changes to the composition of board committees and may ask for the resignation of a committee chair. Some improvements may be achieved by changing board procedures (such as holding meetings more frequently or changing the dates of meetings to give management more time to prepare the information required).

Governance checklist

- Does the board perform the leadership functions expected of an effective board?
- Does it develop strategy and promote behaviours consistent with the culture and values it has defined for the organisation?
- Is there an effective process in place to allow the organisation to make well-informed and high-quality decisions based on a clear line of sight into the business?
- Does the board know what the balance of skills, experience, knowledge and personality it requires currently and in the medium to long term? Does it have that balance?
- What consideration has the board given to equality and diversity with regard to its own composition?
- Is the nomination committee actively involved in developing the recruitment and appointment process for new board members? Is there a focus on competencies rather than experience?
- Is there an open and positive interplay between the nomination and remuneration committees?
- Is there a clear and informative report from the nomination committee in the annual report?
- Are the terms of reference for the nomination committee available publicly and subject to regular review?
- Does the board have a succession plan and is it kept under regular review?
- What plans does the board have for annual self-evaluation of itself, its committees and individual directors?
- How are external assessors for evaluation appointed so that their independence is assured?

Summary

- There is a fine balance to be maintained in assessing the effectiveness of a board. There should be quantitative evidence of outcomes achieved and processes followed, yet there must also be a more subjective and qualitative approach that considers the individual skills, experience and personalities that are represented in the board. How do these people work together to make a cohesive unit?
- This chapter has sought to demonstrate that there is guidance to outline best practice in processes and procedures though at the same time posing

questions or challenges about behaviour and culture, which each board and each individual board member must consider in its or their own development.
- As John Deffenbaugh says in his 2012 *British Journal of Healthcare Management* article, 'It's the People in the Boardroom': 'In a world requiring a high-performing board, the knowledge derived from this insight to behaviour and relationships can enable the individual components to meld into an effective decision-making body.'

10
The chair of the board

Introduction

Although this chapter explores the role of the chair of the board, it should also be considered in the light of the next chapter and the role of the CEO. This is because these are the two most powerful roles within the board. Consequently, there needs to be a clear distinction between the roles and a clear understanding by the individuals fulfilling them how they are meant to complement and work together.

Much of the friction in board relationships is centred upon this key dynamic; effective boards often demonstrate what the dynamic should be and vice versa. Much of what follows here can also be applied to the role of board committee chairs. Obviously, the focus here on the role of the chair must not distract from the underlying principle of the unitary board, with the chair having the same duties and responsibilities of every other board director. However, the role of the chair in creating the right team dynamic for a disparate group of board directors with varied and strongly held views to reach agreement on strategic direction and corporate objectives is crucial.

As the Financial Reporting Council has commented, 'good boards are created by good chairs'; therefore, the role warrants further examination here.

The role of the chair

Whereas the CEO is responsible for the executive management, the chair's responsibilities relate primarily to managing the board of directors, and ensuring that the board functions effectively. To do this, a chair needs to ensure that the board discusses relevant issues in sufficient depth, with all the information needed to reach a decision, and with all the directors contributing to the discussions and decision making.

The UK Code states that:

'The chair leads the board and is responsible for its overall effectiveness in directing the company. They should demonstrate objective judgement throughout their tenure and promote a culture of openness and debate. In addition, the chair facilitates constructive board relations and the effective contribution of all non-executive directors, and ensures that directors receive accurate, timely and clear information.'

The FRC Board Guide is clear that the chair is pivotal in:

- creating the conditions for overall board and individual director effectiveness;
- setting clear expectations concerning the style and tone of board discussions; and
- ensuring the board has effective decision-making processes and applies sufficient challenge to major proposals.

It goes on to say that it is up to the chair to make certain that all directors are aware of their responsibilities and to hold meetings with the NEDs without the executives present in order to facilitate a full and frank airing of views.

The FRC Board Guide defines the chair's role as:

- setting a board agenda primarily focused on strategy, performance, value creation, culture, stakeholders and accountability, and ensuring that issues relevant to these areas are reserved for board decision;
- shaping the culture in the boardroom;
- encouraging all board members to engage in board and committee meetings by drawing on their skills, experience and knowledge;
- fostering relationships based on trust, mutual respect and open communication – both in and outside the boardroom – between NEDs and the executive team;
- developing a productive working relationship with the CEO, providing support and advice, while respecting executive responsibility;
- providing guidance and mentoring to new directors as appropriate;
- leading the annual board evaluation, with support from the senior independent director as appropriate, and acting on the results; and
- considering having regular externally facilitated board evaluations.

The UK Code and FRC Board Guide emphasise the role of the chair in trying to ensure that all directors, in particular NEDs, contribute effectively to board discussions. There is always a risk that individuals who do not work full-time for the organisation may have difficulty in challenging the views of full-time EDs. The chair should make sure that this does not happen.

The FRC Board Guide states that 'the chair creates the conditions for overall board and individual director effectiveness'. It emphasises that an effective chair is a team-builder, developing a board whose members communicate effectively and enjoy good relationships with each other. They should develop a close relationship of trust with the CEO, giving support and advice while still respecting the CEO's responsibilities for executive matters. They should also ensure the effective implementation of board decisions, provide coherent leadership for the organisation and understand the views of the stakeholders.

The chair also has a role in respect of board committees, and should ensure that sufficient time is allowed at the board for committees to report on the nature and content of discussion, on recommendations and on actions to be taken. Where there is disagreement between the relevant committee and the board, the chair should ensure there is adequate time available for discussion of the issue with a view to resolving the disagreement. The chair should also ensure board committees are properly structured with appropriate terms of reference, which should be published on the company website. The chair should make sure that committee membership is periodically refreshed and that individual independent NEDs are not over-burdened when deciding the chairs and membership of committees.

Responsibilities of a chair in the NHS

The NHSI role description for an NHS trust chair sets out that they are accountable to the SoS through the NHSI, for giving leadership to the NHS trust board and ensuring the trust provides high-quality, safe services, and value for money (VFM) within NHS resources.

The key responsibilities of the chair are to:

- provide leadership to the board, the trust, the other NEDs, the CEO and EDs; and ensure the effectiveness of the board in all aspects of its role and agenda;
- ensure the provision of accurate, timely and clear information to the board and directors to meet statutory requirements;
- ensure effective communication with the board, staff, patients and the public in a changing healthcare environment;
- arrange the regular evaluation of the performance of the board, its committees and individual non-executives, directors, and the CEO;
- plan and conduct board meetings with the CEO;
- facilitate the effective contribution of NEDs and ensure constructive relations within the organisation and between executive and NEDs, and
- share and use relevant expertise of all members of the board.

In particular, the chair will:

- proactively direct and manage the development of major board decisions, ensuring that 'due process' has been applied at all stages of decision making and full and complete consideration has been given to all options during the process;
- hold the CEO to account for the effective management and delivery of the organisation's strategic aims and objectives;
- ensure the board develops and oversees strategies, which will result in tangible improvements to the health of the population and clinical services;
- ensure the board establishes clear objectives to deliver agreed strategies and regularly review performance against these objectives;
- ensure the board maintains its responsibility for the effective governance of the organisation by making the best use of resources including the development of effective risk and performance management processes;

THE CHAIR OF THE BOARD

- ensure the board, and the organisation, observe the SoS's policies and priorities, including the requirements of the Codes of Conduct and Accountability;
- be aware of relevant, regulatory and central government policies;
- play a key role in building strong partnerships with the local authorities, local health economy, and other stakeholders in the community and nationally, including regulators such as NHSI and the CQC. For FTs this includes developing an effective council of governors and promoting harmonious relations with the board;
- ensure that the interests of all stakeholders, and influence of all advisers, are fairly balanced;
- provide the leadership needed by the board to shape the organisation; develop a culture which supports the values of the NHS, and ensure the organisation values diversity in its workforce and demonstrates equality of opportunity in its treatment of staff and patients and in all aspects of its business;
- be an ambassador for the trust with national, regional and local bodies; be knowledgeable and aware of local issues, and recognise the trust's role as a major local employer; and
- where necessary, assist in the appointment of EDs and NEDs and ensure systems of support and appraisal.

Independence of the chair

Generally, the chair should be independent when first appointed. This is a provision of the UK Code for listed companies and of the FT Code. See Chapter 12 for a discussion about independence for NEDs generally and Chapter 15 in CCG appointments. Discussions about independence will also need to factor in the length of tenure of office, which is also addressed in Chapter 11.

It follows that the CEO of an organisation should not subsequently become the chair, as a former CEO will not be independent (although the King IV Code states that a former CEO should not become chair for at least three years after ceasing to be CEO, believing that this is sufficient time in which to become independent). If, exceptionally, it is proposed that the current CEO should become the chair when the existing chair retires, major shareholders should be consulted first. The UK Code also states that the reasons for appointing a former CEO as chair should be explained to shareholders both at the time of the appointment and in the next annual report and accounts.

A governance problem with 'promoting' the CEO to become the chair is that the incoming CEO may find it difficult to run the organisation as they wish because the former CEO is still on the board, monitoring what they are doing. Even so, there have been several cases where a CEO has gone on to become the chair without any serious protest from shareholders or investor groups.

The National Association of Pension Funds (NAPF)'s Corporate Governance Policy and Voting Guidelines (2011) also recommend that if the chair is not independent on appointment, the organisation should consult its shareholders and explain why it considers the appointment desirable. The shareholders should then consider the case on its merits.

The chair's commitments

A problem with non-executive chairs – as with NEDs generally – is that the individual may not have enough time to devote to the role because of a large number of other commitments. For example, the chair of a large company may also be the chair of another organisation, without enough time to fulfil either of these roles adequately.

Chairs need to be able to demonstrate that they have sufficient time to perform their role to the standards expected. NAPF's Corporate Governance Policy and Voting Guidelines state that where a chair has 'multiple appointments', investors will require a 'compelling explanation' of how they will be able to handle all the various appointments without any detriment to the organisation. The Walker Report suggested that the chairs of large banks would need to spend about two-thirds of their time with the organisation.

The UK Code is less specific on the amount of time that a chair should commit to the organisation. However, a provision of the Code is that, when a chair is appointed, the nomination committee (see also Chapter 7) should prepare a job description including an assessment of the amount of time commitment that should be expected and recognise the need for the chair to make themselves available in a time of crisis.

The chair's other commitments should be disclosed to the board before their appointment and included in the next annual report and accounts. If there are changes to the time commitment required from or provided by the chair, these should be disclosed to the board and reported in the next annual report and accounts.

The FT Code also sets out that the board of directors should not agree to a full-time ED taking on more than one NED role within a NHS FT or another organisation of comparable size and complexity, nor the chair of such an organisation.

The criteria for independence are set out in Chapter 12 and the same criteria should be applied to the chair (on appointment) as it is to other NEDs. However, circumstances may change, so the independence of NEDs should be kept under review.

Behaviours of an effective chair

The *Harvard Business Review* in its March/April 2018 issue set out the following principles on how to be a good chair (article by Stanislav Shekshnia).

Principle #1: Be the guide on the side

The article argues that more than 85% of the board chairs studied had been CEOs at one time. They were action and results oriented. However, as chairs they nearly all found that the skills and behaviours that had made them effective CEOs were of little help – and even counterproductive – in a chair's work. The shift is from doing to helping others to do.

The research found that effective chairs displayed three characteristics:

- restraint – they focus on creating conditions that allow other people to shine;
- patience – they focus on getting things done properly not quickly; and
- availability – it might be a part-time contract but good chairs are fully committed and put in the required time no matter what they'd agreed to.

The research indicated that industry knowledge was not necessary to the chair's role and at time could be a handicap as they acted as the expert.

Principle #2: Practice teaming – not team building

Collaboration in the context of a board is what the review refers to as 'teaming': gathering experts in a temporary group to solve problems they may be encountering for the first and only time. To enable it, chairs have to shift away from defining team norms and building trust, and focus on quickly scoping, structuring and sorting the collaborative work.

Principle #3: Own the prep work

The review found that inexperienced chairs often think that the job is all about managing the dynamics in the boardroom. Experienced ones, however, recognised that the meetings were just the tip of the iceberg. A great share of the chair's work goes into setting an agenda and putting together a briefing package. One respondent, for example, started preparing meeting agendas a year in advance, asking for the input of the CEO, other directors and the company secretary.

Principle #4: Take committees seriously

The article recorded that experienced chairs agreed that work on committees was key to a board's success. It could be that nearly three-quarters of the work is carried out in committee meetings. Committees should be small, with members who possess relevant expertise, and discussions should always be candid. By definition, board meetings are more formal. Therefore, it makes sense for the profound and detailed discussions take place at the committee level and for the committees to prepare resolutions for the whole board.

Principle #5: Remain impartial

The research behind the article demonstrated that whilst many new chairs might be keen to put their knowledge and experience to full use, in reality when the chair expressed strong views this hampered collective productivity of the board.

One respondent commented, 'If I want to see the whole picture and facilitate the work of the group, I should not play. I should become an onlooker without any stake in the game.'

Good chairs ask themselves, 'What is the best way to organize a discussion of the problem?' rather than 'What is the best solution for a problem?'

Principle #6: Measure the inputs, not the outputs

The article considered how the effectiveness of the board might be measured and there was strong evidence that given the long-term impact of effective decision-making short-term performance indicators were unhelpful. However, board assessment was still seen to be important with regard to the quality of the board's work. Consequently, considering the quality of inputs leads to quality outputs. The article suggests five inputs as critical: people, board agendas, board materials, board processes and board minutes. A good chair takes responsibility for ensuring all five are first-rate.

Principle #7: Don't be the boss

The article recognised that whilst board chairs may interact frequently with management, particularly the CEO; and may even visit customers or vendors, attend press events, or hold meetings with government officials – this should not lead to the chair perceiving themselves as the CEO's boss.

A good chair will remember that they represent the board and keep the other directors informed about all new developments and insights. They understand that the board is the collective 'boss' of the CEO and that the task of the chair is to make sure the board provides the goals, resources, rules, and accountability the CEO needs.

Principle #8: Be a representative with shareholders, not a player

The article concludes that if a CEO's boss is the board, then the board's boss is the shareholders. The relationship with them is a key concern for the chair, who tends to be their primary interface with the company.

What Makes a Top Chair?, published by Hunter Healthcare in 2015, sets out key skills and attributes for the NHS.

> 'Good chairs understand their role in helping their trusts embrace a large cultural shift [as required by the duty of candour]. They lead by example; they are a critical but supportive friend of the chief executive and make sure they do not get dragged into the detail. The new duty of candour places even more weight on the shoulders of NHS trust chairs. There is no hiding from mistakes and top chairs recognise this and use candour as a driver for improvement. Above all, chairs need to understand that success is about relationships, whether this involves creating the right environment for an effective board meeting, or helping clinicians understand management processes. The best chairs understand this and will invest time in developing and nurturing their board members.'

The report goes onto cite the following as key characteristics: courage, strength and agility, curiosity, tenacity, approachability, emotional resilience and integrity. Good communication skills were also seen as key alongside an ability to listen effectively.

The appointment and evaluation of the chair

In an FT, the responsibility for appointing the chair lies with the council of governors and this is set out in more detail in Chapter 14. For CCGs, the appointment of the chair is an appointment from amongst the members of the governing body. More details are provided in Chapter 15. For NHS trusts, the appointment of the chair is carried out by NHSI.

The UK Code states that the NEDs, led by the senior independent director (SID), should be responsible for the performance evaluation of the chair, 'taking into account the views of executive directors'. However, for some organisations, the actual performance review of the chair may be conducted for the NEDs by external consultants.

The chair's performance should be assessed by comparing their responsibilities with their achievements, and asking whether they have been successful in providing the board leadership that should be expected of them.

In an FT, the responsibility for the performance evaluation of the chair lies with the council of governors and this is set out in more detail in Chapter 14. For CCGs the evaluation of the chair is carried out by the lay members of the governing body. Further details are provided in Chapter 15.

Overall responsibility for the NHS trust chair appraisal process rests with the chair of NHSI. Given the number of NHS trust chairs to appraise, it is not possible for the NHSI chair to conduct all NHS trust chair appraisals personally. Therefore, some of this activity is delegated to directors of NHSI.

The initial assessment for all appraisals will be prepared by the relevant Director within NHSI. This will inform the appraisal meetings that will be undertaken. At the end of the appraisal exercise, when all of the appraisals are complete, the chair of NHSI will review all of the appraisal reports to ensure that the exercise has been conducted in a way that is fair and consistent. The final appraisal form will be copied to the chair and a copy put on their personal record by NHSI. In the event of a disagreement between the chair and the appraiser on any element of the appraisal, including the overall assessment, further discussions will take place between the chair and appraiser. If, however, it is not possible to reach agreement, the appraisal will stand as drafted by the appraiser but the chair will be invited to provide comments that will be held on file with the appraisal.

The level of remuneration for NHS chairs is generally considerably lower than that of chairs in the private sector. For NHS trusts, the SoS sets the level of remuneration. All NHS trusts are allocated to one of three remuneration bands, dependent on their turnover. These bands are available on the NHSI website. The remuneration of an FT chair is set by its council of governors.

Separating the role of chair and chief executive officer

A report from Directorbank Group makes it clear that:

> 'The success of a chair undoubtedly hinges first and foremost on the relationship the chair has with the CEO. This is a relationship which should be centred on honesty, trust and transparency, and the success of this relationship is based on mutual understanding by both parties of the distinction between their two roles. One of the main faults identified in chairs deemed to be ineffective is their failure to comprehend that they are not there to run the business; that their role is instead to coach, support and guide.'

As leader of the management team and leader of the board of directors, the CEO and chair are the most powerful positions on the board of directors. It is important, therefore, for the proper functioning of the organisation that the chair and CEO work well together. Acting in alliance, the chair and CEO can dominate the board and its decision making, particularly if the chair also has executive responsibilities in the organisation's management.

More specifically, the Healthy NHS Board report sets out some pointers for chairs and CEOs. The chair should not:

- be too operational, interfere with details of management;
- exceed part-time hours;
- take specific strategic decisions alone; or
- adopt a bullying, macho 'hire and fire' culture.

Chief executives should not:

- be too controlling or autocratic towards the chair;
- get too involved in NED role (e.g. no consultation on shaping board agendas);
- break the fundamental rule of 'no surprises'; or
- be too entrenched in the organisation.

Table 10.1 sets out the key distinctions in role for the chair and CEO.

When the same person holds the position of both chair and CEO, there is a possibility that they could become a dominant influence in decision making in the organisation. As leader of the executive management team, a chair-cum-CEO may be reluctant to encourage challenges from NEDs about the organisation's performance or to question management proposals about future business strategy. In some countries (including the USA), it is common to find organisation leaders who are both chair and CEO, although separation of the roles has become more common there. The UK Code states as a principle that the roles should be separated:

> 'There should be a clear division of responsibilities at the head of the organisation between the running of the board and the executive responsibility

	Chair	**CEO**
Formulate strategy	Ensures board develops vision, strategies and clear objectives to deliver organisational purpose	Leads strategy development process
Ensure accountability	Holds CEO to account for delivery of strategy	Leads the organisation in the delivery of strategy
	Ensures board committees that support accountability are properly constituted	Establishes effective performance management arrangements and controls
		Acts as accountable officer
Shape culture	Provides visible leadership in developing a positive culture for the organisation, and ensures that this is reflected and modelled in their own and in the board's behaviour and decision making	Provides visible leadership in developing a positive culture for the organisation, and ensures that this is reflected in their own and the executive's behaviour and decision making
	Board culture: leads and supports a constructive dynamic within the board, enabling contributions from all directors	
Context	Ensures all board members are well briefed on external context	Ensures all board members are well briefed on external context
Intelligence	Ensures requirements for accurate, timely and clear information to board/directors (and governors for FTs) are clear to executive	Ensures provision of accurate, timely and clear information to board/directors (and governors for FTs)
Engagement	Plays key role as an ambassador, and in building strong partnerships with: • patients and public • members and governors (FTs) • clinicians and staff • key institutional stakeholders • regulators.	Plays key leadership role in effective communication and building strong partnerships with: • patients and public • members and governors (FTs) • clinicians and staff • key institutional stakeholders • regulators.

Table 10.1: Distinctions between NHS chair and CEO roles

for the running of the organisation's business. No one individual should have unfettered powers of decision.'

The UK Code therefore states that the roles of chair and CEO should not be performed by the same individual. In addition, the division of responsibilities between the chair and CEO should be set out clearly in writing, to prevent one of them from encroaching on the area of responsibility of the other. The FT Code makes a similar statement.

When an individual holds the positions of chair and CEO, they could exercise dominant power on the board, unless there are strong individuals on the board, such as a deputy chair or a SID, to act as a counterweight. If the individual also has a domineering or bullying personality, the situation will be even worse, because a chair-cum-CEO who acts in a bullying manner will not listen to advice from any board colleagues, and the board would not function as an effective body. There is even a risk that the individual will run the organisation for their own personal benefit rather than in the interests of the shareholders/stakeholders. The only way to prevent a chair-cum-CEO from dominating an organisation is to have an influential group of directors capable of making their opinions heard. However, it is important to distinguish between the position of 'unfettered power' that is created when the roles of chair and CEO are combined and given to one individual and the ability to act in a dominant or tyrannical way, possibly out of self-interest.

Combining the two roles increases the risk that the organisation and its board will be dominated by a tyrannical individual, but this does not happen every time.

There might occasionally be situations where it is appropriate for the same person to be both chair and CEO. When an organisation gets into business or financial difficulties, for example, there is an argument in favour of appointing a single, all-powerful individual to run the organisation until its fortune has been reversed.

The combination of the roles of chair and CEO might have been necessary in the short term to give an organisation strong leadership to get it through its difficulties.

The chair and the company secretary

Though the role of the company secretary is set out more fully in Chapter 13, it is worth highlighting the key dynamics in the relationship between these two roles. The essential criterion is a relationship of mutual trust, with the chair having full confidence in the company secretary and vice versa.

In particular, there are a number of key areas where the two roles will work very closely together. The first is governance. The company secretary should be responsible for advising the board through the chair on all governance matters (UK Code). This should include the evaluation of the board and the periodic review of governance processes, including the effectiveness of board committees.

A second area where the chair and company secretary need to work together is on the development and implementation of training and development programmes for board members, which may include both individual training and board development sessions. Though this remains the chair's responsibility, in practice this is often delegated to the company secretary.

A further area is that of obtaining a good flow of information within the board and its committees, and between senior management and the NEDs. The UK Code sets this out as a responsibility of the company secretary under the direction of the chair. Other areas of work might include agenda planning, quality control of board papers; overseeing the production of accurate minutes; induction programmes for all board members and for FTs; and supporting the work of the council of governors.

The chair and the senior independent director

The UK Code recommends that the 'board should appoint one of the independent NEDs to be the senior independent director to provide a sounding board for the chair and serve as an intermediary for the other directors and shareholders. Led by the SID, the NEDs should meet without the chair present at least annually to appraise the chair's performance, and on other occasions as necessary'.

The FRC Board Guide expands the role as follows:

> 'The senior independent director should act as a sounding board for the chair, providing them with support in the delivery of their objectives and leading the evaluation of the chair on behalf of the other directors. The senior independent director might also take responsibility for an orderly succession process for the chair, working closely with the nomination committee. It is a good idea for the senior independent director to serve on committees of the board to improve their knowledge of company governance.'

The role of the SID has also been taken up by the FT Code and has been adopted as good practice in NHS trusts. The lay members in a CCG governing body have a similar role, in particular, the lay member for governance. The FT board of directors appoints one of the independent NEDs to be the SID in consultation with the council of governors. The SID is then available to members and governors if they have concerns that contact through the normal channels of chair, CEO or finance director have failed to resolve or for which such contact is inappropriate. Both the UK Code and the FT Code state that the SID may also be the deputy chair. In NHS trusts, the board appoints the SID and they are available to all stakeholders where concerns cannot be addressed through the normal channels. In the NHS, the SID often has a key role to play in the organisation's whistleblowing procedures.

Having a SID is a key element of an effective board. The FRC Board Guide sets this out quite clearly, making a distinction between the role of the SID in 'normal times' and when the board is undergoing 'a period of stress'.

At normal times, the role of the SID is to:

- provide support for the chair;
- ensure that the views of other directors, particularly the other NEDs, are conveyed to the chair;
- ensure that the views of the shareholders, particularly matters that concern them, are conveyed to the rest of the board;
- ensure that the chair is giving sufficient attention to succession planning; and
- carry out the annual review of the performance of the chair, in conjunction with the other NEDs (see Chapter 12).

At times of stress for the board, the role of the SID should be to take the initiative to resolve the problem, working with the other directors and stakeholders and/or the chair, as appropriate. Examples of problems where intervention by the SID may be appropriate include situations where:

- there is a dispute between the chair and the CEO;
- shareholders or the NEDs have expressed serious concerns that are not being addressed by the chair or CEO;
- the strategy pursued by the chair or CEO is not supported by the rest of the board;
- there is a very close relationship between the chair and the CEO;
- decisions are being taken without the approval of the board; and
- succession planning is being ignored.

Issues where intervention may be required should be considered when defining the responsibilities of the SID and should be set out in writing. The FRC Board Guide makes it clear that the SID should work alongside the chair and other board directors but requiring intervention by the SID will also mean at times acting to challenge custom and practice and demonstrating significant people skills to find a solution.

Critics of the SID concept argue that the chair should be able to resolve difficulties between an organisation and its shareholders/stakeholders, and the position of SID should therefore be superfluous. Opening up the possibility of an additional channel of communication for shareholders/stakeholders is perhaps more likely to undermine organisation–stakeholder relationships than improve them.

However, the International Corporate Governance Network (ICGN)'s ICGN Global Corporate Governance Principles put forward reasons why a 'lead independent director' or independent deputy chair is necessary:

- If the chair is the CEO or former CEO or was for another reason not independent when first appointed, the SID should provide independent leadership for the

board, and should have a key role in setting the agenda for board meetings and acting as spokesman for the independent members of the board.
- Even when the chair was independent when first appointed, the role inevitably brings them closer than the NEDs over time to the views of the CEO and executive management.
- The SID should provide leadership to the independent members of the board when this situation creates a problem.

The ICGN Principles also recognise the role of the lead independent director as an alternative conduit for communication with the shareholders/stakeholders.

Although not specifically set out in the UK Code, in the event that the chair had to be removed, it would be the SID's job to lead that process. In the NHS, this would also involve NHSE or NHSI.

Under the UK Code, a further responsibility of the SID is to chair the annual meeting of NEDs, without the chair's presence, and to appraise the chair's performance as well as any other meeting as appropriate. In the NHS, this will happen to some extent, but will be bound by the specific appraisal structures for NHS trusts, FTs and CCGs.

The role of the SID is most effective when there is a strong working relationship between the chair and SID, which is often why the SID will also be appointed as the deputy chair.

The chair and stakeholders

The UK Code is very clear that the chair must make sure that the board listens to the views of shareholders, the workforce, customers and other key stakeholders. As outlined earlier, this engagement with stakeholders has become more focused in the latest UK Code (2018) and has been covered extensively in Chapter 6.

The dissemination of information about the performance of the board and the organisation to stakeholders is also important and the chair has a key role to play in that dissemination. This may be through the formal route of publicly available information or more informal meetings to discuss issues with key stakeholders.

The annual report

From a formal perspective, the Preface to the UK Code encourages chairs to report personally in their annual statements how the principles of the Code relating to the role and effectiveness of the board have been applied. This is one way in which the chair is held to account in a very public and personal way for their ability to oversee the role and effectiveness of the board. There is also a requirement for the annual board evaluation to be set out in the annual report, including the evaluation of the board committees and its individual directors. External evaluation should also be declared in the annual report.

From an informal perspective, regular briefing meetings or board to boards with key stakeholders are another useful way of engaging with stakeholders at which the chair will play a vital role. For NHS organisations, this is a key role for the chair as such meetings can help to support the development of an active and collaborative local health economy.

The annual meeting

The chair also has a key role to play in the organisation's annual meeting. For companies this will be the annual general meeting with its institutional and individual shareholders in attendance; for NHS trusts, this will mean the annual public meeting.

The NHS Trusts (Public Meetings) Regulations 1991 require NHS trusts to present their audited accounts, annual reports and any report on the accounts to a public meeting on or before 30 September every year. They also provide that an NHS trust shall hold a public meeting to consider an auditor's report other than a report on the audited accounts as soon as practicable, and in any event not later than three months after the date on which the NHS trust received that report.

Governance checklist

- Does the chair have the necessary personal attributes to create the right conditions for the board and its directors to be effective?
- What leadership, decision making and governance skills does the chair possess?
- Does the process for appointing and appraising a new chair follow the best practice outlined here?
- Does the chair set the board agenda and chair meetings effectively?
- Do the chair and the CEO work together effectively? Do they complement each other's roles and personalities?
- Is the company secretary available to the chair and do they work together effectively? Is there a clear delegation of tasks to the company secretary from the chair?
- Is there evidence of high quality, timely information, access to external advice, successful induction programmes and effective annual evaluation?
- Has a SID been appointed with a clearly defined role and with the necessary personal attributes to deal with potentially conflicted situations?
- Has the chair developed clear lines of communications, both formal and informal, with key stakeholders?

Summary

According to the Directorbank Group annual survey, *Life in the Boardroom 2013*:

> 'The role of the chair and NED has never been more important nor more challenging and, though the financial rewards are generally not comparable

to those for executive roles, the ideal non-executive is one who does not need the position for money and has chosen the company as much as vice versa.'

The survey, which also looks at chair and NED remuneration, commented on the levels of remuneration within the public sector:

'The public sector is paying substantially less than listed companies; and for many small public sector organisations no fees are paid. We suspect this is an area for concern – it is difficult to insist on the highest standards of competence, contribution, conduct and performance when directors are not paid a fair reward. If people are paid fairly, then they expect to be held to account. With increasing pressure on costs and value for money in the public sector, this problem can only grow.'

These comments are very perceptive given the current challenges faced by NHS organisations, both financially and reputationally. The NHS organisations with largest challenges and the most fraught relationships with stakeholders will need to be able to command the kind of leadership from their chairs set out here as prerequisites. Consequently, the need for effective selection and appointment processes is hugely important, as is clarity on how the role of the chair complements other key roles within the board.

11
Executive directors

Introduction

EDs combine their role as director of the board with their position within the executive management of the organisation. NEDs perform the functions of director, only without any executive responsibilities. The interests of EDs are therefore likely to differ from those of NEDs.

The focus in this chapter on the role of the CEO and EDs must not distract from the underlying principle of the unitary board. EDs have the same responsibilities and duties as NEDs; these extend to the entire business of the organisation, not just their own specific portfolio.

The role of executive directors

Unlike NEDs, outside of their board role EDs are full-time employees of the organisation, with executive management responsibilities. Management is responsible for running the business operations and is accountable to the board of directors and the CEO.

For the EDs, there is a tension between their role as members of the board, 'one step down from the stakeholders' and their role as senior operational directors, 'one step up from management'.

This can manifest in different ways. There will be times when individual EDs and/or the CEO are held to account for their executive performance by fellow EDs, acting alongside NEDs as a unitary board. This can raise tensions – especially if the CEO is being held to account – and highlights the critical role of the chair in maintaining an effective board.

On the other hand, EDs and the CEO may want to present a united front to the rest of the board to justify what the management team has done and achieved, or what it would like to do. However, if the EDs come together with a united opinion, this raises doubts in their ability to provide effective challenge in discussions on strategy. Independent NEDs should not have this problem, which is why they should be more effective in providing effective challenge in board discussions, encouraged by the chair.

The issues for EDs are, therefore, that they may be inclined to support the views of the CEO on all matters, including strategy, and they may mistrust the NEDs as 'outsiders' who do not know much about the organisation and its business.

In recognition of this problem, the FRC Board Guide suggests that EDs should welcome constructive challenge from NEDs as an essential aspect of good governance, and encourage their non-executive colleagues to test proposals in the light of their wider experience outside the company.

ICSA: The Governance Institute's guidance note, the Governance Challenge for the NHS Executive Director, sets this out quite neatly by suggesting EDs ask, 'Which hat am I wearing?' to retain an appropriate balance between the varying roles for which they are being paid. These include:

- leadership and management of their particular section or department;
- being a member of the senior operational management of the organisation;
- wider leadership and management responsibility within the operational environment;
- ensuring the organisation remains focused on delivering its core business objectives; and
- governance and strategic responsibility from the board perspective.

The governance role is different to the management role. An ED's governance role along with the other members of the board is to:

- ensure that sufficient assets are aligned against the operational objectives being set though also guarding, maintaining and nurturing those same assets;
- debate, determine and set the strategy for the organisation; and
- monitor progress towards its fulfilment.

In contrast, the management role is to utilise the assets of the organisation in the fulfilment of the operational objectives of the organisation and to deliver the strategy determined by the board. The publication *New Voices, New Accountabilities: A guide to wider governance in foundation trusts* states:

> 'Boards of directors will increasingly have to operate as corporate entities, not sounding boards, in a world of contestable service provision ... Executive directors must make the transition from operating as functional heads of service to members of a corporate board, bearing the full weight of the fiduciary responsibility that falls on their shoulders and contributing fully to the strategic decision making of the trust.'

The appointment of executive directors

The nomination committee has a key role to play in the appointment of EDs, as discussed in Chapter 7. The CEO will bring recommendations to the committee on succession planning and appointment, but the board will delegate the responsibility for appointment to these committees (which are essentially composed of NEDs). The key principle about the appointment of EDs is that it is the responsibility of the chair and the NEDs, acting under the remit of the nomination committee. The exception worth noting relates to the appointment of the NHS CEO, which is covered below.

Induction of an executive manager as an executive director

The induction process for a new ED who is already an executive manager of the organisation needs a specific focus. A senior executive of the organisation should already be familiar with many aspects of the organisation's operations (although their induction might include visits to parts of the organisation they have not worked with before).

An executive manager 'promoted' to the board is more likely to lack knowledge and experience about being a director and governance, although some larger organisations try to give their senior executives experience as a director by allowing them to take a position as a NED in another organisation.

An induction programme for an ED may therefore need to focus on matters such as:

- the role of the board, including matters reserved for the board and oversight of management;
- the powers and duties of directors, and the rights of shareholders/stakeholders (the new director should be given a copy of the organisation's constitutional documents);
- the role of board committees and their membership;
- the role of the board in monitoring risk and internal control (see also Chapter 16);
- membership of the board and its committees, how the board operates and the role of the company secretary;
- frequency of board meetings;
- what the new director will be expected to contribute;
- who the major shareholders/stakeholders are and their relationship with the organisation;
- compliance with governance requirements;
- the potential liabilities of directors;
- directors' liability insurance;
- organisation policy on public involvement and sustainability; and
- arrangements for monitoring the performance of board members.

NHS Providers offers an ED induction programme, which was developed following requests from new board EDs for a deeper understanding of their board role as part of a unitary board and of the wider context within which the role is set. The programme includes:

- understanding the developing NHS environment and what that means for the leadership of foundation trusts and trusts;
- governance, risk and assurance in the provider sector;
- what your chief executive expects of you;
- the Care Quality Commission (CQC) and regulation;
- NHS Improvement (NHSI) – the way forward;
- your board role vs your ED role;
- working with commissioners; and
- your responsibilities and accountabilities.

This list is not exhaustive, although in some cases it might be considered too long. The main point is that an executive manager appointed as a director needs to learn about the differences in the roles of manager and director, and that they have not been appointed as a director simply to be a 'high level' executive of the organisation.

The role of the CEO

The FRC Board Guide says the CEO is the most senior ED on the board, with responsibility for proposing strategy to the board and for delivering the strategy as agreed.

Consequently, the CEO's relationship with the chair is a key relationship that can assist board effectiveness. The CEO leads the executive team, is responsible for the executive management of the organisation's operations and is the senior executive to whom all other executive managers' report. Other executive managers might also be directors of the organisation, but the CEO is answerable to the board for the way the business is run and its performance.

The CEO has, with the support of the executive team, primary responsibility for setting an example to the organisation's employees and communicating to them the expectations of the board in relation to the organisational culture, values and behaviours. The CEO is also responsible for supporting the chair to make certain that appropriate standards of governance permeate through all parts of the organisation and will make certain that the board is made aware, when appropriate, of the views of employees on issues of relevance to the business.

In order to improve the standard of boardroom discussion, the CEO should also act as a spokesperson for the executive team in board discussions, explain the views of the executive team to the rest of the board and explain in a balanced way any differences of opinion within the executive team.

The chief executive is also responsible for ensuring that management fulfils its obligation to provide board directors with:

- accurate, timely and clear information in a form and of a quality and comprehensiveness that will enable it to discharge its duties;

- the necessary resources for developing and updating their knowledge and capabilities; and
- appropriate knowledge of the company, including access to company operations and members of the workforce.

The UK Code states that the differing responsibilities of the chair and the CEO should be set out in writing and agreed by the board. Particular attention should be paid to areas of potential overlap.

The role of the accountable/accounting officer in the NHS

At a macro level, the DHSC accounting officer (AO), as principal AO, has overall responsibility in government for the proper and effective use of resources as voted by Parliament for the health and care system, including the NHS.

The majority of resources are allocated annually to NHSE. Its CEO, as AO, is responsible for the effective use of these resources. There is a robust system in place to allow the AO to discharge their responsibilities by providing assurance about the commissioning of NHS care and the provision and regulation of services. This system entails the appointment of accountable officers (for NHS trusts and CCGs) and AOs (for FTs).

For NHS trusts, the accountable officer is the CEO, who is accountable to Parliament via the DHSC AO and the SoS. The NHSI AO is responsible for the appointment of accountable officers for each NHS trust. In clinical commissioning groups (CCGs), the accountable officer is either the chief officer or the chief clinical officer (CCO). They are accountable to Parliament via NHSE's AO (the CEO, as designated in the Health and Social Care Act 2012 (HSCA 2012)) and the SoS. In NHS FTs, AOs are directly responsible to Parliament.

The accountable officer memorandum for chief executives of NHS trusts sets out the responsibilities as follows:

- ensuring there are effective management systems in place to safeguard public funds and assets and assisting in the implementation of corporate governance;
- ensuring value for money (VFM) is achieved from the resources available to the trust;
- ensuring the expenditure and income of the trust has been applied to the purposes intended by Parliament and conform to the authorities which govern them;
- ensuring effective and sound financial management systems are in place; and
- ensuring annual statutory accounts are prepared in a format directed by the Secretary of State, with the approval of HM Treasury, to give a true and fair view of the state of affairs as at the end of the financial year. This should include the income and expenditure, recognised gains and losses and cash flows for the year.

The CCG accountable officer is responsible for ensuring that the CCG fulfils its duties to exercise its functions effectively, efficiently and economically

– thus ensuring improvement in the quality of services and the health of the local population though maintaining value for money. They will ensure that the regularity and propriety of expenditure is discharged, and that arrangements are put in place to ensure that good practice is embodied (as identified through the head of the National Audit Office, the Comptroller and Auditor General). They will also ensure that funds are safeguarded through effective financial and management systems.

The CCG accountable officer, working closely with the chair of the governing body, will ensure that proper constitutional, governance and development arrangements are put in place to assure the members of the CCG's ongoing capability and capacity to meet its duties and responsibilities. This will include arrangements for the ongoing development of its members and staff. The individual who takes on the accountable officer role for a CCG will be proposed by the governing body of the CCG and formally appointed to the role by NHSE in accordance with the NHSE guidance CCG Guidance on Senior Appointments including Accountable Officer (2017). In circumstances where the lead clinician undertakes the accountable officer role, they will be known as the CCO. When a manager undertakes the role, the individual will be known as the chief officer. The accountable officer may not be the chair of the governing body or the chief finance officer (CFO). The involvement of NHSE does not create an employment relationship between the accountable officer and NHSE; instead, the accountable officer is an employee of the individual CCG.

Each FT has an AO, who has responsibilities for ensuring regularity, propriety and value for money, including signing the trust's accounts, annual governance statement and annual report. The National Health Service Act 2006 designates the CEO of an NHS FT as the AO. The NHS Foundation Trust Accounting Officer Memorandum (2015) sets out the role as responsibility for the overall organisation, management and staffing of the NHS FT and for its procedures in financial and other matters, and ensuring:

- there is a high standard of financial management in the NHS FT as a whole;
- the NHS FT delivers efficient and economical conduct of its business and safeguards financial propriety and regularity throughout the organisation; and
- financial considerations are fully taken into account in decisions on NHS FT policy proposals.

The FT AO has a particular responsibility to see that appropriate advice is tendered to the board and to the council of governors on all matters of financial propriety and regularity and, more broadly, as to all considerations of prudent and economical administration, efficiency and effectiveness. The NED-led appointments committee appoints the AO and the appointment is approved by the council of governors.

In all three settings, if the board or the chair is contemplating a course of action that the accountable/accounting officer considers would infringe the requirements of propriety and regularity, they should set out their objections (and the reasons for it) in writing to the chair and the board. If the decision is still taken to proceed, a written instruction to take the action in question should be issued. The audit committee, which has specific terms of reference and delegated powers to inquire into matters of propriety and regularity, should receive a copy of the objections.

If the board is contemplating a course of action that affects the responsibility for obtaining VFM from the organisation's resources, then the accountable/accounting officer should draw the relevant factors to the attention of the board. If the accountable/accounting officer is overruled, despite clear advice to the contrary, then the accountable/accounting officer should refer their concerns to their appointing body. In all such cases, the accountable/accounting officer should, as a board member, vote against the course of action rather than merely abstain from voting.

The accountable officer, together with the director of finance, is responsible for ensuring that the accounts of the trust presented to the board for approval are prepared under principles and in a format directed by the SoS with the approval of HM Treasury (as set out in the NHS Finance Manual and in 'The Role of the Director of Finance in the NHS' – EL(94)18). These accounts must disclose a true and fair view of the trust's income and expenditure; cash flows; gains and losses; and of its state of affairs. The accountable officer will sign these accounts, along with the director of finance/CFO, on behalf of the board.

In FTs, the CEO, as the AO, should sign and date the statement of financial position and annual report after adoption by the board as evidence of this. As AO, the CEO should also sign the foreword to the accounts, the annual governance statement and the remuneration report. Once the annual report and accounts have been approved by the external auditors, the AO or director of finance must sign a certificate that states that the FT consolidation (FTC) schedules are consistent with the annual accounts.

The role of the director of finance or chief finance officer

NHS trusts and FTs are required to have a director of finance (DoF) on the board and CCGs are required to have a CFO on their governing body.

Though financial management is the corporate responsibility of the board, and the individual responsibility of the CEO/CO as the accountable officer, the DoF has both a professional and corporate role as a board member. The DoF ensures that systems are in place so that the organisation is properly governed in terms of financial transactions, financial reporting, financial performance, financial planning and in securing value for money. They also must also maintain assurance processes to ensure that internal controls and checks are working properly (such as engagement with clinical and non-clinical staff holding delegated financial budgets). These systems also include ensuring that 'treasury management' systems are in place to manage cash flow and liquidity.

The key responsibilities for finance directors are to provide business and commercial advice for the board as well as financial governance and assurance, and to fulfil their corporate responsibilities as a board member. A key requirement for NHS organisations is sustainable financial viability; the DoF has to involve and inform the board in assessing all the options in terms of strategic financial risk, including a 'worst case' scenario.

The DoF should be a professional accountant, and as such is required to behave with confidentiality, integrity, objectivity, professional competence and due care as mandated in the International Federation of Accountants (IFAC)'s Code of Ethics. They must also comply with professional quality standards, especially those relating to professional ethics, continuing professional development, and national and international external reporting requirements. The conduct and behaviour of a DoF must be within the law and, as a professional accountant, they also have a 'public interest' role. However, as a board member, the DoF's contribution is not, and should not be, limited to finance as a specialist area.

The National Health Service (Clinical Commissioning Groups) Regulations 2012 require that the CCG's governing body must also include an employee who has a professional qualification in accountancy and the expertise or experience to lead the financial management of the CCG, to be known as the CFO. If the governing body's membership includes two or more individuals of that description, the CCG must designate one of them as the CFO. They should be an individual with a recognised professional accounting qualification, as well as significant experience and skills. The CFO cannot be the chair of the governing body nor may they undertake the accountable officer role. The role may, however, be combined with that of chief operating officer (COO) in circumstances where a CCG has a COO (for instance, in CCGs where the clinical leader is also the accountable officer). In these circumstances, the role is known as 'chief finance and operating officer'.

Other executive director roles

There are several other key ED roles that are an important part of an NHS board.

The roles of medical director and director of nursing (or chief nurse or executive nurse) are mandatory roles for a legitimately constituted board. Again, as board members, these roles should not be limited to their areas of professional expertise and they are required to contribute across the breadth of the organisation.

In a CCG, the lead clinician is the individual recognised by the CCG as the clinical voice of its members. This individual is either the chair of the governing body or undertakes the role of accountable officer as chief clinical officer. In circumstances where a CCG chooses to appoint a clinician to the chair of the governing body and nominate a clinician for the role of the accountable officer, then the CCG should identify one of them to be known as the lead clinician.

The remuneration of executive directors

The remuneration of EDs and other senior executives in the corporate sector is a contentious issue, partly because of the amounts paid to top executives in some companies and partly because remuneration for senior executives has generally risen by a much larger percentage than increases in pay for other employees.

While remuneration packages should be sufficient to attract and retain executives of a suitable calibre, they should not be excessive. Such packages should also reward executives for successful performance, in both the short term and the longer term, because pay incentives are expected to encourage executives to perform better. A further area of concern to the corporate sector (and to the NHS) is the payment of large 'rewards for failure'. Contracts of employment for senior executives should try to minimise the risk of these severance payments when a senior director fails to perform to a satisfactory standard and is dismissed.

The remuneration committee is the critical mechanism for governing executive remuneration.

Remuneration in the corporate sector

This has become a hot topic concerted focus of government and industry discussion. Total pay for the CEOs of FTSE 100 companies quadrupled between 1998 and 2015, according to the Department for Business, Energy and Industrial Strategy (BEIS) analysis, largely due to the growth in annual bonus payments and long-term pay incentives. It far outstripped growth in average pay in the UK in the same time period. According to the High Pay Centre, in 1998 the ratio of average FTSE 100 CEO pay to the average pay of full-time employees in the UK was 47:1. This ratio increased to 132:1 in 2010 and stood at 160:1 in 2018.

The remuneration of EDs and senior executives was not seen as a major problem of corporate governance until the 1990s in the UK and early 2000s in the US. A sense that something might be wrong began when the general public, alerted by the media, criticised some top executives for being paid far more money than they were worth and investment institutions criticised directors for receiving ever-increasing rewards even when their company performed badly.

In many listed companies in the UK during the 1980s and early 1990s, the CEOs and executive chairs were involved in deciding their own remuneration package. Concern about remuneration has grown in other countries, particularly with regard to the banking crisis in 2007–09 and the high rewards earned by senior bankers in spite of the large amounts of public funds provided to prevent banks from financial collapse.

As can be seen from the statistics above, the remuneration of top corporate executives rose rapidly regardless of company performance, the effects of global recession, and at a faster annual rate than the remuneration of other company employees. This seemed counter to the principle of good corporate governance that remuneration should be linked to some extent to company performance, so that a director will earn more if the company does well, but less if it does badly.

Government reforms in 2013 introduced new shareholder controls and oversight over executive remuneration. The reforms gave shareholders a binding vote on pay policies (at least once every three years) and an annual advisory vote on the actual pay awards made to directors under the shareholder-approved pay policies. They also introduced greater clarity in the reporting of executive pay. There are concerns, however, that these reforms have not had sufficient impact.

The Government Green Paper on Corporate Governance Reform (November 2016) includes a section on further reforms to executive remuneration and sets out the following options for further discussion:

- Make all or some elements of the executive pay package subject to a binding shareholder vote.
- Introduce stronger consequences for a company losing its annual advisory vote on the remuneration report.
- Require or encourage quoted company pay policies to (a) set an upper threshold for total annual pay (from all elements of remuneration), and (b) ensure a binding vote at the annual general meeting (AGM) where actual executive pay in that year exceeds the threshold.
- Require the existing binding vote on the executive pay policy to be held more frequently than every three years.
- Strengthen the Corporate Governance Code to provide greater specificity on how companies should engage with shareholders on pay, including where there is significant opposition to a remuneration report.

The Enterprise and Regulatory Reform Act 2013 (ERRA 2013) contains amendments to the Companies Act 2006 relating to quoted companies' disclosure of directors' remuneration and shareholder approval of quoted company directors' remuneration reports. The key changes made by ERRA are as follows:

- The directors' remuneration report must include a forward-looking remuneration policy report.
- Shareholders have been given a new binding ordinary resolution vote on the remuneration policy report (and retain their existing advisory ordinary resolution vote on the implementation report).
- Any subsequent changes to the remuneration policy must be agreed by shareholders and, even if no changes are made to the remuneration policy, it must be approved by shareholders at least every three years.
- If shareholders did not approve the advisory vote on the implementation report at the company's previous AGM, the remuneration policy must be put to shareholders at the next AGM.

- All remuneration and loss of office payments to directors must be consistent with the approved remuneration policy.
- Unless a payment has been separately approved by shareholders in advance, any unauthorised payment is held on trust by the party that received it (usually this will be the director themselves). Directors who authorised the payment will be liable for any loss to the company unless they can demonstrate that they acted honestly and reasonably.

A directors' remuneration report in the new format must be put to shareholders in the first financial year to begin on or after 1 October 2013. Though these regulations apply to companies, not to NHS organisations, the principles they contain are applicable and should still be considered by NHS boards.

NHS remuneration

NHS organisations are subject to a greater level of remuneration regulation than the corporate sector but pay levels for senior management have still come under close public scrutiny – especially as all public sector wage rises have been seriously constrained since April 2013. Indeed, on 2 June 2015, the SoS wrote to the chairs of all NHS trusts, FTs and CCGs urging restraint over very senior managers (VSM) pay and announcing a range of initiatives, including:

- a requirement for ministers to see all proposals for VSM pay above £150,402 before appointments are confirmed (£150,402 being the salary of the Prime Minister);
- the development of a national framework for VSM pay in the NHS; and
- the introduction of a limit on the daily rate payable to an off-payroll interim VSM and request for rigorous compliance with Her Majesty's Treasury guidance on off-payroll engagements.

The Secretary of State set out their expectation that there should be no significant difference in the terms and conditions of senior leadership teams and those working on the front-line and their view that it is not acceptable that some senior managers experience high levels of pay, with year-on-year increases, as a matter of course.

Guidance on pay for very senior managers in NHS trusts and foundation trusts issued in March 2018 requires the approval of NHSI and the DHSC and Her Majesty's Treasury for all VSM pay review decisions.

This process covers:

- all on-payroll appointments (substantive and fixed term) for VSM roles in NHS ambulance and community trusts until this is replaced by the new pay framework;
- on-payroll VSM appointments (substantive and fixed term) in all other NHS trusts and in all NHS foundation trusts where the annual salary is £150,000 or above (irrespective of whether or not the new salary is an increase);

- acting-up arrangements, promotions/pay rises for individuals already in post and earning £150,000 or above, and NHS secondments and conversion of off-payroll interims into on-payroll arrangements;
- directors who by virtue of their qualifications and the requirements of the post are eligible to be on the standard NHS consultant contract; and
- CEOs or EDs who plan to resign and take their pension benefits when they reach pensionable age, and then return to work.

There are established pay ranges for all such appointments in the NHS. Examples for a CEO are given in Table 11.1.

Chief executives	Lower quartile	Median	Upper quartile
Small acute NHS trusts and foundation trusts (£0–£200 million turnover)*	£141,000	£167,500	£182,500
Medium acute NHS trusts and foundation trusts (£200–400 million)*	£160,000	£182,500	£202,500
Large acute NHS trusts and foundation trusts (£400–£500 million)	£190,000	£197,500	£230,000
Very large acute NHS trusts and foundation trusts (£500 million +)	£195,000	£225,000	£267,500

Note: * Specialist trusts can apply for a 15% premium.
(NHSI, 2018)

Table 11.1: Pay ranges for CEOs

The framework, when published, will be informed by the Rose Review (June 2015). Sir Stuart Rose, the former Chairman of Marks & Spencer, was commissioned by the SoS to review the NHS leadership challenge and identified the following three areas of concern:

1. **Vision:** There is a lack of One NHS Vision and of a common ethos.
2. **People:** The NHS has committed to a vast range of changes; however, there is insufficient management and leadership capability to deal effectively with the scale of challenges associated with these.
3. **Performance:** There is a need for proper overall direction of careers in management across the medical, administrative and nursing cadres.

Consequently, CCGs, NHS trusts and NHS FTs are no longer free to determine their own rates of pay for VSMs – CEOs, EDs and others with board-level responsibility who report directly to the CEO.

VSM pay in DH arm's-length bodies (ALBs) such as NHSE, Monitor, the CQC and the NHSI is subject to two national pay frameworks, one set in 2006 and the other in 2012. Performance-related pay is available to VSMs within ALBs on either of the existing national pay frameworks, although it is currently restricted by the government to the top 25% of performers and to a maximum of 5% of reckonable pay.

Pay data for CCGs analysed by e.reward.co.uk in 2015 identified that more than two-fifths (43%) of chief officers in CCGs servicing the largest populations (more than 500,000 people) collected pay above the £120,000 to £130,000 recommendations. These decisions were taken despite strong encouragement from NHSE to make lower pay awards to senior executives. NHSE had proposed three pay ranges for chief officers and CFOs, based on the population sizes of CCGs (see Table 9.2).

CCG level	Population size	Pay range for chief officer	Pay range for CFO
Level 3	At or over 500,000	£120k–£130k	£95k–£110k
Level 2	150,000 to 499,000	£105k–120k	£85k–£95k
Level 1	149,000 or below	£90k–£105k	£75k–£85k

(NHSE, 2018)

Table 11.2: CCG pay ranges

All other posts within the NHS are governed by the Agenda for Change system, which allocates posts to set pay scales using a job evaluation scheme. All FTs have the freedom to use local terms and conditions when setting pay for all employees, yet continue to be guided by VSM and to operate Agenda for Change for their staff.

The ongoing period of austerity for the public sector will restrain remuneration levels in the public sector; however, corporate sector remuneration will also influence NHS remuneration levels, as suggested by the response of the NHS Confederation:

> 'NHS organisations are large and complex in nature and require the right managerial skills to be led effectively. A large city hospital could have a budget of between £500 million and £1 billion and employ as many as 10,000 staff – comparable to many FTSE 250 companies. Because of the challenging nature of a chief executive's role, NHS boards must consider a range of factors, including pay, to encourage the best candidates in to these positions. The NHS is looking to involve more clinical staff in top management positions. Given that a number of hospital doctors will be paid more than NHS chief executives, this factor must be taken into consideration when making a decision on pay.'
>
> David Stout, Deputy CEO, NHS Confederation

Public attitudes

Public attitudes about remuneration within the NHS are somewhat contradictory. This fact was recognised, although not specifically, in the Hutton Review of Fair Pay (2011) in the public sector (covered in more detail later):

> 'Success [of the public sector] would be a fundamental building block in supporting economic growth and social well-being, but it cannot be done without motivated, high calibre public servants, along with managers to lead them.
>
> But while the British public is very sympathetic to front line delivery staff, it is hostile to the public sector managers responsible and accountable for the effective deployment of resources – and even more hostile to their pay. In the eyes of some, they are the quintessential "burdens" on the rest of us.'

The review set out that some of this public reaction is quite reasonable, since public sector managers have also benefited from significant earnings growth at the top remuneration levels, particularly in the early 2000s. However, some balance is required. As the Hutton interim report demonstrated, only £1 of every £100 earned by the top 1% of earners in the UK is earned by public sector employees.

Even so, the perception remains that the public sector is no less awash with 'fat cats' than the private sector; indeed, in one poll, a quarter of respondents thought that public sector executives earned more than their private sector counterparts. Regardless, Hutton maintains that: 'the public has the right to know that pay is deserved, fair, under control and designed to drive improving public sector performance'.

Rewards for failure

In the UK, there was institutional investor concern, supported by widespread media coverage, about large remuneration packages for senior corporate directors where the size of the reward did not seem sufficiently linked to performance, and large severance payments (payments on dismissal) to outgoing senior executives who had been ousted from their job following poor company performance.

High severance payments to unsuccessful directors were seen as 'rewards for failure'. Following the global banking crisis of 2007–09, there was also widespread criticism of remuneration in banks, whereby top executives and traders received large bonuses even though their bank may have been close to collapse or in need of government financial support to remain in business.

Similar problems of rewards for failure have been seen in the NHS and raises very clear issues of health service governance.

The problem of inappropriate remuneration policies for senior executives is now well recognised within both the NHS and the corporate sector, but a satisfactory solution has not necessarily been found. However, a distinction should be made between the unethical 'corporate greed' of some senior executives, and a reasonable desire by senior executives to be well remunerated for what they do. Similarly, it is important to make the distinction between high rewards that are justified by performance, and high rewards that are earned in spite of poor performance.

■ Why is remuneration a governance issue?

Remuneration of senior executives is a governance issue for several reasons.

- Excessive remuneration for senior executives that is not clearly linked to good performance breaches the requirement for economy, efficiency and effectiveness which underpins the NHS.
- Executives should not be rewarded for failure.
- Large organisations need to attract and retain talented professionals to provide them with effective leadership. Top executives are attracted and retained by the remuneration packages they are offered.
- Organisations need effective boards and senior executive management. Remuneration incentives can be used to motivate executives to perform better and to achieve better results, however, remuneration incentives should be designed carefully to align the interests of the organisation and executives as much as possible, in both the short term and the longer term.
- The remuneration of senior executives may antagonise employees (and employee representatives), when it appears that senior executives are paid excessive amounts in comparison with their own pay. A sense that benefits or rewards are unfairly distributed could lead to industrial unrest within the organisation.

A further reason relates to the stability and continuity of the board. A study by Income Data Services in February 2016 found that while median salary levels had flatlined, boardroom turnover across all parts of the NHS was running at high levels. Overall, the attrition rate stood at around 30% with some variations according to country and trust type. In fact, turnover in non-FT boardrooms was 35% in the year to March 2015 and 27% in foundation trusts. This contrasts with March 2012 when board turnover levels were around 25% and this was considered substantial because they followed the initial stages of change that resulted from the Health and Social Care Bill 2011. Additionally, Will Hutton identified in his 2011 review on fair pay that there were real concerns about director tenure in the NHS, where the average tenure of NHS acute trust chief executives was just two years and four months, compared with the average tenure for FTSE 100 chief executives at 5.9 years. He went on:

> 'Such short tenures not only compare unfavourably with the private sector (average tenure for FTSE 100 chief executives is currently 5.9 years) but are also not conducive to successful management: business management research suggests that most chief executives need an average of 30 months to complete their learning curve upon taking up a new role.'

This is backed up by research by the King's Fund in 2018 that found that the median tenure of an NHS provider chief executive was three years and the mean average was four years. Previous research has suggested that there are positive links between how long senior leaders remain in organisations and the performance of the organisations they lead. The NHS Leadership Academy has suggested that chief executives should ideally stay in post for at least five years to give organisations the stability they need for effective strategic planning. The impact of a high turnover can be strategic paralysis, a loss of organisational memory and diminished credibility of leaders.

Principles of executive director remuneration

Principles of remuneration are now included in the corporate governance codes of many countries. In a system of good governance, the remuneration of directors and key senior executives should be sufficient to attract and retain individuals of a suitable calibre. At the same time, the structure of an individual's remuneration package should motivate the individual towards the achievement of performance that is in the best interests of the organisation and its stakeholders, as well as those of the individual.

The UK Code states as a principle that:

> 'Remuneration policies and practices should be designed to support strategy and promote long-term sustainable success. Executive remuneration should be aligned to company purpose and values and be clearly linked to the successful delivery of the company's long-term strategy.'

It is widely accepted that senior executives should be able to earn a high level of remuneration in return for the work they do and the responsibilities they carry. If a company does not offer an attractive package, it will not attract individuals of the required calibre. It is also generally accepted that the level of remuneration should be linked in some way to satisfactory performance. If an executive performs well, they should receive more rewards than if they perform only reasonably well.

The central issue for good corporate governance is concerned with the link between pay and performance. In the corporate sector, the remuneration package should include a performance-related element. If the director successfully achieves predetermined levels of performance, they will be rewarded accordingly. There could be some debate as to how much remuneration should be performance related, but there is a view that a substantial part of a director's total potential remuneration should be linked to performance. Linking remuneration, wholly or in part, to performance is not an easy task, however, as the following shows.

- Unsuitable measures of performance may be selected, so that although the individual executive succeeds in achieving targets that earn high rewards, the organisation does not obtain a comparable benefit.

- Many performance measures are based on the short term, possibly linked to annual results. This may not be in the interests of the organisation's longer-term development and performance.
- Remuneration systems are normally designed to provide the reward after the performance has been made. This time delay means that if the organisation has poor results in the current year after having done well in the previous year, an executive may be paid high remuneration (for the previous year) at a time the organisation is doing badly.

The UK Code requires that the responsibility for setting the remuneration of EDs (and possibly other senior executives) should be delegated by the board to a remuneration committee. The remuneration committee is explained in more detail later in this chapter and the FRC Guidance on Board Effectiveness (2018) sets out provisions for the design of the performance-related elements of a remuneration package that the remuneration committee should apply. These provisions offer a useful insight into how incentive schemes may be structured and approved.

If it is not an easy task for corporate governance, then it becomes even more difficult for health service governance. As this handbook has already demonstrated, there is significant diversity and complexity amongst stakeholders and their objectives for NHS organisations. Finding suitable measures of performance is a challenge that was highlighted in the Hutton Review (see below). For health service governance, a key principle relates to the public scrutiny and transparency of the remuneration package and the accountability of the ED.

Hutton Review of fair pay in the public sector

The Hutton Review was published in March 2011 and sets out a Fair Pay Code for senior pay, to be adopted by all organisations delivering public services, on a 'comply or explain' basis based on the principle of fairness as due desert – namely, reward should be proportional to the weight of each role and each individual's performance. The Code also required pay levels to be set according to a fair process, though recognising that an organisation's success derives from the collective efforts of the whole workforce.

The review also set out 12 recommendations to the government that together form the framework for fairness.

1. Using pay multiples to track executive pay against that of all employees: the government should not cap pay across public services but should require that from 2011–12 all public service organisations publish their top to median pay multiples each year to allow the public to hold them to account.
2. Informing the public debate through annual Fair Pay Reports: to support citizen accountability, the government should commission the Senior Salaries Review Body to publish annual Fair Pay Reports, starting from 2011–12.
3. Re-calibrating the pay of non-departmental public body chief executives.

EXECUTIVE DIRECTORS

4. From disclosure to explanation – ensuring complete transparency over executive roles and remuneration: to enable citizens to understand executive remuneration and the nature of executive responsibilities, from 2011–12 the government should require that all organisations delivering public services disclose in precise numbers the full remuneration of all executives, alongside an explanation of the responsibilities of each role and of how executives' pay reflects individual performance.
5. Enabling citizen analysis of executive pay: from 2011–12, the government should require public organisations to submit executive pay data through an online template, and make this data available on data.gov.uk, to allow citizens to access and analyse this data and thus have the information required to hold public service organisations to account.
6. Abandoning arbitrary benchmarks for public service pay: once this framework of recommendations is in place, the government should refrain from using the pay of the Prime Minister or other politicians as a benchmark for the remuneration of senior public servants, whose pay should reflect their due desert and be proportional to the weight of their roles and their performance.
7. Preventing rewards for failure through earn-back pay for senior public servants: to allow pay to vary down as well as up with performance, all public service executives should have an element of their basic pay that needs to be earned back each year through meeting pre-agreed objectives with excellent performers who go beyond their objectives eligible for additional pay.
8. Extending earn-back pay to high performing middle managers.
9. Sharing the rewards of greater productivity: to prevent executives monopolising the rewards of productivity increases, and allow all employees who have contributed to share the benefits, government departments should identify ways of offering gainsharing schemes linked to achievement of the efficiency aspects of their business plans.
10. Opening up opportunities for future generations of public service leaders: to increase the supply of candidates for top positions and reinforce public service management as a career, the government should facilitate greater opportunities for managers to move across different public services.
11. A Fair Pay Code: to embed fairness principles and ensure fair process in executive remuneration, all public service organisations should adopt the Fair Pay Code proposed by this Review. Government departments should, by July 2011, bring forward proposals for the application of this code to all bodies and sectors in which they have an interest.
12. Tracking pay multiples across the economy: to make tracking pay multiples normal practice across the economy, as part of its commitment to improve corporate reporting, the government should require listed companies to publish top to median pay multiples in their annual reporting from January 2012.

The component elements of executive directors' remuneration

The remuneration package for a senior executive in the corporate sector is likely to consist of a combination of: a fixed-pay element – remuneration received regardless of performance, such as a fixed salary and payments made into a salary-related pension scheme – and a variable pay element. This might consist of performance-related incentives, which might be tied to short-term performance such as an annual bonus, and longer-term incentives such as share option awards. In addition, executives might enjoy a number of other perks such as free private medical insurance, a company car and the use of a company plane or apartment. The major issue for the corporate sector in negotiating a remuneration package with an executive is deciding on the balance between the fixed and the variable elements, and to agree on measures of performance as the basis for deciding on how much the performance-related payments should be. Short-term incentives are based on annual performance targets. Long-term incentives may be awarded each year but are linked to performance over a longer period of time, typically three years (or longer). Another problem in deciding a remuneration package is to find a suitable balance between short-term and longer-term incentives.

Admittedly, this is less of an issue for the NHS, where a senior executive remuneration package usually consists of a fixed salary and a final salary-related pension. The FTN Remuneration Survey of executive pay confirms this, although some FTs are now adding a car allowance or lease car to their remuneration packages.

There is also evidence that some FTs offer a performance-related pay scheme in connection with the achievement of trust corporate objectives. These schemes, however, are still in their infancy and small in number.

The remuneration committee

It is a well-established principle of 'best practice' in governance that there should be a formal procedure for deciding on remuneration for directors and senior executives, and no individual should be involved in setting their own remuneration. This is made clear in the UK Code. This means that EDs should not be involved in setting their remuneration packages (although they can negotiate with the individuals who make the decision) and NEDs should not decide their own fees.

The remuneration of EDs was recognised as an important governance issue in the UK in the 1990s with the work of the Greenbury Committee, whose recommendations were subsequently incorporated into the UK governance code in 1998. Health service governance has adopted these principles, either in the constitution of an FT or the founding regulations and statutory instruments of other NHS organisations. It is therefore worth considering the provisions of the UK Code, as they underpin the provisions of health service governance. Specimen terms of reference for NHS Remuneration Committees can be found on the ICSA website.

The requirement for a remuneration committee

The UK Code states that 'the board should establish a remuneration committee ... [which] should make available its terms of reference, explaining its role and the authority delegated to it by the board'.

The remuneration committee is responsible, therefore, for both developing remuneration policy and for negotiating the remuneration of individual directors. Although these two matters are related, they are different. According to the UK Code, the remuneration committee in the corporate sector should consist entirely of independent NEDs. In larger companies, the committee should consist of at least three members, and in smaller companies (i.e. companies below the FTSE 350) at least two members. The company chair may be a member of the committee, but not the committee chair, provided that they were considered to be independent on appointment as company chair. The remuneration committee should have delegated responsibility for setting the remuneration for all EDs and the chair (including pension rights and any compensation payments or severance payments). The remuneration committee should also recommend and monitor the level and structure of remuneration for senior management. The definition of 'senior management' is a matter for the board to decide, but it will normally include the first level of management below board level.

The composition and main duties for a remuneration (and terms of service) committee for are set out more fully in Chapter 7.

Evaluation and appraisal of executive directors

Both the FT Code and the UK Code state as a main principle that the board should undertake a 'formal and rigorous annual evaluation of its own performance and that of its committees and individual directors'. This includes the EDs in their board member roles. The performance of individual EDs as executive managers is not dealt with by a governance code, because individual executive performance is not a governance issue. For governance purposes, the evaluation of performance relates to performance as a director.

Good workforce management would require the EDs to undergo an annual appraisal with the CEO as their line manager in respect of the portfolio of management responsibilities that they undertake. However, this appraisal should also take into account the board level responsibilities that they carry, and the chair of the board should be asked to participate in this aspect of their appraisal.

The chair of the board will appraise the CEO, and this appraisal will include both their management and board role responsibilities. The remuneration committee should then consider the appraisals of the EDs in considering any annual pay review decisions.

Use of remuneration consultants

Companies and NHS organisations often use remuneration consultants, who give advice to the remuneration committee on remuneration packages, including basic salary levels for senior executives. Consultants should not be given responsibility for deciding remuneration; this responsibility should remain with the remuneration committee of the board. Consultants may use competitive pay data to recommend a basic package for senior executives. Competitive pay data is simply information about the rewards that are being paid to senior executives in other top companies. It is essential that there is a robust tendering exercise for the appointment of such consultants in order to demonstrate their independence and objectivity.

Practice and process

There is no set requirement for the frequency of meeting of the remuneration committee; however, it needs to meet at least annually to approve the remuneration report for the annual report and accounts. Other meetings are likely in order to consider the remuneration policy required by ERRA 2013, any annual reviews of executive remuneration, and decisions on individual EDs as they are appointed. It is routine practice for non-members to be invited to attend the committee as required by the business of the meeting (e.g. the CEO, director of workforce or employment lawyer). The company secretary (or someone from the company secretary's department) should act as secretary to the remuneration committee, because it is the company secretary's responsibility to ensure that the board and its committees are properly constituted and advised. The company secretary can also play a role as intermediary and co-ordinator between the committee and the main board.

The FRC Board Guide makes it clear that whilst the board may make use of a committee to assist its consideration of remuneration, it still retains responsibility for, and makes the final decisions on, all of these areas. The chair should ensure that sufficient time is allowed at the board for discussion of these issues and for allowing the remuneration committee to report on its activity and decisions. As with all board committees, the effectiveness of the committee and its terms of reference should be reviewed annually.

Severance payments

Most EDs have employment contracts with their organisation that provide for an annual review of their remuneration and a minimum period of notice in the event of dismissal. When an organisation decides to dismiss a director, it is bound by the terms of the employment contract. There are various reasons why an individual might leave the company – for instance, they might be regarded as having failed to do a good job, and someone else should do the job instead. In this instance, a high severance payment would be seen as 'rewarding failure'. Alternately, there may have been a disagreement or falling out between directors, resulting in one or more of them being asked to leave; in this instance any severance payment needs to be fair and not calculated to prevent whistleblowing disclosures or reputational damage.

The employment contract of a director might provide for the payment of compensation for loss of office. Alternatively, an organisation might be required to give the individual a minimum period of notice, typically one year or six months in the UK. If an individual is asked to leave, they might be paid for the notice period without having to work it out. In addition, the individual may be entitled to further bonus payments under the terms of their remuneration package – in spite of being considered a failure in the job.

Shareholder concerns, and the wider public concern in regard to public sector organisations, arise particularly where the severance payment is paid even though an individual is being dismissed for having performed badly. In the past, severance payments have been high for executives who have been seen to have failed. A large compensation payment can seem annoying, because it seems that the individual is being rewarded for failure. Large severance payments reduce company profits and returns to shareholders; in the public sector, they are viewed as the improper use of public sector monies.

Remuneration committees should consider whether the organisation should retain an entitlement to reclaim bonuses if performance achievements are subsequently found to have been materially mis-stated. Contracts of employment should not provide for compensation payments to senior executives in the event of a change of control over the organisation (a takeover).

Remuneration committees should also ensure that the benefits of mitigation are obtained when an individual is dismissed. This should include a contractual obligation of the dismissed individual to mitigate the loss incurred through severance by looking for other employment. The contract should provide for the severance payment to be reduced in circumstances where the individual finds alternative employment.

The former NHS TDA (now NHSI) published guidance in June 2014 set out the processes NHS Trusts are required to follow in agreeing severance payments. The guidance aims to ensure appropriate governance to protect the reputation of the NHS and ensure probity and value for money. It does not cover FTs who should seek guidance directly from NHSI.

This guidance applies to:

- all severance payments (contractual or non-contractual) to CEOs and EDs of NHS Trusts;
- non-contractual severance payments to all staff; and
- contractual payments over £100,000 to all staff including CEOs and EDs.

Severance payments in excess of or outside of statutory or contractual entitlements or payments that are novel and/or contentious should be exceptional and require HM Treasury approval. HM Treasury define a 'special severance payment' as one paid to employees, contractors and others above normal statutory or contractual requirements when leaving employment in public service whether they resign, are dismissed or reach an agreed termination of contract.

Once such approval has been obtained and the employer is satisfied that termination of the employee's employment, together with making a severance payment, is in the best interests of the employer and represents value for money, then a proposal for the remuneration committee, as appropriate and in line with its terms of reference, should be prepared containing the business case for the severance payment.

This document should be created in order to take legal effect and should be marked as such. In addition to the preparation of the proposal, the following steps should be taken:

- Written advice from the trust's auditors and legal advisers should be taken on the proposed business case and severance payment. Advice should also be sought on the proposal and, if appropriate, a settlement agreement should be drafted.
- The legal advice about the draft proposal, together with the audit advice and the proposal itself, should be put before the remuneration committee of the employer for approval.

In the event the remuneration committee approves the business case, further approval should be sought from NHSE or NHSI (as applicable). If a settlement agreement is to be used, the approving body and HM Treasury will need reassurance that it does not include a confidentiality clause which prohibits an individual raising a concern covered under the Public Interest Disclosure Act 1998 (PIDA 1998). If the appropriate national body approves the business case, it will seek HM Treasury's approval on behalf of the employer.

The remuneration committee, operating in accordance with its terms of reference, should satisfy itself that it has the relevant information before it to make a decision and should conscientiously discuss and assess the merits of the business case. It should then consider the payment or payment range being proposed and address whether it is appropriate, taking into account the issues set out under initial considerations. The committee should only approve such sum or range which it considers value for money, the best use of public funds and in the public interest. A written record must be kept summarising its discussions and its decision (remembering that such a document could potentially be subject to public scrutiny in various ways – such as by the Public Accounts Committee (PAC)).

It is only once all of the above steps have been taken, and the necessary approvals received, that the employer should enter into the appropriate agreement to terminate the employee's employment and make the severance payment. In addition, the Small Business, Enterprise and Employment Act 2015 legislated that highly paid public sector executives who receive redundancy payments only to return to work within a year will need to repay some or all of it. In brief, the

Act means that individuals earning more than £100,000 who take a new job in the same part of the public sector within 12 months of being made redundant will have to repay all of it. The proposals will mainly affect NHS and local government administrators, many of whom have taken redundancy payments only to go back into the public sector. The precise amount of the repayment will be pro-rated depending on the length of time between exit and re-employment. The legislation will require the old employer to inform the individual of their obligation to repay the exit payment. Any new employer would be unable to engage with the individual until recovery arrangements for the money have been agreed.

Disclosure of directors' remuneration details

Directors' remuneration report

Under ERRA 2013, companies are required to publish a remuneration report, which includes three sections:

- a statement from the chair of the remuneration committee;
- a forward-looking remuneration policy report (not subject to audit); and
- an annual report on remuneration (audited) which includes both how the policy has been implemented in the year under review and how it will be implemented in the forthcoming year.

Shareholders have a binding vote on the policy report at least every three years, or whenever any changes are made, in addition to an annual advisory vote on the annual remuneration report. The report must set out the total remuneration of individual executive members disclosed as a single figure in the financial statements (including base pay, bonuses, dividend equivalents, pensions etc). The Act does not, however, make a distinction between EDs and NEDs and information about both must be included in the report.

The remuneration report must be approved by the board and signed on its behalf. A copy must be circulated to shareholders in the same way as the annual report and accounts, and it is normal for the remuneration report to be included in the same document. The auditors must state whether in their opinion the report has been prepared properly in their audit report (see Chapter 19). For companies, a signed copy of the report must also be filed with the Registrar of Companies, in the same way as the annual accounts, directors' report and auditors' report.

The remuneration committee should also be available at the annual general meeting to assist in answering any questions put to the board on any aspect of the remuneration report or generally on remuneration principles and practice.

Items to be included in the committee chair's statement include the key messages on remuneration, the context in which decisions were taken and any major changes during the year. This places the chair of the remuneration committee in the spotlight with regard to the organisation's approach to executive remuneration.

The remuneration policy must include an explanatory table, with detailed notes, setting out the approach taken to directors' remuneration in the period covered by the policy. This must be supplemented with a bar chart showing illustrative scenarios. It must also include a section on the approach to remuneration for new directors recruited to the board, as well as details of the policy on payments for loss of office. An explanation of the extent to which the views of employees' and shareholders have been taken into account is also required.

The annual report then sets out how the remuneration policy was implemented in the previous financial year. A new requirement in this report is the obligation to include a single total figure for the remuneration of each director. The aim is to provide comprehensive disclosure on all types of remuneration – fixed and variable elements, as well as pension provision – in a consistent format. There is also a focus on including a breakdown of payments for loss of office. Any such payment, in addition to being included in the annual report, will also need to be published on the company's website 'as soon as practicable' after the payment has been agreed. These details will need to be kept available until the next annual report is published.

The NHS FT annual reporting manual (NHS FT ARM) and the NHS Finance Manual both require a similar report to be made in the organisation's annual report. This report should include all exit packages, including those paid to senior managers.

Governance checklist

- Are the EDs aware of their wider role as a board member? Does their induction and ongoing development support them in their board role?
- Does the CEO or chief officer enhance board effectiveness by ensuring high standards of board/committee reporting?
- Is there evidence of the CEO implementing board decisions and lead on delivering best practice in governance across the organisation?
- Is the DoF an effective partner with the CEO with the required professional and corporate experience to both support and challenge the CEO?
- Does the remuneration committee have the necessary skills for its role and is it sufficiently independent of the EDs?
- Is there evidence of the committee eliciting the appropriate professional advice as and when required?
- If remuneration consultants are retained, then has there been a robust rendering process to ensure their independence and objectivity?
- Has the committee determined a coherent policy on directors' remuneration, which is regularly reviewed to ensure it remains 'fit for purpose' and in line with best practice?

EXECUTIVE DIRECTORS

- Does the committee apply the policy to its decisions, taking account of appropriate benchmarking information?
- Do the EDs' employment contracts address issues relating to rewards for failure on termination?
- Does the committee fulfil its responsibilities with regard to the reporting requirements on remuneration?
- Does the committee make itself available at the annual meeting or on other occasions for scrutiny and challenge by the shareholders/stakeholders?

Summary

- The matter of executive remuneration will continue to be a contentious issue both in the corporate and public sector. Ongoing debate and discussion continue to surround shareholder voting on executive remuneration in the annual round of corporate AGMs.
- It is clear that the greater degree of regulation in the NHS, combined with the attitude of largely well-motivated public servants – including senior managers – is currently providing control and restraints on NHS ED remuneration. Public perception is unlikely to reflect this; however, therefore boards and their remuneration committees will continue to have to balance the need to attract high calibre appointments, the morale of the wider workforce and the reputation of their organisation.

12
Non-executive directors

Introduction

A non-executive director (NED) is a member of the board of directors without executive responsibilities in the organisation. NEDs should be able to bring judgement and experience to the deliberations of the board that the executive directors (EDs) on their own would lack.

To be effective, a NED has to understand the organisation's business, but there appears to be general consensus that the experience and qualities required of a NED can be obtained from working in other industries or in other aspects of commercial and public life. NEDs may therefore include individuals who:

- are EDs in other public companies;
- hold NED positions and chair positions in other public companies;
- have professional qualifications (e.g. partners in firms of solicitors); or
- have experience in government, as politicians or former senior civil servants.

NEDs are expected not only to bring a wide range of skills and experience to the deliberations of the board, particularly in the area of strategy and business development, but also to ensure that there is a suitable balance of power on the board. A powerful chair or CEO might be able to dominate other EDs, but in theory at least, independent NEDs should be able to bring different views and independent thinking to board deliberations. Decisions taken by the board should therefore be better and more in keeping with the aims of good corporate governance.

The role and effectiveness of NEDs has been the subject of much scrutiny and challenge since the publication of the Higgs Report in 2003, with doubts being expressed at the level of balance they are able to bring to the board. The role of the NED was also considered as part of the Walker Review (2009), following the banking crisis. The review found firmly in favour of the NED role, stating that the NED contribution was materially helpful in financial institutions that had weathered the storm better than others.

In broad terms, the role of the NED, under the leadership of the chair is to:

- ensure that there is an effective executive team in place;
- participate actively in the decision-taking process of the board; and
- exercise appropriate oversight over execution of the agreed strategy by the executive team.

The appointment, induction and evaluation of non-executive directors

The appointment of the chair and NEDs is the responsibility of the nomination committee, and its composition and role generally is set out in more detail in Chapter 7.

In the NHS, such appointments are overseen by NHSI for NHS trusts. FT chairs and NEDs are appointed by the council of governors (Chapter 12), and the appointment processes for clinical commissioning group (CCGs) are covered in Chapter 15. Even so, the best practice guidance set out below benchmarks best practice for those fulfilling the role of NED in all types of NHS organisation.

Practical aspects of board appointments: time commitment

In practice, a nomination committee is likely to carry out its responsibilities by:

- using a firm of headhunters to find individuals outside the firm who might be suitable for appointment (as NED, CEO, finance director, and so on);
- vetting the candidates put forward by the headhunters; and
- making a selection and recommendation to the full board.

When an individual is appointed to the company board, the appointment may be for a fixed term. This is usually the case with NEDs: in the UK, NEDs are typically appointed on a fixed three-year contract, which may then be renewed at the end of each term. EDs are commonly appointed for an indeterminate length of time, subject to a minimum notice period (typically six months in the NHS). At present, the more usual term of office being offered to NEDs by the NHSI is two years (four years for chairs).

The UK Code states that 'all directors must be able to allocate sufficient time to the company to discharge their responsibilities effectively'. EDs are full-time appointments, so the problem of time commitment is not usually significant for them (unless the executive is also appointed as NED for another organisation). The main problem is ensuring that the chair and NEDs give sufficient time to the company. More time will probably be required from the chair than from a NED, and some NEDs (such as the chair of the audit committee) will be expected to commit more time than others.

When the nomination committee prepares a job description for the position, this should include an estimate of the time commitment expected. A NED should undertake that they will have sufficient time to meet what is expected of them. This undertaking could be written into the NED's letter of appointment.

Governing the NHS (June 2003) had this to say about likely time commitments.

> 'In our view a [NHS] non-executive serving on a board, which is properly focused on its governance responsibilities and which is properly supported by papers and information from the executive team, should be able to fulfil the

role in 2.5 days per month. This may be regarded as the minimum acceptable commitment. Clearly some individuals will be able to give more time to the organisation and where this is helpful, we are not suggesting that it should be discouraged. However, these additional duties should not be regarded as an extension or part of their board role or cross the boundaries set out above.'

NHS NED posts are usually advertised as a minimum time commitment of two-and-a half days per month, and a commitment for an NHS chair of two to three days per week. If an individual who is proposed to the board as chair or NED has significant time commitments outside the organisation, this should be disclosed to the board before the appointment is made.

An organisation should also protect itself against the risk that an ED is unable to commit sufficient time to the organisation because of NED appointments with other organisations. The UK Code states that the board should not allow one of its own EDs to take on more than one NED post in a FTSE 100 company, or the chair of a FTSE 100 company.

Accepting an offer of appointment as a NED

The formal procedures for appointing a new NED are the same for the appointment of an ED, with the exception of the close involvement of the NHSI. In addition, a newly appointed NED is likely to be less familiar with the organisation than a senior executive manager and they should not accept an appointment unless they are satisfied that there are no matters of concern.

An individual should only be willing to accept an appointment as NED if:

- the organisation does not use unethical business practices and has a good reputation;
- the organisation is a going concern and is not in financial difficulties;
- they can commit to the role the time that the organisation expects;
- the individual believes that they can contribute positively to the effectiveness of the board;
- there is no risk that the directors of the organisation could be held liable for any breach of duty, or that there is sufficient directors' and officers' liability insurance as protection against this risk; and
- the fee that the organisation has offered is adequate.

As ICSA has commented: 'by making the right enquiries, asking the right questions and taking care to understand the replies, a prospective director can reduce the risk of nasty surprises and dramatically increase the likelihood of success.'

Guidance from ICSA on the due diligence that a prospective NED should undertake recommends asking questions about:

- the business (e.g. its nature and size, and the organisation's market share, financial performance and financial position);

- governance and stakeholder relations – who the major stakeholders are, and about the structure of the board of directors and its committees;
- the role that the NED would be expected to perform, including membership of board committees. The prospective NED should be satisfied that they have the necessary qualities or experience to make an effective contribution to the work of the organisation's board;
- the organisation's risk management systems and controls; and
- ethical issues, and whether there are any ethical matters that might give cause for concern.

NHS NEDs may also want to ask questions about the impact of any health reform legislation. Answers to many of these questions can be obtained from published documents that are available to the general public, in paper form or on a website. These include the annual report and accounts of the organisation, the organisation's constitution, standing orders, any quality accounts, sustainability report or social and environmental report that the organisation publishes, regulator inspection reports or reviews and press reports about the organisation.

Terms of engagement

If a prospective NED decides to accept the offer of the appointment, terms of engagement should be agreed with the organisation (either with the board as a whole or its nomination committee). The terms that must be agreed are as follows.

- The initial period of tenure in office.
- Time commitment: the organisation must indicate how much time the NED is expected to commit to the organisation, and the NED should make this commitment. This should be included in the formal letter of appointment. Typically, NEDs of listed companies are expected to commit between 15 and 30 days each year, and possibly more for a committee chair. NHS NEDs are expected to commit a minimum of 30 days each year, with more for a committee chair.
- Remuneration: the annual remuneration of the NED should be agreed. This is usually a fixed annual fee. It is generally considered inappropriate for NEDs, including the chair, to be remunerated on the basis of incentive schemes linked to organisation performance, because this would undermine their independence.

The terms of engagement should be set out in a formal letter of appointment. As well as including details of the role that the NED will be required to perform (including initial membership of board committees), the expected time commitment, the tenure and the remuneration, the letter of engagement should also:

- specify that the NED should treat all information received as a director as confidential to the company;
- indicate the arrangements for induction;
- give details of directors' and officers' liability insurance that will be available;
- indicate the need for an annual performance review process for directors; and
- state what organisation resources will be made available to the NED (e.g. desk, computer terminal and telephone).

A sample letter of appointment for a NED can be found on the ICSA's website (www.icsa.org.uk).

Induction for non-executive directors

The FRC Guidance on Board Effectiveness (2018) provides useful guidance on induction of NEDs.

> 'A NED should, on appointment, devote time to a comprehensive, formal and tailored induction that should extend beyond the boardroom. Initiatives such as partnering a NED with an executive board member may speed up the process of him or her acquiring an understanding of the main areas of business activity, especially areas involving significant risk. The director should expect to visit, and talk with, senior and middle managers in these areas.'

The chair is responsible for making sure that all NEDs have such a tailored induction programme, although in practice this is often undertaken and overseen by the company secretary.

Evaluation of non-executive directors

Both the FT Code and the UK Code state as a main principle that the board should undertake a 'formal and rigorous annual evaluation of its own performance and that of its committees and individual directors'.

Chairs of NHS trusts are responsible for ensuring that NEDs receive performance appraisals at least annually. Trusts can determine the approach to appraisal that is most relevant to their own circumstances. An NHSI good practice guide to appraisal, as well as copies of the chair and non-executive role descriptions and behaviour frameworks, are also available to support an effective appraisal and appointment process.

NHS trusts should retain copies of NED appraisal forms, and share copies with those who have been appraised. This meets the requirement of the Office of the Commissioner of Public Appointments that all performance reviews must be formally recorded in the event of an investigation into a complaint. These copies may be needed to support future re-appointments, as evidence of poor performance. NHSI does not intend to collect NED appraisals routinely but may request them as and when required.

The key board level competencies for a NED set out by NHSI are as follows:

- **Patient and community focus:** a high level of commitment to patients, carers and the community, and to tackling health inequalities in disadvantaged groups.
- **Strategic direction:** the ability to think and plan ahead, to develop a clear vision and enthuse others, balancing needs and constraints.
- **Holding to account:** the ability to accept accountability for board performance, and probe and challenge constructively.
- **Effective influencing and communication:** a high level of ability to gain support and influence, political acumen.
- **Team working:** be committed to working as a team member, self-belief and drive – the motivation to improve NHS performance and confidence to take on challenges.
- **Intellectual flexibility:** the ability to think clearly and creatively, make sense of complexity and clarify it for other people.
- **Application of standards of public life:** uphold the highest standards of conduct set out in The Seven Principles of Public Life (see Chapter 1).

Key questions for independent NED evaluation include the following.

- How many board meetings has the director attended, and how many times have they been absent?
- How well prepared has the individual been for meetings (e.g. have they read the relevant papers in advance)?
- What has been the quality of contributions of the individual to board meetings (e.g. on strategic development and risk management)?
- Has the individual shown independence of character, or have they tended to go along with the opinions of certain other board members?
- How many board committee meetings has the director attended and how many have they missed?
- What has the individual contributed to committee meetings?
- Has the time commitment of the director been sufficient? Has the time commitment been as much as expected, or as much as stated in the director terms of appointment?
- Does the NED continue to show interest in and enthusiasm for the organisation?
- Are there reasons why the director may no longer be considered independent?
- Does the director communicate well with the other directors and with senior executives of the organisation?

The performance evaluation of NEDs in FTs is carried out by the council of governors and is set out in more detail in Chapter 9. The performance evaluation of CCG general practitioner (GP) members, lay members, secondary care and nurse members is carried out by the governing body: more details on this can be found in Chapter 15.

Independence of non-executive directors

NEDs are either independent or non-independent. A NED is not independent if their opinions are likely to be influenced, in particular by the senior executive management of the organisation or by a major stakeholder. What follows is an exploration of the importance of independence and the criteria for making that judgement.

Although this applies directly to CCGs, NHS trusts and FTs alike, the implications are somewhat different for CCGs as they are essentially membership organisations. These are explored more fully in Chapter 15.

Independent NEDs are supposed to bring an independent view to the deliberations of the board. However, they are in a difficult position, as they are legally liable in the same way as EDs. For example, they owe the same fiduciary duties to the organisation, as well as an obligation to exercise the duty of skill and care. As fellow directors, they might also be reluctant to blow the whistle on their executive colleagues. If they have been selected and appointed by the chair or the CEO, they will be less likely to ask tough questions about the way the organisation is being run.

The UK Code does not suggest that all NEDs should be independent. Non-independent NEDs are permissible, although the majority of the total board should consist of independent NEDs. If there are NEDs on the board who are not considered independent, this could create problems with the size and composition of the board. It may be considered necessary to appoint independent NEDs to act as a counterbalance to the NEDs who are not independent. Similar principles apply to the NHS.

The FT Code states that:

> 'The board of directors should identify in the annual report each NED it considers to be independent. The board should determine whether the director is independent in character and judgement and whether there are relationships or circumstances which are likely to affect, or could appear to affect, the director's judgement. The board of directors should state its reasons if it determines that a director is independent notwithstanding the existence of relationships or circumstances which may appear relevant to its determination.'

What is meant by 'independent'? It is easier to answer this question by specifying what is not independent. A NED is not independent if their opinions are likely to be influenced by someone else, in particular by the senior executive management or by a major stakeholder. The independence of a NED could be challenged, for example, if the individual concerned:

- has a family connection with the CEO – a problem in some family controlled public companies;
- until recently used to be an ED in the organisation;

- until recently used to work for the organisation in a professional capacity (e.g. as its auditor or corporate lawyer); or
- receives payments from the organisation in addition to their fees as a NED.

A person cannot be independent if they personally stand to gain, or otherwise benefit substantially, from income from the organisation (in addition to their fee as a NED) or from the organisation's reported profitability and movements in its share price.

A NED cannot be properly independent if, for example, they accept a fee from the organisation for consultancy work. Consultancy involves the individual in the operational aspects of the organisation, and by implication puts them on the side of the executive team. Nor can an individual be independent if they have been awarded a large number of share options by the company. Holding share options gives the individual a direct interest in the share price of the company around the time the options can be exercised. They might therefore favour decisions that improve the reported profitability of the company in the short term, because good financial results are likely to be good for the share price.

Occasionally, NEDs are appointed to represent the opinions of a major stakeholder (e.g. the appointment of a NED from a related university or dental school in NHS teaching hospitals). In such cases, the individual can be expected to voice the wishes of the stakeholder, and so could not be regarded as independent.

To ensure that NEDs should not rely for their tenure in office on one or two individuals, the UK Code recommends that they should be selected through a formal process. EDs cannot be independent. Not only are they involved in the running of the organisation's operations and report (and are accountable) to the chief executive officer (CEO) for this aspect of their work, they also rely on the organisation for most (if not all) of their remuneration.

Criteria for judging independence

The UK Code, and as quoted above, the FT Code, both require the board to identify in the annual report each NED it considers to be independent. Although this is a matter for the board's judgement, both codes set out the circumstances in which independence would usually be questionable.

- The director has been an employee of the organisation within the last five years.
- The director has a material business relationship with the organisation (or has had such a relationship within the last three years). This relationship might be as a partner, shareholder, director or employee in another organisation that has a material business relationship with the organisation.
- The director receives (or has received) additional remuneration from the organisation other than a director's fee, is a member of the organisation's pension scheme or participates in the organisation's share option scheme or a performance-related pay scheme.

- The director has close family ties with any of the organisation's advisers, directors or senior employees.
- The director has cross-directorships or has significant links with other directors through involvement in other companies or organisations. A cross-directorship exists when an individual is a NED on the board of Organisation X and an ED on the board of Organisation Y, when another individual is an ED of Organisation X and a NED on the board of Organisation Y.
- The director represents a significant shareholder or stakeholder.
- The director has served on the board for more than nine years since the date of his first election (six in the case of FTs).

These criteria of independence should be applied to the chair (on appointment) as well as other NEDs. Circumstances may change, and the independence of NEDs should be kept under review.

Independence of serving directors

As stated above, NEDs are typically appointed in the UK for a fixed period of three years, but it is now a requirement of the UK Code that directors of FTSE 350 companies should stand for re-election annually. The three-year contract may be extended at the end of that time for another three years and so on. There is a general view that the independence of a NED is likely to diminish over time as the NED becomes more familiar with the organisation and executive colleagues. The risk is that the NED will take more of the views of executive colleagues on trust and will be less rigorous in their questioning. This is noted in the UK Code, the King IV Code and the FT Code.

There will be circumstances where NEDs, having served their full terms, may exceptionally remain on the board. Indeed, the UK Code is pragmatic in its approach to the nine-year rule. If the board considers that a director is still independent even after nine years' service, they may still be considered 'independent' for the purposes of the corporate governance provisions. The FT Code takes a similar approach, although restricting the length of tenure to six years, stating that:

> 'Any term beyond six years (e.g. two three-year terms) for a NED should be subject to particularly rigorous review and should take into account the need for progressive refreshing of the board. NEDs may in exceptional circumstances serve longer than six years (e.g. two three-year terms following authorisation of the NHS FT), but subject to annual re-appointment. Serving more than six years could be relevant to the determination of a NED's independence.'

NHSI takes a slightly different approach, however, and NEDs generally serve no more than eight years in one post although, depending on individual circumstances, they may remain in post for a maximum of ten years.

The effectiveness of non-executive directors

The Higgs Report of 2003 is helpful in identifying the behaviours and attitudes that will make for an effective NED.

'Non-executive directors should constantly seek to establish and maintain confidence in the conduct of the company. They should be independent in judgement and have an enquiring mind. To be effective, non-executive directors need to build a recognition by executives of their contribution in order to promote openness and trust. To be effective, non-executive directors need to be well-informed about the company and the external environment in which it operates, with a strong command of issues relevant to the business. A non-executive director should insist on a comprehensive, formal and tailored induction. An effective induction need not be restricted to the boardroom, so consideration should be given to visiting sites and meeting senior and middle management. Once in post, an effective non-executive director should seek continually to develop and refresh their knowledge and skills to ensure that their contribution to the board remains informed and relevant.'

The key recommendations on the role and effectiveness of NEDs from Higgs and the UK Code are as follows:

- NEDs should 'constructively challenge and help develop proposals on strategy'.
- NEDs should also scrutinise the performance of management in meeting agreed goals or targets of performance, and they should monitor the reporting of performance (to ensure that this is honest and not misleading).
- NEDs should satisfy themselves about the integrity of the financial information produced by the organisation, and that the financial controls and systems of risk management are 'robust and defensible'.

Another aspect to the effectiveness of the NEDs is to ensure that there is a diversity of background and experience. This encourages a diverse range of views to be expressed in consideration of proposals being brought to the board. Being less closely involved in the day-to day running of the organisation enables NEDs to bring a fresh perspective to the discussion – highlighting shareholder/ stakeholder concerns is a vital role that NEDs can play. This supports the board in avoiding the 'group-think' tendencies that can develop in any group that works closely together.

'Even where the NED composition on the board is well balanced between financial industry experience and deep experience from elsewhere, the effectiveness of the overall NED contribution will be enhanced by a combination of appropriate induction and, thereafter, regular training programmes, adapted to the needs of the individual director; and dependable access for NEDs to support from within the company, for example from a dedicated capability in the company secretariat and greater time commitment.'

The rigour that the NEDs bring to the independent scrutiny and challenge of board decisions is equally important; it is therefore essential that NEDs have the necessary people skills. Exercising influence rather than a 'command and control' role requires very particular interpersonal skills of diplomacy and persuasion.

The Walker Review highlighted that NEDs sitting on the boards of highly complex businesses needed to ensure that they had the right mix of industry specific experience as well as a diverse range of other backgrounds to ensure there was an external critique of the business being considered. It further recognised that:

- NEDs should be responsible for deciding the remuneration of EDs; and
- NEDs should have a significant role in the appointment (and where necessary removal) of EDs and in succession planning for the major positions on the board.

The UK Code recognises there are matters that the NEDs should discuss without EDs being present, and a provision of the UK Code is that the chair should hold meetings with the NEDs without EDs being present. In addition, NEDs should meet at least once a year to discuss the performance of the chair, without the chair and led by the senior independent director (SID) (see Chapter 9). They should also meet on other occasions if this is considered necessary or appropriate.

The FRC Board Guide makes the following recommendations on the role of NEDs:

- NEDs need to make sufficient time available to discharge their responsibilities effectively.
- Their letter of appointment should state the minimum time that the NED will be required to spend on the organisation's business. IT should also indicate the possibility of additional time commitment when the organisation is undergoing a period of particularly increased activity, such as an acquisition or takeover, or as a result of some major difficulty with one or more of its operations.
- NEDs should insist on receiving high-quality information sufficiently in advance so that there can be thorough consideration of the issues prior to, and informed debate and challenge at, board meetings. High-quality information is that which is appropriate for making decisions on the issue at hand – it should be accurate, clear, comprehensive, up-to-date and timely; contain a summary of the contents of any paper; and inform the director of what is expected of them on that issue.

The Walker Report (2009) suggested that the role of NEDs is crucial to the effectiveness of a board in formulating and implementing business strategy. The report included the following comments.

- Stakeholders have a right to expect that there should be a material input from the NEDs in a unitary board to decisions on strategy and oversight of strategy

implementation. It should also be expected that when there is such shared decision making between EDs and NEDs, the organisation should perform better in general and over time than if strategy were determined exclusively by the executive management. This expectation appeared to have been justified by the banking crisis in the US and Europe.
- NEDs should provide a 'disciplined but rigorous challenge on substantive issues'. This should be seen as the norm, not an exception and, if any NED has insufficient strength of character to participate in providing a challenge, their continued suitability to remain as a board member should be thrown into question.

The Walker Report did add a note of caution on the extent to which NEDs should challenge the executive team, however:

'This does not, of course, mean open season for challenge to the executive team. Appropriate balance will only be achieved where the ED expects to be challenged, but where the board debate surrounding such challenge is conducted in a way that leaves the executive team with a sense of having drawn benefit from it.'

Barriers to effectiveness

There are differing views about the effectiveness of NEDs. The accepted view is that NEDs bring experience and judgement to the deliberations of the board that EDs on their own would lack.

An alternative view is that the effectiveness of NEDs can be undermined by lack of knowledge about the business operations of the organisation, insufficient time spent with the organisation, the weight of opinion of the EDs on the board and that NED involvement leads to delays in decision making.

Insufficient knowledge

The quality of decision making depends largely on the quality of information available to the decision-maker. The UK Code states that the board as a whole should be 'supplied in a timely manner with information in a form and of a quality appropriate to enable it to discharge its duties'. However, the senior executives in an organisation control the information systems, and so control the flow of information to the board. It is quite conceivable, for example, that the CEO and other EDs might have access to management information that is withheld from the board as a whole, or that is presented to the board in a distorted manner. Lacking the 'insider knowledge' of EDs about the business operations, and having to rely on the integrity of the information supplied to them by management and the EDs, restricts the scope for NEDs to make a meaningful contribution to board decisions.

Insufficient time

NEDs often have executive positions in other companies and organisations, where most of their working time is spent. As a general rule, NEDs do not have an office at the organisation headquarters and may spend at most two to three days per month on the organisation's business. A further criticism of NEDs is that some individuals hold too many NED positions, with the result that they cannot possibly give sufficient time to any of the organisations concerned. It could be argued, for example, that an individual cannot be an effective NED of an organisation if they are also the CEO of another public organisation and hold four or five other NED positions in other organisations.

The UK Code states that all directors should be able to allocate sufficient time to the organisation to discharge their responsibilities effectively. Although this principle of the code applies to all directors, the main concern is with NEDs (since EDs are usually full-time employees) and in particular the chair. The UK Code requires that when a chair or NED is appointed, the nomination committee should prepare a job specification that includes an assessment of the expected time commitment and in particular for the chair, recognising the need to be available to the organisation in times of crisis. When a NED or a new chair is appointed, the letter of appointment should set out the expected time commitment. In addition, the Code requires all new chair or NED appointments to disclose any other significant commitments they already have.

Overriding influence of executive directors

Yet another criticism of NEDs is that if a difference of opinion arises during a meeting of the board, the opinions of the EDs are likely to carry greater weight, because they know more about the organisation. NEDs may be put under pressure to accept the views of their ED colleagues. This potential problem provides an argument for the role of a strong SID, to ensure that the opinions of the independent NEDs are properly considered.

Delays in decision making

It may be argued that NEDs delay decision making within an organisation. Major decisions should be reserved for the board; therefore, to implement an important new strategy initiative it may be necessary to call a board meeting. The time required to hold the meeting, giving the NEDs sufficient time to reach a well-informed opinion about the matter, may delay the implementation of the proposed strategy. It has also been argued that NEDs may be conservative in outlook, whereas the board of directors needs to be 'entrepreneurial'.

One counter-argument is that when a major new strategy or initiative is proposed, it should be given full and careful consideration before a decision is made. NEDs, with their range of skills and experience, can contribute positively to this decision-making process.

The 'inherent tension'

The Cadbury Report – published in 1992 – first raised the issue of the balance for the NED role between monitoring the performance of the executive team against the contribution to the strategic direction of the organisation.

In a heavily regulated sector like the NHS, this can be a particularly challenging balance to achieve. This was covered again in 1998's Hampel Report, which noted that though NEDs are normally appointed to the board primarily for their contribution to the development of the company's strategy, there was also a general acceptance that NEDs should have both a strategic and a monitoring function.

This dual role was supported by the Higgs Report, which recommended that the NED role should not be forced to decide between these two perspectives. For the NED role to be overly concerned with monitoring would be for the NED to take on 'an alien policing influence on the board' whereas being overly concerned with identifying the strategic direction could lead to the NED over-identifying with the executive team.

Keeping these two aspects of the role in 'tension' is what helps NEDs provide a valuable contribution. Though the FRC Board Guide has overtaken the Hampel and Higgs reports, these reports still offer helpful insights and demonstrate the balance between the role of monitoring and providing strategic direction very clearly. For example, Higgs listed the key elements of the NED role as follows:

- **Strategy:** NEDs should constructively challenge and contribute to the development of strategy.
- **Performance:** NEDs should scrutinise the performance of management in meeting agreed goals and objectives and monitor the reporting of performance.
- **Risk:** NEDs should satisfy themselves that financial information is accurate and that financial controls and systems of risk management are robust and defensible.
- **People:** NEDs are responsible for determining appropriate levels of remuneration of EDs and have a prime role in appointing, and where necessary removing, senior management and in succession planning.

Non-executive director remuneration

The level of remuneration appropriate for any particular NED role should reflect the likely workload, the scale and complexity of the business and the responsibility involved.

Where a NED has extra responsibilities (such as membership of or chairing a board committees), the total remuneration should reflect these. The Higgs Report recommended that NED fees should be clearly built up using an annual fee, meeting attendance fees (to include board committee meetings) and an additional fee for chairing a committee (typically a multiple of the attendance fee) or role as senior independent director. In addition, organisations should expect to pay additional reasonable expenses in addition to the director's fee to cover related costs incurred by their NEDs (such as travel and administrative costs). Any significant support of this kind should be agreed in advance.

The principle that individuals should not decide their own remuneration applies to NEDs as well as to EDs. This means that a remuneration committee should not decide the fees of the NEDs. In the corporate sector, deciding the remuneration of the NEDs should be the responsibility of the chair and the EDs (or the shareholders if required by the articles of association). Where permitted by the articles, the board may delegate this responsibility to a committee, which might include the CEO. A provision in the UK Code is that the level of remuneration for NEDs should reflect the time commitment and responsibilities of the role.

NEDs are not employees. They receive a fee for their services, not a salary. In the UK corporate sector, it is usual for NEDs to receive a fixed annual fee, typically in the region of £20,000 to £60,000 (or possibly more), for attending board meetings, some committee meetings and general meetings of the company. This is substantially less in the health service sector, although the annual NED fees are increasing in larger FTs.

The NHS Providers Remuneration Survey of chairs and NEDs revealed average annual NED remuneration in FTs of £11,350 and in NHS trusts of £6,000. The average for FT chairs was £43,465, with an average monthly time commitment of 11 days. The difference in fees is tied to the size of trust turnover or number of staff in the trust, as these are usually the indicators used to benchmark individual trusts when assessing the level of non-executive fees.

The remuneration for chairs and NEDs in NHS trusts is set by the SoS and overseen by the NHSI. In FTs, the council of governors decides their remuneration. This provides the same protection as in the corporate sector, preventing individuals from setting their own remuneration. However, in CCGs the fees for GP members, lay members, secondary care and nurse members are set by the CCG itself. The CCG remuneration committee therefore needs to set clear parameters to ensure that individuals are not allowed to participate in decisions about their own fees. This is explored further in Chapter 15.

In the corporate sector, NEDs may receive other forms of remuneration or reward from the organisation alongside the basic fee (such as payment for additional services); however, this can raise questions about their independence. For example, a NED might be paid additionally as a 'consultant' to the company. No matter how genuine and useful these consultancy services are, they put the NED's independence at risk because executive management decides the size of a consultancy fee. Management also decides whether to extend or renew a consultancy agreement. This kind of arrangement is very unusual in the NHS.

The UK Code makes specific provisions about performance-related rewards for NEDs, including the award of share options to NEDs.

- As a general rule, the remuneration of NEDs should not include share options or any other performance-related reward.

- In exceptional cases, share options may be granted. However, the approval of the shareholders should be obtained in advance, and if the NED subsequently exercises options to acquire shares in the company, these shares should be held until at least one year after the NED leaves the board.
- Holding share options could affect the determination of whether or not the NED is independent.

Resignation

Some of those who responded to the consultation for the Higgs Report described the resignation of a NED as being the ultimate sanction at their disposal. Higgs believed that resignation should be regarded very much as a last resort once other efforts to resolve problems have failed. Indeed, NEDs may be constrained from resigning by their fiduciary duty to act in the organisation's best interests. Where NEDs have real concerns about the way in which an organisation is being run or about a course of action proposed by the board, the first step should be to raise their concerns with the chair and their fellow directors. NEDs should, as a matter of course, ensure that their concerns are recorded in the minutes of the board meeting if they cannot be resolved.

If the NED feels that resignation is the only course of action left, a written statement should be provided to the chair, for circulation to the board, setting out the reasons for resignation. Higgs also recommended that a NED should explain their reasons for resigning when they leave in other circumstances.

Governance checklist

- Do the NEDs contribute to the strategic direction of the organisation, the performance of management, review the risk management system and both appoint and set the remuneration of the EDs?
- Are the NEDs provided with timely and sufficient information and resources to fulfil their role?
- Do the NEDs have the right attributes, skills and diversity of experience to provide sufficient and credible challenge to board debate and discussion?
- Do they have the intellectual capacity to test management proposals and the right influencing skills to suggest alternatives where appropriate?
- Are at least half of the board members judged to be independent, taking account of the criteria in the UK code?
- Do the NEDS have clear terms of appointment in writing, which include independence, time commitment, duties, and fees?
- Is there a comprehensive and formal induction programme on appointment tailored to the needs of the individual?
- Is there ongoing development for each NED based on the findings of the annual evaluation process?

- Do the NEDs give sufficient commitment to such development activities and acknowledge the value of engaging in them?

Summary

- The role of the NED is a vital link in the chain of governance and a key part of the principle of the unitary board.
- In balancing the tension between monitoring and setting strategy, the NED acts as an important check and balance to the power and authority of the executive team.
- It is important for the board to understand the nature of the role and for the chair to develop a good working relationship between the NEDs and the EDs on the board.
- Clarity as to the independence of each individual NED will provide a robust framework in which to manage any potential conflicts of interest that might arise.

13
The company secretary

Introduction

'All directors should have access to the advice and services of the company secretary, who is responsible to the board for ensuring that board procedures are complied with.'

(UK Code, 2018)

This is repeated in the King IV Code, which suggests that even for those companies not required by the CA 2006 to employ a company secretary, it is good practice to do so.

With the spotlight firmly fixed on corporate governance issues in the banking sector in recent times, the profile of the company secretary has been increasing. The All Party Parliamentary Corporate Governance Group commissioned research into the role and their report in May 2012, *Elevating the Role of the Company Secretary*, highlighted the important role that the company secretary can play in ensuring effective corporate governance. The report recognised that there was a potential for the administrative duties laid on the company secretary to undermine the potential to be seen as a high-level adviser to the board; this was also affected by the use of the term 'secretary' in the title, with a common suggestion that an alternative of corporate governance director be used.

A recurring theme of the review was the unique position of the company secretary as the interface between the board and management. The review considered that this could be developed further, so that the company secretary could coach management to help them understand the expectations of, and value brought by, the board. Interestingly, the review went on to consider that company secretaries might make good non-executive directors (NEDs) due to their insights from observing and advising a number of boards during their career.

In 2013, ICSA: The Governance Institute worked with Henley Business School to explore how company secretaries help organisations create trust through governance, and the skills and knowledge that they need. The key findings of the study, *The Company Secretary – Building Trust through Governance*, published in November 2014:

'illustrate how high-performing company secretaries ultimately help build trust, which results in good governance. Many company secretaries acknowledge that their individual discretion, freedom of choice, personal morals and ethics are important in positively impacting corporate judgement. Other respondents note how effectiveness is achieved through more than fixed administrative capabilities or technical knowledge.'

The study was also clear about some of the challenges that are faced by company secretaries. These included:

- being considered 'traitors' by the executive team;
- supporting chairs exhibiting poor performance;
- acting as the third person in a CEO–chair relationship;
- becoming the pivotal contact for insurmountable problems; and
- maintaining independence from other executives and board members.

More recently, the Institute of Directors (October 2018) stated that with 'the increasing focus in recent years on corporate governance, the role of the company secretary has grown in importance. In many ways, the secretary is now seen as the guardian of the company's proper compliance with both the law and best practice.' Interestingly, the recent scandals had led to the responsibility for developing and implementing processes to promote and sustain good corporate governance being largely within the remit of the company secretary. This is reflected in the Institute of Chartered Secretaries and Administrators forthcoming name change to 'The Chartered Governance Institute' and their creation of a new chartered governance professional designation.

To use the official ICSA terminology, company secretaries are governance professionals. They are valued strategic advisers with in-depth knowledge of law, taxation, finance and management who give independent, impartial advice and support to directors, trustees and other key decision makers across the private, public and not-for-profit sectors. They support and advise the boards of organisations and ensure that the organisation they work for is complying with regulatory standards. In an increasingly regulated world, this is no mean feat.

The role of the company secretary is less developed within the NHS. Therefore, this chapter will outline the role within the corporate sector to give a richer and more diverse picture of the role, before looking at its development within the NHS.

The skills and knowledge required to be a company secretary

The Henley/ICSA study *The Company Secretary: Building trust through governance* identified three broad areas of skills and knowledge required by a company secretary:

- technical expertise
- commercial and business acumen
- social skills and emotional intelligence.

Company secretaries need technical expertise in law, governance codes and an understanding of financial issues. They need commercial experience in decision-making, problem-solving, analytical skills, attention to detail and ability to get things done properly. Finally, but just as importantly, they need interpersonal skills and relationship management skills including judgement, diplomacy, tact and discretion – along with adaptability and patience.

Company secretaries also need to be incredibly resilient, as without the authority of a board member, they still need to be able to challenge and remain independent of the individual board members while at the same time building good working relationships. Anecdotally, it was once said that the best person to take on the role is someone who has already retired or who is not dependent upon their monthly salary from the organisation, as they can then challenge the chair or CEO when required, without fear of jeopardising their career.

Before setting out the specific responsibilities, it is important to note that the most effective company secretary:

- is regarded by the board as its trusted adviser;
- can be seen as the board's chief of staff; and
- wins the confidence of and acts as a confidential sounding board to the chair and other directors on issues of concern.

Company secretaries provide, where appropriate, a discreet but challenging voice in relation to board deliberations and decision making, drawing in particular on their professional experience and historical knowledge of the organisation. They also keep under review legislative, regulatory and governance developments that may affect the organisation and ensures that the board is appropriately briefed on them.

The Henley/ICSA report went on to describe the attributes of a company secretary as very similar and closest to the role of the chair. A good company secretary requires the leadership qualities of humanity, humility, high intelligence, an understanding of agendas, negotiation and a tough resilience to dealing with everyday issues. The report was originally titled 'the breadth and majesty of the role of the company secretary' – referring to the breadth of competency required and aligned to refined high-level social qualities – majesty.

The company secretary as an officer of the company

The secretary of a public limited company must be appropriately qualified. Under section 273 of the CA 2006, the board must be satisfied that the secretary has the 'requisite knowledge and experience to discharge the functions of the secretary of the company'. In addition, the CA 2006 states they must meet one or more of the following qualifications:

- be a member of any of the following bodies: ICSA; the Institute of Chartered Accountants in England and Wales; the Institute of Chartered Accountants of Scotland; the Association of Chartered Certified Accountants, the Institute of Chartered Accountants in Ireland; the Chartered Institute of Management Accountants (CIMA); or the Chartered Institute of Public Finance and Accounting (CIPFA);
- have held the office of company secretary of a public company for at least three out of the five years immediately before their appointment as secretary;
- be a barrister, advocate or solicitor called or admitted in any part of the UK; or
- be a person who appears to the directors to be capable of carrying out the functions of company secretary, because that person holds or has held a similar position in another body or is or was a member of another body.

This contrasts significantly with the lack of any statutory qualification requirements for a company director. The appointment of a company secretary has to be notified to the registrar of companies, including confirmation of the person's consent to be appointed.

However, like the director, the company secretary is an officer of the company and as such owes fiduciary duties to the company and its shareholders. These duties include acting in good faith in the best interests of the company, avoiding conflicts of interest and not making secret profits from dealings for or on behalf of the company.

The CA 2006 imposes numerous obligations on companies regarding the conduct of their affairs. Most of these requirements are backed up by criminal sanctions so that, in the event of a breach, the company and every officer of it who is in default is liable to a fine and, in some cases, imprisonment. As an officer of the company, the company secretary can be prosecuted for these offences. For example, if the company becomes insolvent, the company secretary may also become liable under the Insolvency Act 1986, which allows an action in damages against any officer of a company for a misfeasance or breach of trust. Responsibility for ensuring compliance with these matters ultimately rests with the directors. However, by making the company secretary liable as an officer, the Act not only recognises that the directors usually rely on the company secretary in this regard, but also provides a strong indication that they should give the company secretary responsibility for (or an involvement in) these matters.

It is clear that, in view of their potential liabilities, the company secretary should not close their eyes to cases of non-compliance even if the directors have purported to make someone else responsible for those matters. At the very least, the company secretary should draw such cases to the attention of the directors and advise on the company's duties and obligations. The company secretary should be in a position to act independently and not be restricted by their reporting line within the company. The company secretary should also ensure that where certain of their responsibilities have been delegated, such tasks are properly executed, since they can still be held accountable in law for any failure by the company to comply.

The responsibilities of the company secretary

Whatever the type of organisation, company secretaries are in a unique position to fulfil an important role in governance. They are not members of the board of directors, and so do not have direct responsibility for governance and accountability to stakeholders. Without being a director, they know about what is taking place at board level in the organisation and can give advice and assistance – not only to the chair, but also to the board as a whole, board committees and individual directors.

Before the specific functions/responsibilities are laid out here, it is interesting to note the areas of influence that a company secretary may exercise. These are set out neatly by David O'Callaghan in his 'The Influential Company Secretary' series as:

- facilitating board effectiveness and performance;
- supporting alignment of the board's focus with strategic and governance priorities;
- making board information management and processes fit for purpose; and
- influencing board composition, diversity and succession planning.

(https://boardexcellence.ie/blog)

Good governance relies on communication and the exchange of information, and the company secretary can help to ensure that this happens. By attending board meetings and committee meetings, they should ensure that relevant information is passed from board to committee or from one committee to the board or another committee. By acting as a point of communication and contact for NEDs, the company secretary should also be able to contribute to the flows of information between NEDs and senior executive managers in the company. The company secretary should have a full understanding of governance requirements, and should be able to identify governance issues that arise and advise the board accordingly:

> 'The company secretary should be responsible for advising the board through the chair on all governance matters.'

(UK Code)

The specific responsibilities of a company secretary for governance matters should be decided by the organisation. The ICSA guidance note the Corporate Governance Role of the Company Secretary (2013) provides a list of responsibilities relating to corporate governance divided into the following areas.

Specific responsibilities derived from the UK Code

Board composition and procedures:

- Establishing a formal schedule of matters reserved for decision by the board and a formal division of responsibilities between the chair and CEO.
- Scheduling board meetings, assisting with the preparation of agendas, providing guidance on board paper content, ensuring good and timely information flows within the board and its committees and between senior management and NEDs; recording board decisions clearly and accurately, pursuing follow-up actions and reporting on matters arising.
- Ensuring that appropriate insurance cover is arranged in respect of any potential legal action against directors.
- Ensuring board committees are constituted in compliance with the UK Code and that the committees have the appropriate balance of skills, experience, independence and knowledge of the company.
- Supporting the board and nominations committee on board succession planning and on the process for the appointment of new directors to the board.

Board information, development and relationships:

- Planning and organising director induction programmes which provide a full, formal and tailored introduction to the board and the business.
- Planning and organising director professional development programmes to refresh the directors' skills and knowledge.
- Arranging for major shareholders to be offered the opportunity to meet new directors.
- Facilitating good information flows between board members, the committees and senior management as well as fostering effective working between EDs and NEDs.
- Establishing and communicating procedures for directors to take independent professional advice at the company's expense if required.
- Developing a proactive relationship with board members, providing a source of information and advice, and acting as the primary point of contact with NEDs.
- Supporting the process for the board to undertake formal annual evaluation of its own performance and that of its committees and individual directors.

Financial and business reporting:

- Having a detailed knowledge of, and advising on, the board's responsibility to present a fair, balanced and understandable assessment of the company's position and prospects in annual and interim reports plus other price-sensitive public reports and reports to regulators and that information required under statute.

- The company secretary should also ensure that the requirements of the Financial Conduct Authority (FCA)'s Listing, Prospectus and Disclosure and Transparency Rules (LPDT Rules) are met and be aware of the guidance available on these areas.

Risk management and internal control:

- Assisting the board in an annual review of the effectiveness of the company's risk management and internal control systems including financial, operational and compliance controls.

Audit committee and auditors:

- Ensuring that the audit committee is fully conversant with the UK Code principles around corporate reporting, risk management and internal control principles. This should include the relationship with the external auditors, in particular as regards audit quality, provisions of non-audit services, recommendations for appointment and renewal of auditors and putting the audit contract out to tender.
- Ensuring the implementation of and monitoring the effectiveness of the procedure for staff to raise concerns about possible improprieties in matters of financial reporting or other matters.

Remuneration:

- Ensuring that the remuneration committee is familiar with the UK Code principles and provisions on remuneration, including the provisions on the design of performance-related remuneration for EDs set out in Schedule A to the UK Code.
- Ensuring that grants of share options and other long-term incentive awards do not contravene the UK Code.
- Ensuring that the provisions in the directors' term of appointment in relation to early termination are in accordance with the UK Code.
- Ensuring that non-executive remuneration is determined in line with UK Code provisions and within the limits set by the articles of association.
- Ensuring that all new long-term incentive schemes and significant changes to existing schemes are submitted to shareholders for approval, in accordance with the Listing Rules.
- Ensuring compliance with the legal requirements in relation to directors' remuneration, including any necessary shareholder approvals, contributing to the drafting of the directors' remuneration report and ensuring its compliance with the full range of disclosure requirements.

Relationship with shareholders:

- Ensuring the board keeps in touch with shareholder opinion on a continuing basis.

- Managing relations with institutional investors on corporate governance issues and board procedures in accordance with the principles established in the UK Stewardship Code.
- Managing the convening and conduct of the annual general meeting (AGM) in line with statutory and regulatory requirements and the UK Code, and using it as an opportunity to communicate with retail investors.

Disclosure and reporting:

- Ensuring that the necessary disclosures on corporate governance and the workings of the board and its committees are included in the annual report. All companies with a premium listing of equity shares in the UK are required under the Listing Rules to report how they have applied the UK Code in the annual report and accounts.
- Ensuring that the requisite types of governance information are made available, as required (e.g. on the company's website).

The FRC Board Guide emphasises the role of the company secretary as:

- ensuring good information flows within the board and its committees and between senior management and NEDs, as well as facilitating induction, arranging board training and assisting with professional development as required;
- arranging for provision of the necessary resources for developing and updating its directors' knowledge and capabilities consistent with the board evaluation findings; and
- ensuring that directors, especially NEDs, have access to independent professional advice at the company's expense.

There is further guidance available in ICSA's The Duties and Reporting Lines of the Company Secretary (2013) which explains the role in more detail.

Responsibilities for statutory and regulatory compliance

Compliance with laws and regulations is a requirement of good governance. The company secretary is responsible for implementing procedures to help directors discharge their statutory duties as codified in the CA 2006, in particular their specific duties to promote the success of the company, taking account of a wide range of stakeholder interests and to avoid conflicts of interest. Guidance on these particular duties is available in the ICSA guidance note Directors' General Duties (2015).

The company secretary should be responsible for ensuring compliance with all the statutory and regulatory requirements relating to governance. For health service governance, these include the key pieces of NHS legislation and voluntary codes outlined in Chapter 6. For UK corporate governance, these include the requirements of the CA 2006 and the FCA's LPDT Rules.

The company secretary should also be responsible for ensuring proper disclosure of information. For example, these include quarterly disclosures to NHSI. In the case of companies, this includes the dissemination of regulatory news announcements to the stock market, such as trading statements and information about share dealings by directors.

The company secretary should also keep under review all legal and regulatory developments affecting the organisation's operations, and making sure that the directors are properly briefed about them.

In addition, in corporate governance, the Listing Rules require companies to comply with the Model Code, which sets out rules about when directors should not usually be permitted to buy or sell shares in the company. For example, directors should not deal in the company's shares during 'close periods' before an announcement of their financial results. The company secretary is responsible for making sure that directors understand the requirements of the Model Code and comply with them.

Additional duties of the company secretary

In addition to the core duties above, the duties that the company secretary commonly undertakes in areas such as legal, accounting, financial services, personnel and HR, property, risk management, estates and facilities, pensions and insurance management must also be considered. Though these are not seen as core duties, these duties will frequently take up a substantial proportion of the company secretary's time and their importance should not be underestimated, as there is clear evidence that the breadth of competency required by company secretaries is growing.

The professional background, previous work experience and general personal capabilities of the company secretary will generally dictate the nature and scope of these additional responsibilities, as will the nature of the company's business activities. For example, a lawyer is more likely to specialise in litigation and an accountant is more likely to manage a treasury function. A chartered secretary, being specifically trained for the role, is more likely to take on additional responsibilities such as property management, pensions and insurance matters.

The conscience of the company

In the context of business ethics and governance, the company secretary can be described as the 'conscience of the organisation'. There will often be situations where it is in the best short-term interests of an organisation to ignore best governance practice or even act in an unethical way. For example, the board of directors may want to 'window dress' the financial statements and make the performance of the organisation appear better than it really is, or an organisation may wish to bribe a government official in order to win a major contract.

The company secretary should speak out against bad governance and unethical practice and remind the board and senior executives of the appropriate course of conduct and the principles of good governance that they should apply. As the Henley/ICSA report summarises: 'the company secretary has to have the trust of both the board and the executive while at the same time maintaining an independence to act in the "best interests of the organisation".'

In order to act in this way, as a 'conscience' for the directors and senior executives, the company secretary must be independent-minded, and should not be under the influence of any other individual, such as the chair or CEO.

The independence of the company secretary

> 'You're not a member of [the] executive team, you're not a member of [the] board, you're the interface between board and executive, you've got to have independence.'
>
> (Co Sec 04 and 05, Private sector, Henley/ICSA Report, 2014)

The role of the company secretary in governance is such that it is essential to ensure their independence from undue influence and pressure from a senior board member. An ICSA guidance note, *The duties and reporting lines of the company secretary*, comments:

> 'The company secretary is a key member of the executive team appointed by the board of directors as an officer of the company with specific responsibility to the entity as a whole for its sound corporate governance and for the guidance of the board in its responsible and effective execution of its tasks. Boards of directors have a right to expect the company secretary to give impartial advice and to act in the best interests of the company. However, it is incumbent on boards of directors to ensure that company secretaries are in a position to do so, for example by ensuring that they are not subject to undue influence of one or more of the board of directors. If the board fails to protect the integrity of the company secretary's position, one of the most effective in-built internal controls available to the company is likely to be seriously undermined. The establishment of appropriate reporting lines for the company secretary will normally be a crucial factor in establishing that protection. It will also be important for NEDs to have access to the advice and services of the company secretary and for them to support the company secretary in his or her role.'

It is neither practical nor desirable in terms of line management for the company secretary to report on a day-to-day basis to all the directors. However, it is important not to lose sight of the ultimate line of authority when establishing these reporting lines. The company secretary is responsible to the board of directors collectively rather than to any individual director.

The FRC Board Guide states that 'the company secretary should report to the chair on all board governance matters'. This does not preclude the company secretary also reporting to the CEO, or other ED, in relation to their other executive management responsibilities. The remuneration of the company secretary should be determined by the remuneration committee'.

UK Code reinforces this by stating that 'both the appointment and removal of the company secretary should be a matter for the board as a whole'.

The ICSA Guidance on the Appointment of the Company Secretary (November 2014) recommends that the company secretary is responsible to the board and should be accountable to the board through the chair on all matters relating to corporate governance and their duties as an officer of the company (core duties). As the person elected by the directors to act as their leader, the chair is the person to whom the company secretary should report with respect to responsibilities that concern the whole board.

If, in addition to the core duties mentioned above, the company secretary has other executive or administrative duties, they should report to the CEO or such other director to whom responsibility for that matter has been delegated by the board. The company secretary should not report to a director (except the chair) on any matter unless responsibility for that matter has been delegated to that director by the board.

A director who is authorised unilaterally to fix the company secretary's remuneration and benefits could gain undue influence. It is therefore recommended (particularly where the company secretary reports to the chair on all matters) that decisions on remuneration and benefits should be taken (or at least noted) by the board as a whole, or by the remuneration committee of the board on the recommendation of the chair or CEO. In this way, the company secretary is not dependent on one individual, or a small group of board members, for their role or remuneration. Where the company secretary has an additional reporting line to the CEO or other director, the views of that director can be taken into account by the board or board remuneration committee when decisions are taken on the remuneration and benefits of the company secretary.

Similar recommended practice was included in King III (prior to King IV, which does not reference company secretaries), which stated that the board should appoint and remove the company secretary and empower the individual to enable them to fulfil their duties properly. It also recommended that the company secretary should have an 'arm's-length relationship' with the board, emphasising the requirement for independence.

Departures from these guidelines will reduce the ability of the company secretary to perform their core duties in accordance with the standards, which boards of directors should expect.

The company secretary and the in-house lawyer

Many of the governance duties of a company secretary have a legal aspect or involve compliance with regulations or a voluntary code of governance practice.

It could be argued that an in-house lawyer working for the organisation could perform many of these tasks better, since corporate lawyers are specialists in company law and regulations. However, as stated previously, independence is a critical aspect of the governance role of the company secretary; to perform the task effectively, the company secretary needs to be as independent as it is possible for a full-time employee to be. The Henley report in November 2014 stated that 'there is a conflict of interest in the combined "Head of Legal (or General Counsel) and Company Secretary" role. The roles should be separate, as they can be incompatible.'

In their legal work, an in-house lawyer must at times consider the specific interests of the organisation and individual directors and may be required to advise them on the most appropriate way of dealing with legal issues that arise. In performing this role, the lawyer will often have to 'take sides' to represent a particular interest. This would be inconsistent with the requirement to be independent when advising on governance issues.

It would therefore be inappropriate for the organisation's in-house lawyers to take on the governance that is usually given to the company secretary. An individual who has trained and qualified as a professional lawyer could be a suitable candidate to act as company secretary or take on governance responsibilities within the organisation, but only if two key conditions are applied:

- the qualified lawyer does no legal work for the organisation; and
- the independence of the individual can be protected in the same way as for a company secretary, with the board as a whole responsible for appointing and dismissing them and deciding their remuneration.

Appointing a lawyer may increase the company secretary's responsibility and may make them responsible for some of the legal judgements, which is fundamentally not a company secretary role.

The development of company secretaries in the NHS

The Integrated Governance Handbook attempted to establish an equivalent role within the NHS and the authors had discussions with a number of FTSE 100 companies to look at the role of the company secretary, exploring, more importantly, whether these companies could exist without such an adviser. The evidence clearly pointed to the need for such integrated corporate support.

FTs began to establish such a role in their corporate structures and guidance is included in the FT Code. The significance of the role is to ensure that, for the first time in the history of NHS boards, the board per se can confidently assure itself that at the end of the 12-month cycle it has full evidence and is fully appraised before signing off the AGS. The Integrated Governance Handbook also clarifies the point by stating that it is not necessary for the company secretary to be either an accountant or a lawyer.

The Good Governance Institute (GGI) published research into the role, *The Role of the Company Secretary in the NHS*, in July 2016. The research found wide variances in the seniority and scope of the role within the NHS and ultimately, concluded that the role of the company secretary in the NHS is under-appreciated and under-utilised, with a need for clearer guidance from the centre to improve awareness of the role and reaffirm its importance to the workings of the board.

The GGI summarised the responsibilities of the role as follows:

1. **Administrative function:** The company secretary should ensure that all committees are properly serviced (including working with chairs to formulate agendas and business cycles), and should manage information flows between the board, its committees, and senior management.
2. **Conscience of the organisation:** The company secretary should be the interface between different elements of the board, the first point of contact for NEDs and governors, and a trusted advisor to board members, governors and senior management.
3. **Governance:** The company secretary should play a central role in governance advising the board on all current governance matters: reviewing terms of reference and the annual cycle of business; managing the induction and development of board members and governors and enhancing board and committee structures (including co-ordinating effectiveness reviews).
4. **Compliance:** The company secretary should manage procedures to ensure compliance with any relevant regulatory and legal requirements.
5. **Governors:** In the case of FTs, the company secretary should manage the governors, organise and attend the council of governors' meetings (including the AGM) and endeavour to integrate the governors with the rest of the organisation in support of core values and goals.

It also supported the view that the company secretary should be accountable to the collective board in order to retain their position as a neutral, independent advisor. The management of the company secretary, as opposed to the accountability, is to an executive member of the board, usually the CEO or director of corporate affairs.

The difficulty in establishing the role within the NHS has been the misapprehension that the role is purely an administrative role, with many NHS company secretaries still responsible for taking the minutes and circulating board papers as opposed to a recognition of the seniority of the governance professional. The other common misapprehension has been that this is a role to be undertaken by the director of corporate affairs, which although they were often responsible for engagement with stakeholders and the annual disclosure and reporting functions, the role did not fully encompass the corporate governance and board advisory role.

There has also been some difficulty with the terminology for the role as the use of the word 'company' in the job title clashes with the public sector NHS.

Accordingly, the role is sometimes referred to as board secretary, trust secretary or assistant to the board. There has also been some difficulty with establishing the board-level nature of the role through the Agenda for Change (AfC) job evaluation panels as the use of the word 'secretary' has also imbued the role with too much of an administrative flavour. As a result, some posts are advertised on AfC pay bands, while others are advertised as very senior management (VSM) roles.

The creation of the lead governor role in FTs in 2011 demonstrates the limited understanding of the role of the company secretary, and possibly the senior independent director (SID). The lead governor role will be covered in more detail in Chapter 14 but, suffice to say, NHSI already had a direct line of contact with the council of governors through the company secretary and the SID for those situations where it would be inappropriate for NHSI to contact the chair, or vice versa.

As can be seen by the more extensive and wide-ranging role within the corporate sector that establishes the role as part of the executive team, there is significant scope within NHS organisations to adopt a similar board level role. A number of NHS trusts and FTs have recently established a board level role of director of governance, which has encompassed the role of company secretary. The caveat to this arrangement that the independence of the role must be maintained within a direct line of report to the chair for on all matters relating to corporate governance and their duties as an officer of the company. In addition, the appointment and removal of the company secretary should remain a matter for the board as a whole, not just the CEO as the line manager of the executive function carried out by the director of governance. The FT Code departs from this slightly by requiring the appointment and removal of the company secretary to be a joint matter for the CEO and chair.

The other challenge for NHS organisations is to be clear where the boundaries lie between corporate governance and clinical governance. This too can create tensions for the role of the company secretary. The Integrated Governance Handbook helpfully set out the following points to establish the independence of the company secretary.

- The remuneration committee, as opposed to either the chair or the CEO, appoints the company secretary in order to ensure the neutrality of role.
- The company secretary is answerable to the board but will be line managed by the CEO in order to ensure personal development and accountability.
- The company secretary will also work closely with the chair, the CEO and the NEDs.
- The company secretary will be actively involved in or be a member of the executive team to ensure a full understanding of the organisation's business.
- The company secretary will not undertake executive activity in respect of having a specific role, but will be the neutral observer and adviser to the board or executive team.

- An NHS-based company secretary should have sufficient knowledge of the NHS to gain the respect of the doctors in the organisation but need not necessarily be a clinician.
- The company secretary should be appropriately qualified to carry out their role and should ideally be accredited by a professional body such as ICSA.

Whilst current legislation does not specify the need for CCGs to appoint a company secretary, good practice from the corporate sector and experience in FTs suggests that this is also a key role in the governance of an organisation. The company secretary could play a leading role in governance, supporting the chair as well as helping the governing body and committees to function effectively. They could also have a key role in ensuring good communication between the governing body, senior management and committees and helping to ensure compliance with legislation and regulations. It has been interesting to observe the profile of the company secretarial role in the new governing bodies, which have been established. In many cases, although a corporate secretary or head of corporate services seems to be in post, further research needs to be carried out to see whether these appointments are in line with the best practice set out here.

The ICSA has worked alongside the NHS to produce a sample job description outlining the responsibilities of a FT secretary (May 2015), set out below.

Core duties of an NHS foundation trust secretary

The following list includes both those duties, which are legal obligations as well as those which result from best practice. This is not a comprehensive list, and the trust secretary will need to refer to other pertinent legislation and regulation.

Board meetings – directors and governors:

- Facilitating the smooth operation of the FT's formal decision making and reporting machinery.
- Organising board of directors and council of governors meetings along with those of their committees (e.g. audit, remuneration, nomination committees etc).
- Ensuring that there is proper and appropriate co-ordination of boards and committees and an effective flow of information.
- Formulating meeting agendas with the chair (and CEO) and advising management on content and organisation of memoranda or presentations for the meeting.
- Collecting, organising and distributing such information, documents or other papers for meetings.
- Ensuring that all meetings are minutes and that the minute books are maintained with certified copies of the minutes; and that action is taken on matters arising.

- Communicating board decisions to those required to implement them and ensure that actions and tasks assigned are managed appropriately and to the required timetable, reporting back as required.
- Ensuring that the board of directors and council of governors meetings and all board committees are properly constituted and provided with clear reference.
- Managing the FT HQ secretariat ensuring the effective running of the board's support system including the production of board and committee papers.

Annual members' meetings:

- Ensuring that an annual members' meeting is held in accordance with the requirements of the National Health Service Act 2006 (NHS Act 2006) and the FT's constitution.
- Preparing and issuing notices of meetings.
- Obtaining internal agreement to all documentation for circulation to members.
- Preparing directors and governors for any members' questions and helping them create briefing materials.
- Formally minuting those aspects of the meeting that are required to be recorded.

Constitution:

- Ensuring that the FT complies with its constitution and drafting and incorporating amendments in accordance with correct procedures.
- Leading the process of non-financial compliance with the trust's constitution, including management of the public and staff membership and governance reporting requirements with NHSI.
- Reviewing, proposing and implementing approved changes to the trust's constitution.

NHSI requirements:

- Establishing and monitoring procedures to ensure that the FT complies with the requirements of the NHS Act 2006 and its provider licence.
- Ensuring that the requirements of the compliance framework are fulfilled appropriately and in a timely manner.
- Submitting the annual risk assessment to NHSI.
- Ensuring quarterly submissions are accurate and timely.
- Acting as initial point of contact between the FT, NHSI and other regulators.

Statutory registers:

- Maintaining the following statutory registers and responding to appropriate requests concerning the information they contain:
  - members, including the constituency they belong to (and class, if relevant);
  - members of the council of governors;
  - governors' interests;

- members of the board of directors; and
- directors' interests.

Statutory returns:

- Ensuring that formal documentation is filed with appropriate bodies, as required, and to report certain changes regarding the FT:
  - annual report and accounts;
  - amendments to the constitution; and
  - notices of removal or resignation of the auditors.

Annual report and accounts:

- Co-ordinating the preparation, publication, distribution and presentation of the annual report (including annual accounts), in consultation with the FT's internal and external advisers, and ensuring its presentation to Parliament.

Membership communications:

- Communicating with the members (e.g. through circulars, newsletters); maintaining good general relations with members and other interested parties.
- In liaison with the communications team, co-ordinating communications with the FT's members.
- Establishing and monitoring the election processes for public and staff governors.
- Supporting the council of governors in reviewing and suggesting proposals for the membership development strategy.
- Ensuring that arrangements are made for the election of public and staff governors including:
  - establishing members entitlement to vote;
  - obtaining the necessary declarations from candidates;
  - arranging the distribution of candidates statements;
  - arranging the issue of voting papers;
  - arranging for the returning of ballot papers and the counting of votes; and
  - declaring the results of the elections.

Corporate governance:

- Continually reviewing developments in corporate governance.
- Facilitating the proper induction of directors and governors into their role.
- Advising and assisting the directors and governors with respect to their duties and responsibilities.
- Advising and facilitating board performance evaluations and any ongoing development matters resulting from that exercise.
- Counselling directors and governors when preparing presentations and memoranda.

- Ensuring the FT has a robust framework for compliance with corporate governance standards, the FT Code and recommended best practice.
- Maintaining and reviewing procedures for the sound governance of the FT and advising on developments in governance issues.
- Ensuring the FT has adequate insurance arrangements.
- Ensuring standing orders, including standing financial instructions, a scheme of delegation, and schedule of matters reserved for the board of directors and associated procedures are reviewed updated and properly discharged.

NEDs and governor development:

- Acting as a channel of communication and information for NEDs and governors.
- Advising the council of governors on an appropriate approach to reviewing board performance and facilitating an annual board evaluation for NEDs and facilitating any ongoing training highlighted.
- Management and development of the governors and their appropriate integration and interaction with the FT, including appropriate organisational development.
- Establishing arrangements for the review of effectiveness of the council of governors and developing ongoing development programme as appropriate.
- Arranging additional training and other support for directors and governors, as required.

Foundation trust seal:

- Ensuring the safe custody and proper use of any corporate seal(s).

Trust identity:

- Ensuring that all business letters, notices and other official publications of the FT show the name of the FT and any other information as required by statute.

General compliance:

- Monitoring and implementing procedures which allow for compliance with relevant regulatory and legal requirements.
- Providing advice on the impact of FT status on the terms and conditions of contracts with NHS bodies.
- Ensuring the FT implements the structures associated with the compliance and board assurance frameworks.
- Co-ordinating and submitting relevant information to other regulatory bodies, as required.
- Arranging for the FT to access a comprehensive legal service, where appropriate.
- Monitoring and reporting on compliance with the NHS Constitution.
- Ensuring any funds held in trust are used and managed appropriately.
- Reporting to the board of directors on any matters of non-compliance.

Subsidiary undertakings

- Ensuring that procedures are in place for the correct administration of any subsidiary undertakings and that correct information is given to the holding company.
- Maintaining a record of the group's structure.

Acquisitions, disposals and mergers

- Participating as a key member of the FT's management team established to implement corporate acquisitions, disposals and mergers.
- Protecting the FT's interests by ensuring the effectiveness of all documentation.
- Ensuring that due diligence disclosures enable proper commercial evaluation prior to completion of a transaction.
- Ensuring that the correct authority is in place to allow timely execution of documentation.

Fit for the future

The latest Grant Thornton research in 2018, *Is the role of company secretary fit for the future?*, identifies that the role of governance is changing and progressing and asks the question whether the role of the company secretary and those tasked with implementing governance is keeping pace. It recognises that the role was traditionally viewed as administrative but that it is now expanding in some sectors with the company secretary viewed as accountable for the embedding of effective governance practices within the organisation. The research concludes that it is clear that there is a demand for the role of the company secretary to become a strategic partner to the organisation; however, these increasing responsibilities are not always being reflected through changing resource or support. Equally, it concludes that if the legacy perception of the role as one associated with company law and administration, rather than as a key shaper of an organisation's governance framework which guides and enables effective decisions, this will undermine the authority and effectiveness of the role, and its ability to address changing expectations in society.

The research offers six questions that boards, chairs and company secretaries should ask themselves to challenge the effectiveness of the company secretary role, and ensure it is fit for the future.

1. Does your organisation support the evolution of the profile of the company secretary?
2. Is there sufficient investment, development and time to support change?
3. How does the structure of the secretarial team or company secretary reporting line influence how they are treated by the board?
4. Are the qualifications in the company secretary team the most relevant and useful to delivering good governance?

5. Could technology be used to support the company secretary in other ways apart from administration?
6. Is the size of the team sufficient for the current responsibilities of the company secretary? Is it scalable?

Governance checklist

- Are the company secretary's role and reporting lines well defined and in line with best practice?
- Does the board understand and promote the role, utilising it to provide support to the board corporately and individual directors?
- Does the company secretary have the trust and confidence of the board and possess the necessary qualifications and personal attributes for the role?
- If the company secretary's role is combined with another executive role, has the board taken steps to ensure that conflicts of interest are addressed and the independence of the company secretary maintained?
- Does the board run efficiently, with high-quality and timely information?
- Does the company secretary support the chair as leader of the board, supporting them with director induction, professional development, training and evaluation?
- Does the company secretary advise the board on all governance matters and in conjunction with the chair, periodically review the board and its committees to ensure they are fit for purpose?
- Does the company secretary take responsibility for the co-ordination of the annual report and accounts and provide quality input to the director's report, annual governance statement and other reports required to be published?
- Is the organisation's stakeholder management strategy in place and implemented by the company secretary?
- Does the company secretary manage and oversee the provision of legal services to the organisation?

Summary

- There are common issues for the role of the company secretary across both the corporate and public sectors – particularly the recognition of the value added to the organisation if the role is appropriately established at board level.
- Chairs and CEOs who have worked with high calibre company secretaries are perhaps the best advocates.
- The understanding of the role of NHS company secretaries still has some way to go in terms of profile and credibility. However, the increasing recognition of the impact of poor governance on the quality and safety of healthcare is lending an impetus to the discussion, and governance practitioners (regardless of job title) are increasingly looked upon to contribute at board level.

- The Henley/ICSA report concluded that as every organisation is different and leadership teams are unique, there is a need to build discretionary capacity into the role of company secretary. However, it went on to make some broad recommendations for large and medium-sized organisations across all sectors.
- The company secretary role should be a direct, primary reporting line to the chair and is most effective as a standalone position.
- The secretariat needs to retain independence to rebalance power as required and demonstrate accountability.
- The profile of the company secretary role needs to be raised among other board members.
- Boards need to have more open internal dialogue, so that strategy can emerge fully and be openly understood.
- Mentoring and succession planning for company secretaries needs to improve to advance junior staff into the top roles.
- The broader ICSA-qualified professional is best placed to fulfil the needs of effective boards.

14
NHS foundation trusts

Introduction

The introduction of NHS foundation trusts (FTs) in 2006 represented a significant change in the way in which hospital services were managed and provided in England. FTs were part of the government's plan for creating a patient-led NHS. The aim of the reforms was to provide high-quality care, with devolved decision-making so that they were more responsive to the needs and wishes of patients and local communities.

Whilst FTs are not, legally, subject to direction from the SoS, in recent times this has begun to shift quite significantly, with FTs coming under increasing levels of central control. The NHS Planning Guidance (December 2015) made it clear that the core elements of the Health and Social Care Act 2012 (HSCA 2012) of competition and autonomy for FTs have now been set aside. Centrally it would seem that it has now been accepted that the widespread levels of deficits, which have resulted from focusing on quality and safety in the aftermath of the Francis Report and the deteriorating financial situation both within the health service and more widely across the economy could not be resolved by provider organisations alone.

The planning guidance set out that creating a sustainable financing model would need all parts of the health economy (e.g. commissioners, providers (primary and secondary) and local authorities, working together). Consequently, this change of policy and direction, at present being fulfilled by the STP process, has led to a significant change with national bodies re-asserting control in order to get a strong grip on finances and performance. With the amalgamation of the NHS TDA and Monitor into NHSI, both NHS trusts and FTs now have the same regulatory body, which again is another example of the diminishing distinction between FTs and NHS trusts.

It remains to be seen how the FT model will continue to operate under these changes. For now, it remains a legal form of body corporate that is set out in statute (i.e. public benefit corporation) which governance practitioners need to be aware of.

The history of foundation trust status

FTs were established through the Health and Social Care (Community Health and Standards) Act 2003, consolidated into the NHS Act 2006. The other legislation outlined in Chapter 5 also applies to FTs, but should always be considered in the light of these two primary pieces of legislation. The 2006 Act provided that FTs would not be directed by government and that they would have greater freedom to decide, with their governors and members, their own strategy and the way services are run. Consequently, they had significantly greater freedoms over the way they conducted their finances. Unlike NHS trusts, FTs were able to build up operational surpluses, retain proceeds from asset sales, raise capital in the public and/or private sectors, and manage their organisations and their resources – free from central government control.

FTs are not required to break even each year, although they must be financially viable. They can borrow money within limits set by the regulator, retain surpluses and decide on service developments and innovations for their local community. The Prudential Borrowing Code, which determined the amount FTs could borrow, was repealed by HSCA 2012 with effect from 1 April 2013. This has, however, been significantly diminished as a consequence of the NHS Planning Guidance (2015) referred to above as it has established a planned health economy with centrally fixed control targets for individual parts of the NHS and where sustainability is achieved by moving money around local NHS organisations.

From 2010 onwards, it was government policy for all NHS trusts to become, or become part of, a FT by 2014. The pipeline for authorisation was overseen by Monitor during this time and this responsibility for this was taken over by the NHS TDA in 2012 with the deadline for authorisation extended to 2016. The Dalton review (see Chapter 3), published in December 2014, concluded that many of the remaining 93 NHS trusts would 'not reach the required standards in their current organisational form'. It identified new organisational forms that had the potential to be adopted by these remaining NHS trusts as an alternative to the FT model. It added that the DHSC should hold the NHS TDA (now NHSI) to account for 'meeting the trajectory and milestones for each of the 93 organisations'.

A number of NHS trusts remain, and the FT pipeline has been on indefinite hold as these trusts explore their route to sustainability through the Sustainability and Transformation Partnership process rather than the imperative to become an FT.

Local accountability and foundation trust status

The advantage of local accountability offered by the FT model is set out in the legally defined constitution FTs are obliged to adopt. It requires FTs to establish stronger connections with their local communities by encouraging people living locally to become members of the trust. The membership of each FT is therefore made up of local people (including patients and carers) and staff.

The model envisaged that FTs will be run locally, whilst remaining fully part of the NHS. They were set up as public benefit corporations, with a primary purpose to provide NHS services to NHS patients and users according to NHS principles and standards – free care based on need and not ability to pay. This is a unique legal form based on the traditions of mutuality.

FTs are accountable to:

- their local communities through their members and governors;
- their commissioners through contracts;
- Parliament (each FT must lay its annual report and accounts before Parliament);
- the CQC (through the legal requirement to register and meet the associated standards for the quality of care provided); and
- NHSI (as their regulator).

Figure 14.1 outlines the FT accountabilities as set out in the legislation.

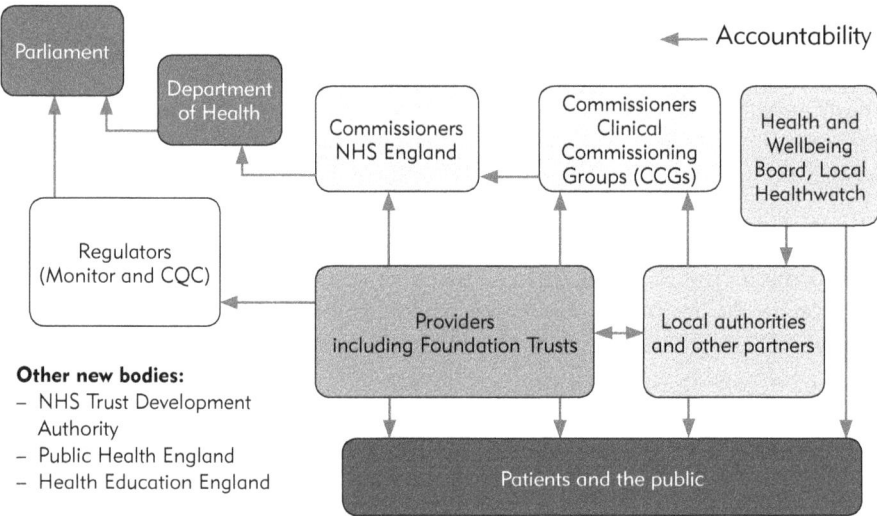

Source: NHS Providers

Figure 14.1: FT accountabilities

The legal and regulatory framework for FTs

The provider licence and reporting requirements

The HSCA 2012 also resulted in FTs becoming subject to the provider licence, the new licensing regime for health and adult social care. This replaced the earlier system of issuing terms of authorisation. In addition to the new licence conditions for all regulated services, it included an additional four conditions for FTs, which are now monitored by NHSI:

NHS FOUNDATION TRUSTS

- provision of information that the regulator has a duty to maintain on the register of NHS FTs;
- payment to the regulator in respect of any registration and related costs;
- an obligation to provide information requested by the advisory panel established by the regulator; and
- a condition that enables the regulator to continue its oversight of the governance of NHS FTs.

This fourth condition sets out the regulator's expectations that an FT has effective board and committee structures, reporting lines and performance and risk management systems. FTs did not need to apply for a licence, as the regulator agreed to license existing FTs from 1 April 2013.

Foundation Trust Licence Condition 4 allows NHSI to use reasonable evidence, from disclosures made about FTs, to determine if there is a risk of a breach of the licence condition and make a decision regarding intervention. The information NHSI will receive includes:

- a forward-looking disclosure on corporate governance (the corporate governance statement);
- a backward-looking disclosure on corporate governance (statement on compliance with the FT Code); and
- a backward-looking statement on internal control, risk and quality governance (the annual governance statement).

It is important to factor in to planning timetables that under the FT Code, the council of governors can 'expect to be consulted on the development of forward plans for the trust and any significant changes to the delivery of the trust's business plan'. The role of the council is to ensure that the interests of the FT's members are considered when establishing the strategic direction for the FT.

Other reporting requirements include the annual report and accounts and the quality account. FTs must submit its annual report and accounts to NHSI and lay them before Parliament. They cannot be presented to the FT annual members' meeting until they have been laid before parliament.

Foundation trust model core constitution

Every FT has a constitution that has been approved by the regulator upon authorisation. The constitution will set out the governance arrangements for the FT. Although each FT's constitution will be unique, there are legal requirements that apply to all FTs set out in Schedule 7 to the NHS Act 2006. These requirements are set out in FT's model core constitution, on which all FT constitutions must be based.

The constitution sets out that the principal purpose of the trust is the provision of goods and services for the purposes of the health service in England and that the trust does not fulfil this purpose unless, in each financial year, its total income from the provision of goods and services for the purposes of the health service in

England is greater than its total income from the provision of goods and services for any other purposes. The constitution also covers:

- who may be a member;
- the makeup of the council of governors and the board of directors;
- how elections of governors will be carried out;
- the statutory duties of the council and board directors;
- the grounds and procedures for the disqualification and removal of members, governors and directors;
- the requirement for open meetings of the council of governors and board of directors;
- the management of conflicts of interests;
- requirements for the disclosure of public documents and the statutory registers; and
- the management of mergers and significant transactions.

The constitution also includes a number of annexes as follows:

- the public constituency;
- the staff constituency;
- the patient constituency (if any);
- composition of the council of governors;
- the model election rules;
- additional provisions – council of governors;
- standing orders – council of governors;
- standing orders – board of directors;
- further provisions; and
- annual members' meeting.

Any changes to the constitution after authorisation must have the approval of both the board and the council. Where the amendments relate to the powers or responsibilities of the council, the constitution must also be approved by the members at a members' meeting. Amendments no longer need to be submitted to NHSI for approval.

The FT Code of Governance (FT Code)

Although the other health service governance codes and corporate governance codes set out in Chapter 6 set out best practice that FTs should consider, the primary governance code for an FT is the FT Code. Key aspects of FT governance emphasised in the Code include:

- the unitary nature of the board of directors and the collective responsibility for all aspects of the performance of the FT, including financial performance, clinical and service quality, management and governance;
- the need for at least 50% of board members to be independent NEDs;
- a recommendation to appoint a senior independent director (SID);

- an emphasis on actively developing the effectiveness of the board of directors through performance evaluation of the board, its committees and individual directors;
- clarification on the committee structure of the board of directors and the council of governors;
- clarification on the roles of the remuneration, audit and nomination committees, including a recommendation for a clear nominations process and for all members of the audit committee to be independent;
- a recommendation for evaluation of the board should be externally facilitated at least every three years. The evaluation now needs to be carried out against the Well-Led Framework;
- clarification of the need for high-quality information tailored to the board's duties and availability of access to external advice;
- a recommendation to appoint a secretary of the board of directors and the council of governors;
- the statutory duty of the council to hold the NEDs individually and collectively to account for the performance of the board of directors;
- the role of a nominated lead governor;
- the duty of the board to take steps to ensure that governors are equipped with the skills and knowledge they need to discharge their duties appropriately;
- board meetings and the annual meeting to be open to the public, with members of the public only to be excluded for special reasons; and
- recommendations to be clear on the purpose and outcomes of the relationships of the FT with other stakeholders including members, patients, the local community, commissioners and other NHS and non-NHS bodies with an interest in the local health economy.

FTs are required to set out a complete set of disclosures in respect of the FT Code within their annual report and accounts.

Foundation trust membership

Members of FTs do not receive any special treatment as NHS patients and users. They have the same access to NHS services as anyone who chooses not to become a member. The eligibility for membership of a FT is open to constituency residents, patients, and carers and staff employed by the trust, in the terms provided in each trust's constitution. All FT members can expect to receive regular information about their local trust and be consulted on plans for future development.

The model constitution sets out that an FT membership will consist of two main groupings, namely staff and public members. In addition, a third grouping of members may be included to represent patient members. These groupings are known as constituencies. Within each constituency, there may be a number of classes, which differentiate between geographical areas for public members or between staff categories for staff members. For the public constituency, the constitution must specify the area or areas; each of these areas must be an electoral area for the purposes of local government elections in England and Wales or an area consisting of two or more areas. The constitution may provide for automatic membership of the staff constituency by default.

It is for FTs to ensure they have a representative membership and sufficient members so that they can mount credible election processes. Governance arrangements for FTs need to be reflective of local conditions and proposals that work best for them.

It is this membership body made up of residents, patients and carers and staff employed by the trust, which are able to vote in the elections to appoint the council of governors of the FT. Each member, if nominated, can stand for election as a governor.

The FT Code sets out the key responsibilities of the council and the board in respect to members as follows. The board should:

- keep in touch with the opinion of members, patients and the local community in whatever ways are most practical and efficient. There must be a members' meeting at least annually;
- ensure the council has the mechanisms in place to secure and report on feedback that will enable them to fulfil their duty to represent the interests of members and the public; and
- monitor how representative the trust's membership is and the level and effectiveness of member engagement and report on this in the annual report. This information should be used to review the trust's membership strategy, taking into account any emerging best practice from the sector.

Elections

Members are able to stand as, and vote to elect, representatives to serve on the council of governors. New model council election rules were published in August 2014. The new rules allow members to vote for FT governors using e-voting technology (internet, telephone or text), initially in tandem with paper-based voting. They also set out that the Independent Elections Arbitration Panel, rather than the regulator, would determine challenges to the conduct of FT elections. The rules make provision for both first-past-the-post and single transferable voting systems.

The constitution of each trust sets out a number of criteria for disqualification for standing as a governor. For example, a person cannot be an FT governor if they are bankrupt or have served a prison sentence of three months or more during the last five years. Other grounds include, in the case of an elected governor, ceasing to be a member of the constituency they represent or, in the case of an appointed governor, the sponsoring organisation withdrawing their sponsorship of them.

Governors may not stand for election if they have previously served as a governor of the trust for a total of six years (whether such years were served consecutively or not) or if they have within the preceding two years been dismissed, otherwise than by reason of redundancy or ill health, from any paid employment with a health service body. The following persons are also not eligible to stand:

- a director of the FT itself; or
- a governor, ED, NED, chair or CEO of another health service body or a body corporate whose business involves the provision of healthcare services, including (for the avoidance of doubt) those who have a commercial interest in the affairs of the trust.

Governors are elected for a maximum of a three-year term of office under Schedule 7 to the NHS Act 2006 but there is some debate about whether they should be allowed two or three terms of office. Some FT constitutions allow for two terms so that the six-year tenure is in line with the terms of office available to NEDs, whereas others allow for three terms of office (i.e. nine-year tenures so that they are in line with the UK Code recommendations for independence of NEDS and refreshing of the board).

The latter FTs would argue that the induction and development of governors is a costly exercise and so it is a better use of taxpayers' money. They also argue that the governors are at arm's length from the FT and therefore likely to stay independent of the FT longer. This obviously depends upon the individual governor and the time commitment they make to being a governor.

All elected governors should be submitted for re-election at regular intervals.

The FT Code states:

> 'Elected governors must be subject to re-election by the members of their constituency at regular intervals not exceeding three years. The names of governors submitted for election or re-election should be accompanied by sufficient biographical details and any other relevant information to enable members to take an informed decision on their election. This should include prior performance information such as attendance records at governor meetings and other relevant events organised by the NHS FT for governors.'

Where a governor stands down mid-term, an election process for a by-election takes place meaning that the newly elected or appointed governor completes the existing term of office. The constitution will often allow a vacancy to remain until the next scheduled election process in order to minimise costs.

Foundation trust council of governors structure and its committees

The council is made up of elected governors and appointed governors. Elected governors are those members elected by the membership to represent the staff, patient and public constituencies that make up the membership of a FT. The appointed governors are the representatives from certain key stakeholders, such as local authorities that commission services from the FT. These representatives are appointed to the council to represent those stakeholder groups.

Council of governors

The primary duties of the council are to hold the NEDs individually and collectively to account for the performance of the board of directors, and to represent the interests of the members of the corporation as a whole and the interests of the public. The requirement for the council to hold the NEDs to account arises from the fact that they can appoint and remove the NEDs but not the EDs.

The council is responsible for representing the interests of the local community in the management and stewardship of the FT, and for sharing information about key decisions with other FT members. It is not responsible for the day-to-day management of the organisation such as setting budgets, staff pay and other operational matters – the oversight of that management is a matter for the board of directors. However, the council allows local residents, staff and key stakeholders to influence decisions about spending and the development of services.

The council typically meets as a full council four or five times a year. The meetings are held in public and are open to all members and the general public. The council is required to hold an annual members' meeting to receive the annual report and accounts and any report of the auditor. This meeting is often used to provide an overview of the year from the CEO.

FTs are allowed some local flexibility over the size and composition of their council. However, every council must have the following.

The chair

The chair of the FT is responsible for leadership of both the board of directors and for the council of governors. The FT Code sets out that it is the chair's responsibility to ensure that the board and the council work together effectively, but that the governors also have a responsibility to make these arrangements work. The council should take the lead in inviting the CEO or other board members to their meetings, where they may raise questions about the affairs of the trust of the chair or other board members.

The lead governor

NHSI and the FT Code recommends that the council appoint a lead who has a role in certain circumstances where it would not be appropriate for the chair to contact NHSI, or NHSI to contact the chair (e.g. in relation to appointment of the chair). Communication would instead take place between the lead governor and NHSI in such circumstances. Routine communication from NHSI to governors is disseminated through the FT secretary.

The main circumstances where NHSI will contact a lead governor are where the regulator has concerns as to the quality of the board leadership at an FT, which may lead to the use of its formal powers to remove the chair or NEDs. As the council appoints the chair and NEDs, NHSI would want to consult with the governors as to the capacity and capability of these individuals to lead the trust, to rectify any issues successfully, and for the governors to understand NHSI's concerns. The other situation where NHSI may wish to contact the lead governor is where it has concerns that the process for the appointment of the chair or other members of the board, or elections for governors, may not have complied with the FT's constitution, or alternatively may be inappropriate. NHSI suggests: 'The lead governor should take steps to understand NHSI's role, the available guidance and the basis on which NHSI may take regulatory action. The lead governor will then be able to communicate more widely with other governors.'

The existence of a lead governor does not, in itself, prevent any governor from contacting NHSI directly if they feel it is necessary. The term lead governor is used to prevent confusion with the deputy chair of the board of directors who is a NED. The council should choose the lead governor, who should not deputise for the deputy chair of the board of directors.

Public governors
More than half of the members of the council are to be elected by members of the trust other than those who come within the staff constituency. Therefore, there must be a majority of public and patient governors.

Staff governors
At least three governors should represent staff.

Appointed governors
At least one member of the council is to be appointed by one or more local authorities which covers the whole or part of an area specified in the constitution as a public constituency. If any of the trust's hospitals includes a medical or dental school provided by a university, at least one member of the council is to be appointed by that university. An FT may also specify other organisations within its constitution as a partnership organisation who may also appoint a member of the council.

The HSCA 2012 abolished the requirement for a primary care trust (PCT) governor and there is no requirement for a CCG representative to be appointed as a governor. Trusts may wish to nominate a specified commissioner as an organisation for the purposes of appointing a governor.

The nomination committee
The council has a similar committee structure to that of the board of directors to fulfil its role of appointing (or removing) the chair and other NEDs. The FT Code sets out that the council is responsible at a general meeting for the appointment, reappointment and removal of the chair and the other NEDs. It should agree with the nominations committee a clear process for the nomination of a new chair and

NEDs. Once suitable candidates have been identified the nominations committee should make recommendations to the council.

The FT Code describes two scenarios for the role of the council in the appointment of NEDs:

> 'In FTs there may be one or two nominations committees. If there are two committees, one will be responsible for considering nominations for EDs and the other for NEDs (including the chair) ... Where a FT has two nominations committees, the nominations committee responsible for the appointment of NEDs should consist of a majority of governors. If only one nominations committee exists, when nominations for NEDs, including the appointment of a chair or a deputy chair, are being discussed, there should be a majority of governors on the committee and also a majority governor representation on the interview panel.'

The chair or an independent NED should chair the nominations committee(s). At the discretion of the committee, a governor can chair the committee in the case of appointments of NEDs or the chair. A person may only be appointed as a NED or chair if they are a member of the public constituency (or the patient constituency, if there is one). Where the trust has a university medical or dental school, a person may be appointed as a NED if they exercise functions for that organisation.

Upon receiving a recommendation to appoint, the council should consider the qualifications, skills and experience required: for the appointment of a chair; they should also consider the time commitment required. The FT Code stipulates that 'no individual, simultaneously while being a chair of an NHS FT, should be the substantive chair of another NHS FT'.

In accordance with the FT's constitution, appointment is by a majority of the governors attending the relevant meeting. Removal requires the approval of three-quarters of the members of the council, not just those in attendance.

Remuneration committee

The council is also responsible for setting the remuneration of NEDs and the chair. The council should consult external professional advisers to market-test the remuneration levels of the chair and other NEDs at least once every three years and when it intends to make a material change to the remuneration of a NED. Levels of remuneration for the chair and other NEDs should reflect the time commitment and responsibilities of their roles. The 2018/19 NHS Providers research shows that the average salary for an FT chair is £43,465 and for an FT NED it is £11,350.

The council may delegate the task of market testing to a remuneration committee consisting solely of governors. Chairing this committee would often be the responsibility of the lead governor if one has been appointed; if not, the council may appoint a chair. The committee then makes its recommendation back to the council for decision.

The committee is required to make a report of its activities in the FT's annual report and accounts. This is in line with the reports required of FTs and NHS trusts; likewise, the report must include the relationship between the remuneration of the highest-paid director in their organisation and the median remuneration of the organisation's workforce, in line with the Hutton Fair Pay Review.

Appointment of auditors

The council should take the lead in agreeing with the audit committee the criteria for appointing, re-appointing and removing external auditors. The council will need to work hard to ensure they have the skills and knowledge to choose the right external auditor and monitor their performance. However, they should be supported in this task by the audit committee, which provides information to the governors on the external auditor's performance as well as overseeing the FT's internal financial reporting and internal auditing.

As part of the appointment process, the FT is required to ensure the appointed auditors meet the criteria set out by NHSI. The auditors must agree the terms of engagement with the FT in a letter of engagement. The auditors must resign if they fail to meet or have cause to believe that they will not be able to comply with, the criteria set out in the terms of authorisation at any point during their appointment. FTs must provide NHSI with details of their auditors on authorisation and whenever a change to the auditors is made. This information should include the name and address of the organisation. When an auditor's appointment ends, the auditor is required to write to the FT and to NHSI giving notice of resignation and setting out a statement of the circumstances or stating that there are none.

As an important independence point for FT auditors, no member of the audit team may be a member or governor of the FT (Audit Code 2011). The board of directors' audit committee should make recommendations to the council about the appointment, re-appointment and removal of the external auditor, as well as the approval of the remuneration and terms of engagement of the external auditor. The council may delegate the work involved to an auditor appointments committee, made up of governors and could be chaired by the chair of the audit committee, before making its recommendation to the council for decision.

If the council does not accept the recommendation, it should include in the annual report a statement from the audit committee explaining the recommendation and should set out reasons why the council has taken a different position. When the council ends an external auditor's appointment in disputed circumstances, the chair should write to NHSI informing it of the reasons behind the decision.

Approval of the appointment of the CEO

It is for the NEDs to appoint and remove the CEO; however, the appointment of a CEO does require the approval of the council. The guide Your Statutory Duties: A reference guide for NHS foundation trust governors (August 2013) which reflects the roles and responsibilities of governors as set out in the HSCA 2012 sets out a clear process for engaging with the council to reduce the likelihood of the governors not giving their approval.

The NEDs should make sure that the governors are kept informed about the appointment process, ensuring that the governors are satisfied with the various stages of the process such as use of advertisements, the criteria for selection and how selection was carried out.

To give their approval, the council needs to be confident that the appointment process has identified a candidate with sufficient experience to fulfil all essential aspects of the job description and that the process has been fair, open and transparent. The council should receive a report setting out that due law and process has been followed, as well as detailing how the proposed candidate's skills and experience meet the agreed role and person specification. The primary responsibility for the appointment lies with the NEDs, and the council should only withhold its approval with good cause.

If approval is withheld, the council must set out their reasons to the chair and the other NEDs. The reasons for withholding approval must be justifiable, as there are likely to be financial consequences. The process, the decision and the reasons for the decision should be set out in the FT's annual report, whatever the outcome.

Liabilities of the council of governors

NHSI has recognised that councils may be concerned about the level of liability they are taking on, particularly when it exercises powers in relation to significant transactions. Councils may be concerned that they will be held responsible if a transaction damages the trust, financially or otherwise.

Although the NHS Act 2006, as amended, does not make explicit reference to governors' liability in this regard, the regulator has made it clear in its guidance on transactions that the council's duty to 'hold the NEDs, individually and collectively to account for the performance of the board of directors' does not mean that councils are responsible for the decision itself, or the operational detail behind it. Responsibility for a decision remains with the board of directors, acting on behalf of the FT. FTs are not required to provide an indemnity for the council, or insurance to cover a governor's individual service on the council.

Duties, rights and powers of the council of governors

The statutory duties of the council are set out in the NHS Act 2006 and HSCA 2012. They are further expanded in the guidance *Your Statutory Duties: A Reference*

NHS FOUNDATION TRUSTS

Guide for NHS Foundation Trust Governors. It should be recognised that these publications set out the baseline in terms of duties, rights and powers; how these are fulfilled in practical terms is open to a great deal of local interpretation. There is also a great deal of helpful guidance on best practice set out in the Foundation Trust Network (FTN) and DAC Beachcroft publication *The Foundations of Good Governance – A Compendium of Good Practice* (2015). The following sections set out the statutory duties of governors, which are essential as an introduction to the role of the council.

The NHS Act 2006 set out that the statutory duties of the council are to:

- appoint and, if appropriate, remove the chair and NEDs;
- decide the remuneration and other allowances of the chair and NEDs;
- approve the appointment of the CEO;
- appoint and, if appropriate, remove the trust's auditor; and
- receive the annual accounts, auditor report and annual report.

The HSCA 2012 sets out the general duty of the council to hold the NEDs, individually and collectively, to account for the performance of the board of directors. It also has the general duty to represent the interests of the members of the trust as a whole and the interests of the public. HSCA 2012 also gave the council additional rights and powers to:

- require one or more of the directors to attend a governors' meeting for the purpose of obtaining information about the trust's performance of its functions or the directors' performance of their duties (and for deciding whether to propose a vote on the trust's or directors' performance);
- approve 'significant transactions' (i.e. at least half of the governors voting agree with the transaction). The trust may choose to include a description of 'significant transactions' in the trust's constitution (see section below);
- approve an application by the trust to enter into a merger, acquisition, separation or dissolution. In this case, approval means at least half of all governors agree with the application;
- to decide whether the trust's private patient work would significantly interfere with the trust's principal purpose (i.e. the provision of goods and services for the health service in England or the performance of its other functions);
- approve any proposed increases in private patient income of 5% or more in any financial year. Approval means at least half of the governors voting agree with the increase; and
- approve any amendments to the trust's constitution. Approval means at least half of the governors voting agree with the amendments.

In addition, HSCA 2012 created the following additional responsibilities:

- Before each board meeting, the board of directors must send a copy of the agenda to the governors. After the meeting, the board of directors must send a

copy of the minutes to the governors. The trust must take steps to ensure that governors have the skills and knowledge they require to undertake their role.
- The regulator gains the power to establish a panel of persons to which a governor can refer questions as to whether the trust has failed or is failing to act in accordance with its constitution. The council must first approve the referral. Approval means at least half of the governors voting agree with the referral.
- The trust must hold annual members' meetings. At least one of the directors must present the trust's annual report and accounts to the members at this meeting.
- Where there has been an amendment to the constitution which relates to the powers, duties or roles of the council, at least one governor must attend the next annual members' meeting and present the amendment to the members. Members have the right to vote on and veto these types of constitutional amendments.

Foundation trusts and significant transactions

An FT can decide for itself what constitutes a 'significant transaction' and may choose to define this in its constitution. Alternatively, if the governors agree, FTs may choose not to give a definition, but this would need to be stated in the constitution. Examples of a definition include any proposed contract valued over a certain monetary threshold or over a certain percentage of the trust's annual turnover, or alternatively using non-monetary terms. If an FT defines some types of transaction as 'significant' in the terms of their constitution, then the FT will need the consent of more than half of the council to proceed with the transaction. However, the consent of more than half of the governors will always be required for any merger, acquisition or separation of the FT. Unlike 'significant transactions', this is not an optional requirement, and this means that, in practice, responsibility for signing off any merger or acquisition moves jointly to the directors and governors.

An increasing number of FTs may plan transactions (including mergers, acquisitions, significant investments, joint ventures and divestments) as they seek to reorganise or respond to changes required within their STP.

> '[W]hile integration remains the current "buzzword", it need not necessarily imply organisational integration through a transaction such as a merger or acquisition. Improved outcomes may equally be achieved through improved collaboration arrangements between partners. These arrangements may take the form of joint ventures, networks, chains or partnerships. In legal terms these arrangements can be set up either contractually through partners entering into one, a series of contracts with each other or through the creation of new corporate vehicles for service delivery which are jointly owned by the partners.'
>
> (New Care Models – Governance between organisations (Hempsons and NHS Providers))

The latest transactions and mergers guidance from NHSI (November 2017) recognises that potential transactions where the ratio of the gross assets, income or consideration attributable to the transaction exceeds 10% of the trust's gross assets, income or total capital respectively is classified as 'material' or 'significant'. The guidance recommends early engagement with NHSI to support such transactions and set out the processes to be followed.

In addition the Competition and Markets Authority (CMA) reviews certain transactions involving one or more FTs (including mergers between an FT and an NHS trust) to determine whether the transaction is likely to have adverse effects on patients by reducing competition between providers. FTs can also approach the CMA for informal advice on whether the transaction is within its jurisdiction (seeking informal advice from the CMA will not automatically trigger a review of the transaction).

Responsibilities of directors and the council in transactions are shown in Table 14.1. A council should be provided with as much information as reasonably possible for it to be able to make an informed judgement. To ensure that the council has sufficient information and is assured that the board has been through a thorough and comprehensive process before voting on the transaction, the council's formal vote should take place after the finalisation of due diligence reports and soon after the board's approval.

This places the councils' vote shortly before completion in the process, after the full business case stage. The vote should, however, take place before the trust's formal application to NHSI (required for statutory transactions), since council approval must be obtained before NHSI can grant the application. In deciding whether to approve a transaction, the council is deciding whether the board of directors has:

- been thorough and comprehensive in reaching its decision to transact; and
- obtained and considered the interests of foundation trust members and the public as part of the decision-making process.

However, it's important to note that the decision to proceed with a transaction is ultimately determined by the board of directors. It has the power under the foundation trust's constitution to exercise all the powers of the foundation trust and provided appropriate assurance is obtained on the two points above, the council should not unreasonably withhold its approval for the transaction to go ahead.

Where a new organisation is formed as the result of a merger, the timings of making appointments to the new board of that organisation needs to be carefully considered, particularly where governors need to be elected in order for such appointments to be made. Transitional arrangements are likely to be required in FT constitutions to transition the various constituencies and ensure they are reflective of the patients served by the enlarged organisation.

Once the council has approved a transaction and the chair has confirmed that it is not confidential, the council should communicate the result to the FT members and the public. Councils are likely to need the FT's help to do so, for example, through its website or at an advertised drop-in session with the governors. The communication method should be agreed locally.

Executive directors	**Non-executive directors**	**Council**
Executive directors should make proposals for the future of the organisation. They should work with governors by providing them with sufficient information on a proposed transaction for the purposes of considering their required approval. They should explain to the council why they believe the transaction is necessary and provide evidence to support their view.	NEDs should challenge the executives to justify their recommendations, deal with the risks involved and seek assurance that the executive directors' decisions are the right ones.	The council must approve any statutory or significant transactions. The council is responsible for satisfying itself that the board of directors (that is, executive and NEDs collectively) has been thorough and comprehensive in reaching its proposal (that is, has undertaken proper due diligence) and that it has obtained and considered the interests of trust members and the public as part of the decision-making process. Provided appropriate assurance is obtained, the council should not unreasonably withhold its consent for a proposal to go ahead.

Table 14.1: Responsibilities of directors and governors in transactions

The material set out here around significant transactions will become increasingly important as STPs progress with their plans as it should be reasonably clear that STPs will involve some quite significant change for FTs and that their governors will need to be consulted. Substantial and open engagement with the council will be necessary to enable it to fulfil its statutory role of holding to account and representing members and the wider public. Such engagement will of course form part of a much wider public consultation process, but if that consultation is to be meaningful, it must allow for the possibility of plans being changed by that consultation process. One of the very valid criticisms of many STPs has been limited engagement and consultation. FT boards would be wise to include the involvement of their council sooner rather than later.

The implications of these changes will require additional training and development for the council in their new role and a much more effective working relationship between the board of directors and council. Care will also be required in the definition of 'significant transactions', otherwise FTs will find they regularly have to seek council approval on more minor or less significant proposals. Judgement will have to be exercised where a number of minor transactions could in fact warrant the attention of the council as collectively, they represent a 'significant transaction'.

NHS Providers has a developed a national governor training programme called GovernWell to support FTs in their statutory obligation to ensure that the council has the skills and knowledge it requires to carry out its role.

Codes of conduct for governors

The Stewardship Standard for Governors of NHS FTs was developed during 2012 amongst governance practitioners, as part of the North West Company Secretary Network hosted by Hill Dickinson. The standard is not copyrighted and is in free circulation.

This voluntary Stewardship Standard sets out good practice on engagement with FTs and provides an opportunity for the high-quality dialogue needed between councils and boards to underpin good governance. The standard describes actions that councils can take to ensure that they fulfil their statutory duties. For example, at least once every three years the council could seek independent assurance to satisfy themselves, to the extent possible, that the FT board is effective and that NEDs provide adequate oversight of the FT. This is in line with the requirements of the Well-Led Framework, which is set out in more detail later. It also suggests that councils could use a wide range of activities to listen to the views of their local communities and reflect them back to the FT, ensuring these views are considered by the board in the development of the FT's annual plan. It makes it clear that the principal relationships between council and the board are via the chair and other NEDs, in relation to the board being held to account. The council will depend upon the CEO and other EDs for information updates on a regular basis.

Appropriate application of the Stewardship Standard should assist councils of governors to avoid taking on a role in which the council directs management, and therefore it ensures that individual governors do not take on the role of shadow directors unintentionally. There are also several other locally determined codes of conduct and published guidance. For example, there is a sample code of conduct in the aforementioned FTN/Beachcroft publication *The Foundations of Good Governance – A Compendium of Good Practice* (2015).

Foundation trust board structure and its committees

The DH's Guide to NHS Foundation Trusts (2002) sets out that the governance of FTs was to be based on experience in other sectors, as the following extracts demonstrate:

> 'The new governance arrangements for NHS FTs have been modelled on cooperative societies and mutual organisations. These combine community

ownership with accountability. NHS FTs will herald a new form of social ownership where health services are owned by and accountable to local people rather than central Government. In this way, much stronger connections will be established between providers of NHS services and their stakeholder communities ... In a similar way to becoming a member of a co-operative society or mutual organisation, the members of an NHS FT will become its owners, taking on responsibility for their local hospitals from national Government.'

The guidance for FTs establishes that they are to be accountable to their members. This accountability is underpinned by the aforementioned establishment of a council in addition to the board of directors, as shown in Figure 14.2. This not a two-tier governance structure as seen in Germany and discussed in Chapter 7. Rather, it refers to the council' oversight role alongside the unitary role of the board of directors, which is unusual in British public services or in corporate models of governance. There is evidence that the structure has led to confusion and conflict, but there has also been a significant amount of development work to clarify the role and powers of the board and the council, and how they relate to one another.

The HSCA 2012 set out a requirement that all FT board meetings be held in public. Boards need to decide which papers and minutes should be discussed in public session. The ability to meet in closed session is still available for confidential or commercially sensitive matters. Boards should strive to deal with as much business as possible in the public part of the meeting. They should be guided by the exemptions in the FOIA 2000 in deciding where to draw the line with regard to information not in the public domain.

Board composition

Under the NHS Act 2006, the FT is to have a board of directors comprising both EDs and NEDs. The board must have a non-executive chair, [*] other NEDs; and [*] EDs ([*] denotes a number to be inserted at the trust's discretion). One of the EDs must be the CEO and they must be the accounting officer. One of the EDs must be the finance director. One of the EDs must be a registered medical practitioner or a registered dentist (within the meaning of the Dentists Act 1984). One of the EDs must be a registered nurse or a registered midwife.

The general duty of the board of directors, and of each director individually, is to act with a view to promoting the success of the corporation so as to maximise the benefits for the members of the corporation as a whole and for the public. The board is directly accountable through the council to trust membership and the wider community. The authority of the board is derived from Schedule 7 to the NHS Act 2006, as amended by HSCA 2012. Schedule 7 states that the constitution must provide for all the powers of the corporation (the FT) to be exercisable by the board directors on its behalf. Any of those powers may, however, be delegated to a committee of directors or to an ED.

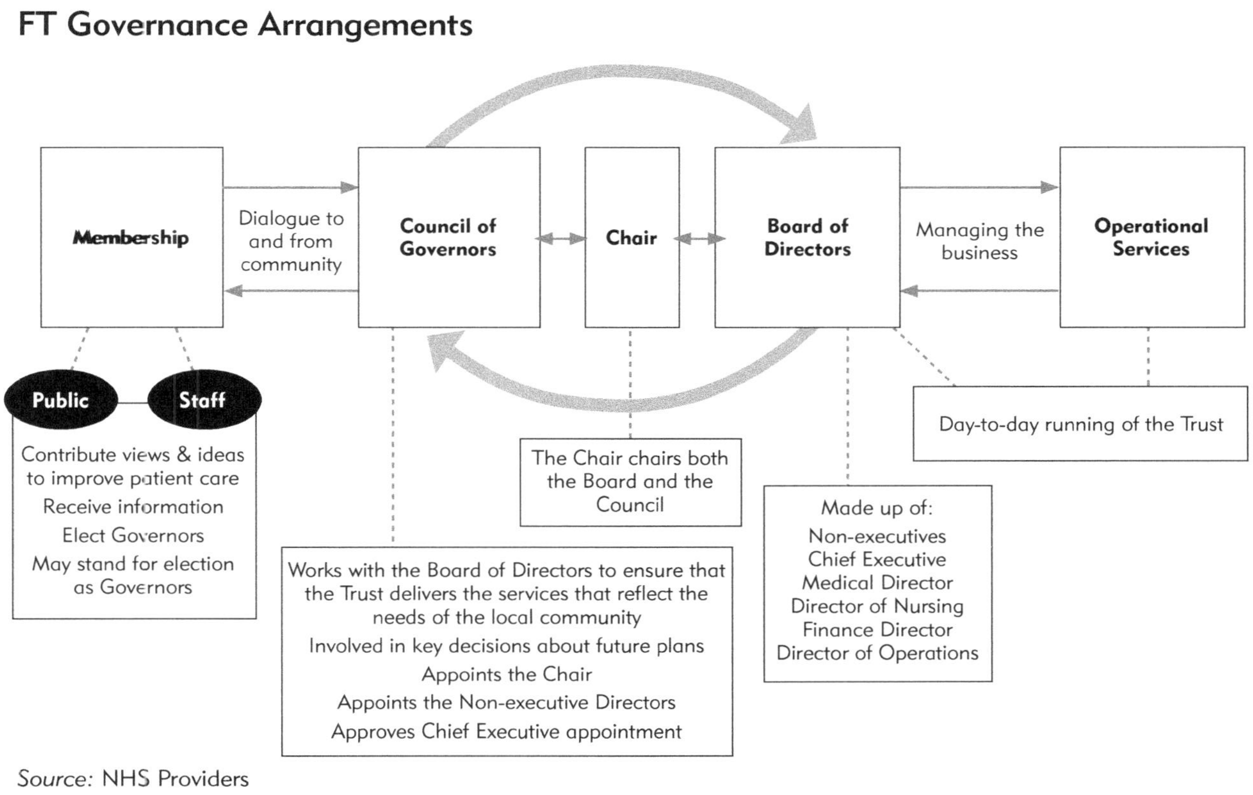

NHS FOUNDATION TRUSTS

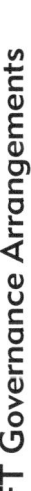

Figure 14.2: Foundation trust governance arrangements

The FT Code recommends that FTs have a schedule of matters reserved for board decision.

Board committees

Under Schedule 7, FT boards may only delegate authority to a committee of directors or to an ED. Committees that have formal memberships that include non-board members cannot have powers delegated to them by the board, and neither can individual NEDs.

FTs are required to establish an audit committee, a nomination committee and a remuneration committee. They may establish other committees as required, such as a quality assurance committee.

The FT Code allows for the establishment of separate NED and governor committees for both nomination and remuneration purposes – dealing with NED appointments and remuneration, and ED appointments and remuneration respectively. Where there is just one nomination and remuneration committee, the membership changes depending upon whether it is considering a NED or ED appointment.

The role of the nomination and remuneration committees for ED appointments/remuneration and the audit committee is in line with the details set out in Chapters 8, 11 and 18 respectively. The role of the nomination and remuneration committees for NED appointments is set out later in this chapter.

The Audit Code for Foundation Trusts (2011) gives the FT audit committee the responsibility for monitoring and ensuring the independence of the external auditors. If the external auditors provide non-audit services to the organisation, the annual report should explain how auditor independence and objectivity are safeguarded.

The auditors of an FT have a primary responsibility to the FT's council. Such auditors may also be responsible to NHSI for the exercise of some functions and will have responsibilities to the members of the FT, as well as the wider public, in the case of public interest reports.

Auditors of FTs are also required to review the organisation's compliance with the FT Code, and to obtain evidence to support the organisation's compliance statement (in the annual report and accounts) of its compliance with the code. In addition, external auditors of FTs are currently required to satisfy themselves that the quality report has been prepared according to the detailed guidance issued by NHSI.

Statutory duties of a foundation trust director

The HSCA 2012 introduced into the NHS Act 2006 provisions on the duties of NHS FT directors. While some of these duties simply amount to a re-statement of the common law in this area, others are new and were intended to address concerns on the need for transparency in the conduct of the business of NHS FT boards. The changes are contained in section 152 of HSCA 2012 and are:

- a general duty of the board, and of each director individually, to act with a view to promoting the success of the corporation so as to maximise the benefits for the members of the corporation as a whole and for the public;
- the duties of NHS FT directors to avoid conflicts of interest and duty, and not to accept benefits from third parties in connection with their directorship;
- the duty to declare any interest that a director may have in relation a proposed transaction with their FT and provides for exceptions to the duty;
- new requirements for an NHS FT board to send a copy of the agenda of its meeting to the council prior to the holding the meeting to which the agenda relates, and send a copy of the minutes of its meeting to the council as soon as practicable after the holding of the meeting to which those minutes relate; and
- the duty of the board to ensure that the constitution of its NHS FT provides for board meetings to be open to members of the public. The provision permits exceptions to be provided for in an NHS FT's constitution in relation to this requirement.

In addition, directors have a role under HSCA 2012 in approving constitutional changes (alongside governors), and a duty to equip governors with the skills they need to do their job.

ICSA welcomed these new duties in its March 2011 memorandum to Parliament 'as [section 152(1) and (2)] makes explicit the step change from being a senior manager to being an ED, and brings the duties of FT directors in line with the private sector'.

The FT Code also specifies that directors on the board of directors, and governors on the council, should meet the 'fit and proper' persons test described in the provider licence and required by the CQC. Developments in this area have been covered in Chapters 8 and 9.

Maintaining an effective foundation trust board

The chair of the board and the council

Under Schedule 7 to the NHS Act 2006, the chair is responsible for leadership of both the board of directors and the council. The governors are also given a responsibility under the FT Code to make the arrangements between the board and the council work. The council should take the lead in inviting the CEO to their meetings and inviting attendance by other EDs as appropriate. In these meetings, other members of the council may raise questions of the chair or the deputy chair, or any other relevant director present at the meeting about the affairs of the FT.

Though the council has a statutory duty to appoint the chair and NEDs, they also have a duty to hold the NEDs (including the chair) to account for the performance of the board. This means that there can be a blurring of the role of the chair, who would normally be responsible for appraising and managing the NEDs. Indeed, the appraisal and line management of NEDs has previously been the responsibility of the chair, and this presents a potential conflict for the chair in their dual role of chair of both bodies. The council is supported in this role by their power to require directors to attend a meeting to obtain information about their organisation's performance and that of its directors. FT chairs and governors will have to consider how they work together to hold the NEDs to account. There is also a clear role for the SID in supporting the council in holding the chair to account.

The dual role of the chair exposes the chair to ongoing conflicts of interest. With the increasing power of the council, the chair's role will be crucial, and it will require high levels of interpersonal and listening skills.

Under the existing powers the council could, if it was dissatisfied with performance, remove the chair or the NEDs. This, however, must be handled sensitively and in accordance with the law. The council should initially liaise informally with NHSI over its concerns after exhausting all informal and internal mechanisms, before moving to a formal dismissal proposal at a council meeting. The council will require the support of the lead governor, SID and company secretary in these circumstances.

The foundation trust company secretary

Most of the conversations around the role of the company secretary (see Chapter 13) are applicable to the FT company secretary. However, some specific aspects of the company secretary role are critical for the FT model.

In the FT Code, NHSI recommends the 'appointment of a secretary to the board of directors and the board of governors' and states that 'a FT secretary has a significant role to play in the administration of corporate governance'. Ham and Hunt's 2008 report, *Membership Governance in NHS Foundation Trusts: A review for the Department of Health*, also argues that 'the company secretary has a key role in governance [for the FT]'.

Specific FT duties include establishing and monitoring procedures to ensure that the trust complies with:

- the requirements of the NHS Act 2006;
- its licence conditions;
- its constitution; and
- its standing orders.

Duties also include acting as the initial point of contact between the board of directors, the council and the regulator as set out above. The role also involves supporting the chair in managing the potential conflicts and tensions created by the duality of their role. FT secretaries provide administrative and governance resources for the effective operation of both the board and the council, including any council committees or working groups.

The role also quite often includes ensuring that arrangements are in place for the board and council to communicate effectively with members through a variety of means and supporting the governors in communicating and engaging with members. The other distinction for the company secretary role is in overseeing the effective arrangements for the election of public, patient and staff governors including by-elections, as required.

The role of the FT company secretary is to be a fundamental support for the FT chair by offering 'a sophisticated understanding of the political dynamics at play within the governance structure'. Equally, the company secretary will be the senior manager to whom the governors and members relate. They will be a useful player in helping to manage the relationships between stakeholders, and act as an early warning for the chair when issues arise.

The FT Code requires that the appointment and removal of the FT secretary is a joint matter for the CEO and chair.

The foundation trust governance challenge

Despite the changing scope and freedom of FTs, the governance structure is still the statutory form required for public benefit corporation and it would seem there is little political appetite at present to unpick the current structure. Understanding the challenges and tensions created by the governance structure of an FT will assist governance practitioners as they navigate STPs and the new models of care.

The ICSA memorandum to Parliament (March 2011) still offers a relevant synopsis of the challenge.

> 'FTs still have to operate a governance framework unique within the UK economy and one that presents its own challenges and costs. The additional layer of governance inherent within the dynamic between the council of governors and the board of directors will impact on financial and non-financial resources. The dual nature of the decision-making process on specific areas of business development disadvantages FTs as their governance and accountability framework is more cumbersome operating an almost two-tier board approach.'

Balancing the tension in the foundation trust board's general duty

The HSCA 2012 states: 'The general duty of the board of directors, and of each director individually, is to act with a view to promoting the success of the corporation so as to maximise the benefits for the members of the corporation as a whole and for the public.' This has been taken by some to mean that FTs cannot engage in the collaborative processes under the STP umbrella since this might require the FT board to put the broader interest of patients and public in direct opposition to promoting the success of the corporation in the short term. However, it can also be argued that the long-term success of the STP will maximise benefits for patients and the public and this requires the board to take a broader approach.

Who owns the foundation trust?

Ultimately, health service governance is concerned with the practices and procedures to ensure that the individual parts of the NHS are run in such a way that they achieve their objectives, as well as being in line with public sector values such as VFM and providing universal and free healthcare benefits to all those in need. This provides an interesting contrast to the objectives of a company in the private sector, where the aim is to maximise the wealth of its owners (the shareholders) subject to various guidelines and constraints and with regard to other groups or individuals with an interest in what the company does.

The question for FTs relates to ownership, and therefore who sets the objectives for the organisation. Who owns the NHS organisation and the healthcare services it provides? The governance structure of FTs has attempted to articulate the answer to this question: the FT is accountable to its members and therefore should be governed according to their interests.

The changes proposed by the HSCA 2012 reinforce this view by further empowering governors (the representatives of the members). This only emphasises the largest health service governance issue for FTs – how to establish an effective relationship between the members and their elected representatives. If a governor is not representing the interests of the members who elected them, then there must be clear procedures about how such a governor might be removed. The constitution currently sets out grounds for disqualification, but these do not include failure to act in the interests of the members.

It is not appropriate to liken the members of an FT to the shareholders of a listed company, as this does not reflect the complexity and breadth of the diversity of interests that are represented by FT members (although there are limited grounds for viewing the governors as proxy shareholders). In other words, the members authorise governors to speak and act for them in respect of the business of the FT. The challenge for FTs has been how to ensure that governors are aware of, and informed by, the healthcare concerns of their respective constituencies and the members they represent.

In addition, there are a considerable number of other arrangements that already exist to provide patient and public involvement and scrutiny of NHS decision making, such as Healthwatch and local government overview and scrutiny committees.

Capacity and capability of governors

The HSCA 2012 significantly extended the role of the council. This raises a number of questions around their capacity and capability; many governors are likely to require significant training to understand and be able to discharge their duties. The increased responsibilities may also reduce or limit the number of people who are willing to fill the role.

ICSA's March 2011 memorandum to Parliament states:

> 'Significant resources will have to be made available to governors in order to hold the board of directors to account and understand the competitive market when asked to vote on significant transactions. The requirements on governors are going to be onerous, and councils of governors will require at least some, if not all, of their number to have the financial and commercial skills to evaluate FT proposals in relation to mergers, acquisitions and other significant transactions ... There is also concern as to how governors can reconcile their role as representatives of the membership and play a significant part in the strategic decision-making process.'

This challenge has become increasingly an issue as discussions progress on STPs, vanguards, new models of care etc. FTs can seize the opportunities for local accountability and community engagement that an active and functional council can offer, however, it does take considerable resources (in terms of management time and capacity) to support and develop the council in this manner, which may not be prioritised by FT boards in the current financial context.

Training and support for governors

NHS Providers delivers the national training programme (GovernWell) for governors as well as a broader range of support for governors and FT staff that work to support governors.

Governance checklist

- Is the board aware of how the FT's compliance with its licence is assessed by NHSI? In particular, does it understand the requirements of FT licence Condition 4?
- Does the board review the requirements of the FT Code to ensure it is compliant?
- Has the FT's constitution been properly approved by the board and council (and members if required)?
- Are the board and council confident that the terms of the constitution are in line with HSCA 2012 and that they are followed? How would they become aware of a breach of the constitution?
- Are all FT board meetings held in public?
- Are the statutory board and council committees properly constituted?
- Are the directors aware of their duties under HSCA 2012?
- How does the board keep in touch with members, patients and the local community?
- How do governors secure and report back on feedback that will enable them to fulfil their duty to represent the interests of members and the public?

- How representative is the trust's membership? Is the representation and effectiveness of member engagement report in the annual report?
- Have all governors been elected in accordance with the model election rules?
- Are the governors actively involved in developing the recruitment and appointment process for new NEDs?
- Are the governors aware of the extent of their authority and powers and the purposes for which they have been granted? Is there an induction and development programme for governors in place?
- When is the Well-Led Developmental Review scheduled?
- Does the board and council business programme allow for the FT reporting requirements to be considered in a timely manner?
- Has the FT defined a significant transaction?

Summary

- The unique governance structure of FTs – the membership, the council and the board – has its own specific role to play in an FT's governance arrangements. However, the closer working together of NHSI and the CQC means that many of the regulatory requirements are now the same for FTs and NHS trusts.
- The original concepts for FTs – increased autonomy, freedom from central government and greater local accountability – are still yet to be fully achieved, rather they seem to be diminishing.
- The creation of FTs has not solved the financial or clinical sustainability challenges that the NHS faces. While the private income cap has been lifted, the complexity and immaturity of the current commissioning structures make it hard for FTs to plan and operate strategically despite NHSI's best efforts.
- The new direction of collaboration brought in by STPs seems to cut completely through the concepts of provider/commissioner split and competitive market of earlier government policy.
- In addition, the regulatory burden continues to grow and the response to challenges such as A&E waiting times and financial deficits results in a somewhat hands-on management approach from the SoS and NHSI.
- Consequently, FTs still continue to look towards their regulator and the DHSC rather than to the local population and its representatives.

15
Clinical commissioning groups

Introduction

CCGs are responsible for commissioning secondary and community care services; they have a legal duty to support quality improvement in primary care. Most of the NHS commissioning budget is now managed by CCGs. These are groups of general practices which come together in each area to enable general practitioners (GPs), working with other health professionals, to commission services for their local communities. CCGs are different entities from previous NHS arrangements, with each GP practice being a member and clinicians leading commissioning decisions. The CCG consists of its member practices; the members are the authority and they appoint a governing body to act on their behalf.

The services that CCGs commission include:

- most community health services;
- mental health services;
- learning disability and/or autism services;
- planned hospital care;
- rehabilitative care; and
- urgent and emergency care (including out-of-hours and NHS 111).

The CCG's overarching duty to involve patients and the public is outlined in Chapter 5. However, the HSCA 2012 imposed further duties on CCGs. In summary, these requirements the duties of the CCG are to:

- exercise its functions effectively, efficiently and economically;
- obtain appropriate advice;
- promote education and training;
- promote integration;
- promote the NHS Constitution;
- promote innovation in the provision of health services (including innovation in the arrangements made for their provision);
- promote patient choice;
- promote research on matters relevant to the health service, and the use in the health service of evidence obtained from research;
- reduce inequalities in respect of access and outcomes; and

- secure continuous improvement in the quality of services provided or in the prevention, diagnosis or treatment of illness (quality is defined as the effectiveness and safety of the services, and the quality of the experience undergone by patients).

A CCG also has a general financial duty to:

- ensure its expenditure does not exceed the aggregate of its allotments for the financial year;
- ensure its use of resources does not exceed the amount specified by NHSE for the financial year;
- take account of any directions issued in respect of specified types of resource used in a financial year to ensure the CCG does not exceed an amount specified by NHSE; and
- publish an explanation of how the CCG spent any payment in respect of quality made to it by the NHSE.

Commissioning decisions can affect numerous services and over wide geographical areas. CCGs are increasingly working together to commission services across their local populations and deliver economies of scale. In many areas, CCGs are now sharing staff or have shared management structures and some have established new governance arrangements to support joint commissioning, such as joint committees or boards. These arrangements are often accompanied by the pooling of commissioning budgets. Engaging with local authorities, the voluntary sector as well as community and social enterprise sector is now the direction of travel for commissioning.

The success of the CCGs rests largely upon their ability to make significant changes that improve the quality and productivity of care. CCGs are taking on this challenge at a time when the wider health and social care system is undergoing significant change and in a context of ever-tightening budgets.

The history of CCGs

The Health and Social Care Act 2012 (HSCA 2012) moved responsibility for commissioning care to clinicians by introducing new statutory bodies called clinical commissioning groups (CCGs) which replaced primary care trusts (PCTs) from April 2013.

NHSE set out the application process for becoming a CCG in the October 2012 publication *Clinical Commissioning Group Authorisation: Guide for applicants*. In order to be authorised, CCGs had to meet the following requirements:

- they must have a geographical area;
- all of England must be covered without overlaps;
- all designated holders of primary care contracts must be members of a CCG;

- there must be a governing body, with an accountable officer and a chief finance officer;
- the governing body has to have at least two lay members,* who have to take specific responsibility for audit and governance and for public and patient engagement; and
- the CCG has to have its constitution authorised by NHSE.

(* Note: The minimum number of lay members is now recommended as three (NHSE, Managing Conflicts of Interest: Revised Statutory Guidance for CCGs).

Since their establishment, CCGs have entered into greater levels of collaboration ranging from informal collaboration to full mergers. This has become even more pressing as the STPs have begun to encourage and foster new models of care. During 2018, a number of CCGs have merged resulting in six larger CCGs that work at the STP level and supports the commissioning of new models of care and at the same time reducing costs. This reduces the total number of CCGs to 195.

Since April 2015, CCGs have also had the option to take on new primary care commissioning functions that were previously the responsibility of NHS England ('co-commissioning'). There are also other integrated approaches to commissioning that have been proposed between the NHS and local government, ranging from greater alignment between commissioners (both health and social care) to full integration and single commissioning agreements.

Clinical engagement and CCGs

CCGs were part of the NHS reform programme that also created FTs, and were created to be GP-led groups that would control the majority of the NHS budget and have the task of using this money to improve health services in their local area. CCGs were intended to ensure that there were clinically led approaches to planning and designing health services. According to the Kings Fund (2015) the challenges to their success have been:

- engaging with all GPs in a local area;
- developing the next generation of GP leaders;
- managing conflicts of interest; and
- using links with GPs to improve the quality of general practice locally.

The debate at the time also considered how clinicians other than GPs might be represented at senior levels. As a result, CCGs were required to have a registered nurse and a secondary care specialist doctor on the governing body to offer an alternative perspective on the delivery of health and care services locally.

A more recent survey in June 2017 (Checkland and Moran) suggests that only a minority of GPs think that commissioning services is an important part of their role, and that many current GP leaders of CCGs intend to quit their roles in the next five years. The survey suggests that in practice CCGs have failed to engage GPs with issues around communication between CCGs and their member practices and concerns about the sustainability of GP leadership.

The legal and regulatory framework for CCGs

CCG model core constitution

CCG governance depends on the CCG model constitution; the guidance and form of which was updated in September 2018.

Having said that, the requirements of the constitution do not always seem to be well understood. The King's Fund and Nuffield Trust publication *Clinical Commissioning Groups: Supporting improvement in general practice?* (July 2013) revealed that:

> 'In-depth knowledge of the constitution was scarce [within CCGs], both in the governing body and the membership ... many GPs who were, nominally, signatories to the constitution expressed little knowledge of its contents.'

All CCG constitutions should contain the following information:

- the title of the CCG and its geographical area of operation;
- the purpose of the CCG and from where it derives its legal duties and powers;
- its powers – the ways in which the CCG can fulfil its duties, the activities it may or may not undertake;
- amendments and variations to the constitution requiring the permission of NHSE;
- membership criteria, list of members, voting rights and responsibilities and details of any removal procedures. It may also include the requirement for any membership rights to be exercised in the best interests of the CCG;
- functions and general duties and an outline as to how those duties and functions will be fulfilled, including any conditions attached to the CCG by NHSE; and
- governance arrangements – the principles to be followed, how the CCG will be administered and how decisions will be made.

Further provisions contained in a well-written constitution will include:

- procedures for appointing governing body and committee members;
- procedures for appointing the chair;
- eligibility conditions for such positions;
- re-appointment, tenure, co-option procedures;
- procedures for the removal of governing body and committee members;
- details of how governing body, committee and member meetings will be run;
- the quorum needed to transact business;
- frequency of meetings;
- a statement and details regarding the management of conflicts of interest; and
- a clause indemnifying GP member practices and governing body members.

In addition, the model NHS CCG constitution features options to include:

- the mission, values and aims of the CCG;
- group committee details;
- joint arrangements;
- transparency arrangements;
- financial policies;
- standing orders;
- schemes of delegation and reservation; and
- checklists.

Careful thought should be given as to what material is included within the constitution, as some aspects of administration and strategy are likely to change with time. Such aspects that may be subject to amendment and change and which are not central to the constitution, should not be included in the constitution – such as naming an individual in the constitution as opposed to a role. The constitution forms part of the CCG's authorisation; any changes to the document must be agreed by NHSE. Any amendments to the constitution will not become valid until that permission has been granted.

A CCG can request an amendment to the constitution at any time. However, any amendments that will affect the financial allocation for the group have to meet a June deadline. NHSE demands assurance from the accountable officer, on behalf of the CCG, that the constitution will continue to meet legal requirements. There is no appeal process against NHSE's decision to approve proposed changes. As soon as an amended constitution comes into effect, the CCG should make arrangements to ensure the document is available to the public.

Codes of governance for CCGs

The NHSE and/or the NHS Clinical Commissioners websites host a substantial amount of guidance on governance in CCGs. Key publications include:

- *Towards establishment: Creating responsive and accountable clinical commissioning groups*;
- *Clinical commissioning group governing body members: Role outlines, attributes and skills*
- *The functions of CCGs*;
- *Procedures for clinical commissioning groups to apply for constitution change, merger or dissolution*;
- *Maximising the lay member role in CCGs*;
- *Clinical commissioning group guidance on senior appointments, including accountable officer*;
- *Integrated Support and Assurance Process (ISAP)*;
- *Managing Conflicts of Interest: Revised Statutory Guidance for CCGs* (June 2017);

- *Patient and public participation in commissioning health and care: statutory guidance for CCGs and NHS England;* and
- *Involving people in their own health and care: statutory guidance for CCGs and NHS England.*

The Good Governance Standard for Public Services (The Good Governance Standard).

Other than the minimum composition and a model constitution set out in HSCA 2012, there are no specific requirements for CCG governance. NHSE advocates adherence with the Good Governance Standard as the guidance for best practice. It builds on the Nolan Principles for the conduct of individuals in public life, by setting out six core principles of good governance for public service organisations as set out in Chapter 1 and illustrated in Figure 15.1.

It is important to note that the standard presupposes a form of leadership that is not based on the principle of a unitary board. This is in stark contrast to most other NHS organisations (such as FTs for whom the unitary board is a core principle of governance). As such, CCGs are unlikely to operate in a way that is entirely consistent with the major codes of corporate governance practice for the NHS (such as the UK Code, King IV, the Higgs Report and the FT Code).

Nevertheless, the Standard states that organisations should be clear about a number of areas that bear a close similarity to the recommendations in the above codes:

- the responsibilities of NEDs and the EDs, and that those responsibilities are carried out (Standard 2.2);
- members of the governing body behaving in ways that uphold and exemplify effective governance (Standard 3.2); and
- engaging stakeholders and making accountability real (Standard 6).

The standard also includes a useful appendix, which sets out questions for members of the public and their representatives to ask if they want to assess and challenge standards of governance.

ICSA Code of Governance for NHS clinical commissioning groups

The ICSA published a governance code for CCGs in November 2013 which offered CCGs an apply or explain approach to its six high-level principles. The objective of the six principles contained within the code is to:

> 'support clinicians, and those that work with them, to perform their commissioning activities and help to maintain public trust in clinicians and the NHS. [Moreover] application of the principles ... should be proportionate and appropriate for each CCG and its governing body'.

The document outlines some suggestions for how a CCG can achieve each of the six principles and poses a set of questions for consideration (see Table 15.1).

CLINICAL COMMISSIONING GROUPS

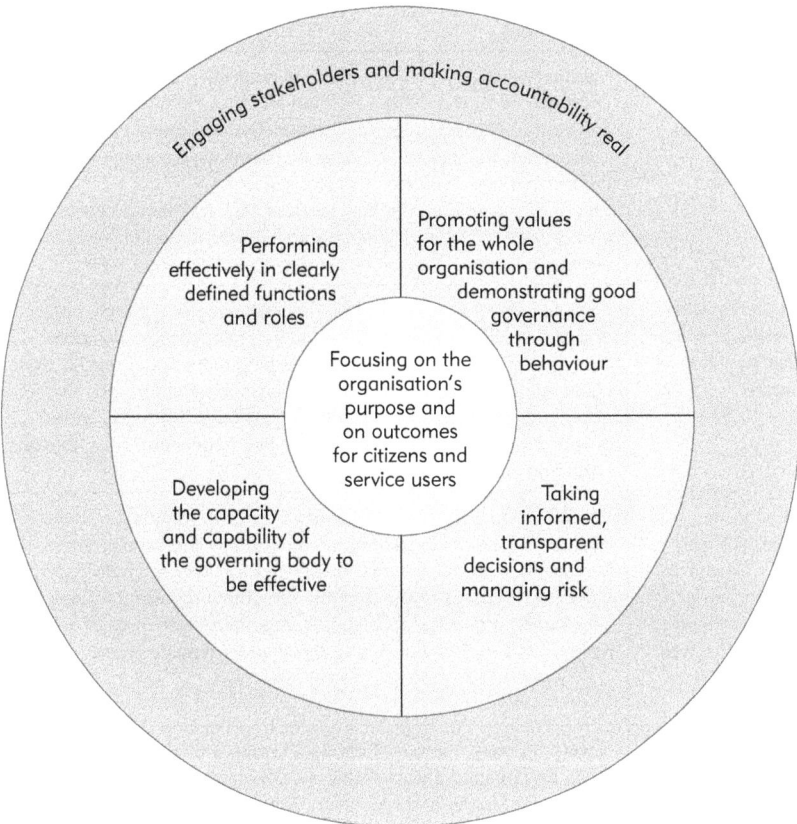

Figure 15.1: The six core principles of the Good Governance Standard

CCG membership

The CCG is made up of its member practices and the governing body is accountable to the members. These member practices must decide how the CCG will operate, through developing the CCG constitution within the legislative framework. They must ensure that the CCG is led and governed in an open and transparent way, which allows them to serve their patients and population effectively.

As a membership organisation, it is the CCG members that must ensure the CCG complies with the full range of regulations and legislation to ensure the group is governed appropriately. Whether it is statutory requirements or NHS guidance, CCG members are legally accountable for meeting these obligations though acting in the best interests of the organisation, patients, their carers and the wider CCG community.

All GP practices are required by law to be a member of a CCG (General Medical Services Contract Regulations 2013). The HSCA 2012 and subsequent regulations require each member of a CCG (each GP practice) to appoint an

Principle	Suggestions
Ensure effective decision-making processes to drive improvements in experience and quality	Member practices and the governing body need a working relationship underpinned by trust, with roles and responsibilities established. Among the suggested mechanisms are: open communication between CCG committees, the governing body and members; transparent approach to resolving any disputes; and clear guidance. The CCG should consider how involved their member practices are involved in its work and whether members understand how to challenge decisions.
Co-operation with 'interested provider parties' to enhance outcomes	This could involve: identification and management of both 'potential and real conflicts of interest'; developing relationships with both 'current and future' providers and keeping them under review; and highlighting outcome improvements in a variety of formats. The CCG also needs to consider how it gathers feedback 'from and about' providers and its processes for responding to concerns from regulators regarding local providers.
Develop strong relationships with other CCGs and regulators to support local and national health systems and contribute to wider policy debate	The CCG and governing body need to ensure clarity around 'the form, level and scope of co-operation required' with the various actors within the system. This can include: guidance for authorised individuals; provision of appropriate information to other organisations; and clear information requests. CCGs should 'maintain full records of delegated decision making' and also keep these under regular review.
Combine collective accountability with 'drawing on the strengths and expertise' from individuals	Governing body members hold equal responsibility for the decisions taken and need to ensure that the CCG invariably complies with relevant legislation and regulation. They must also remain fully aware of relationships and responsibilities with others including patients, member practices and committees. All members should have undertaken a comprehensive induction and clear understanding of aspects such as decision making and collective responsibilities.
The CCG should ensure the views of patients, carers and the public are utilised to inform commissioning and consider consequences of decisions	Among the suggested methods for delivering on this principle are: holding governing body meetings whenever appropriate; effective communication; holding consultations 'on significant changes to services commissioned and policies affecting the wider health economy'; and a system that manages complaints 'constructively, impartially and effectively'. Governing body members need to consider target audience identification, the inclusion of public and patient engagement within CCG annual reports and the publication procedure around learning from complaints.
'Robust and effective processes for decision making' to provide foundations for 'transparency and accountability at every level'	Governing body members are tasked with ensuring their CCG has strong arrangements in place for governance, which could include: adherence to the Nolan Principles; promotion of the NHS Constitution's values; and an updated register of interests. Among the areas for governing body members to consider here are: whether an annual summary of information is publicly available; the regular review of Freedom of Information activity; and feedback in relation to procurement.

Table 15.1: ICSA Code of Governance for NHS clinical commissioning groups

individual to act on its behalf in dealings with the CCG. The intention is that this person has to be a GP or other healthcare professional. Details as to how practice representatives are selected should be set out in the CCG's standing orders and must comply with regulations.

The CCG cannot expel a practice, as they need to have coherent geographical coverage; therefore, there should be no provisions within the constitution that give CCGs the power to expel a practice. The HSCA 2012 does give CCGs the power to apply to NHSE to have a member practice expelled from the group in extreme circumstances. Such circumstances might include refusal to engage or participate with CCG activities, failure to demonstrate active effort to address agreed practice/clinical behaviour, failure to support local plans and/or no commitment to supporting other practices or the CCG by sharing expertise and/or delivery where capacity and resources allow.

Each CCG may also identify a number of other GPs or primary care health professionals from member practices to support the work of the group and/or represent the group rather than represent their own individual practices. Any such role, which is not required by statute, must be set out in the constitution.

Members' Council/Forum

Practice varies across CCGs and many have established a Member Council or Member Forum. Others have established locality arrangements where members within each locality meet on a regular basis and the outcome of such meetings can then be filtered-up into a smaller sub-group of member representatives and ultimately to the governing body. Any such arrangements need to be set out in the CCG's constitution.

Many CCGs have interpreted this as some form of 'member council' comprising either representatives from all practices (in smaller CCGs) or locality representatives (in larger CCGs). The precise responsibilities delegated to these members' councils differ, but the latest guidance on the model constitution (2018) recommends being clear on member's rights and whilst not legally required in the constitution suggests that the CCG has clarity on the following:

- calling and attending a general meeting of the members;
- submitting a proposal for amendment of the constitution;
- putting themselves forward for election to the governing body;
- electing the chair (and/ or other members) of the governing body;
- removing the chair (or other elected members) of the governing body; and
- participating in the development of the CCG's corporate governance documents, including the CCG Handbook.

Most CCGs have agreed some roles that are for the wider membership and the guidance acknowledges that these roles are for local agreement and the relevant processes should be described in the standing orders and/ or the governance handbook as appropriate.

There is no requirement for the members meetings to be held in public, but some CCG councils have voted to do so.

Whilst there is no legal requirement for the members to meet on an annual basis NHSE encourages CCGs to engage with their members on a regular basis and to facilitate some form of annual 'meeting' or stock-take. For instance, it is required that the annual report be presented to a meeting in public and whilst this could be done by the governing body, NHSE suggest that the full membership should also be invited and encouraged to participate. Such a meeting could also be used to enable members to confirm their continued support for the constitution if the members are no longer asked to approve every small change individually.

Some large CCGs have found it to be helpful to include a provision for virtual and electronic gathering of members to ensure the need to travel and disruption to delivery of services in their practices is minimised. This too should be included in the CGG's constitution.

Liability

As the CCG is a body corporate established and existing under the NHS Act 2006 all financial or legal liability for decisions or actions of the CCG resides with the CCG as a public statutory body and not with its member practices. No member or former member is liable for the debts, liabilities, acts or omissions, caused by the CCG in discharging its statutory functions.

The CCG may, however, indemnify any member practice representative or other officer or individual exercising powers or duties on its behalf in respect of any civil liability incurred in the exercise of the CCGs' business, provided that the person indemnified shall not have acted recklessly or with gross negligence.

The position of employees of the CCG is different to that of governing body members, as it is always liable for the actions of its employees in the course of their employment.

CCG governing body and its committees

Whilst all CCGs are legally required to have a governing body by the HSCA 2012 that provides the challenge and assurance that their accountabilities are being effectively met, there can be some variation between each CCG in the arrangements in place for setting strategy and performing its functions.

The governing body is not a committee of the CCG and the constitution must specify the arrangements made for the discharge of functions by the group members or member practices.

Composition

The model constitution framework sets out that the governing body must not have less than six members, consisting of:

- the chair;
- representatives of member practices;
- other GPs or primary care health professionals;
- a minimum of two lay members – one to lead on audit, remuneration and conflict of interest matters and one to lead on patient and public participation matters;
- a registered nurse;
- a secondary care specialist doctor;
- the accountable officer;
- the CFO; and
- any other individuals as required by the CCG.

CCGs may choose to have more than two lay members and other individual roles on the governing body, but this must be specified in their constitution. Indeed, the NHSE's statutory guidance *Managing Conflicts of Interest: Revised statutory guidance for CCGs* (2017) strongly recommends that CCGs appoint a third lay member.

As with all such structures, the numerical size of the governing body needs to be considered: not so large as to be unwieldy, but not so small as to lack the necessary skills and experience. As the governing body is not a committee, it cannot have terms of reference and, therefore details about its composition must be specified in the CCG's constitution. The standing orders of the CCG should also set out:

- how the group will appoint such members of the governing body (e.g. will they be elected?);
- the tenure of office;
- how such a person would resign from their post; and
- the grounds for removal from office.

Elections and appointments

The model constitution does not specify exactly how the governing body should be elected and dismissed. Therefore, the accountability structure can vary in the actual details from CCG to CCG.

One version is where the member practices elect a representative to sit on a member council. The member council then appoints the non-officer members of the governing body, and the governing body appoints the specific officers of the CCG (the chair, accountable officer and chief financial officer (CFO)).

An alternative model sees the member practices directly select and elect or appoint their governing body members and chair. Regardless of the structure used, the governing body is always accountable to the member practices for the running of the CCG in accordance with its constitution.

Appointments are usually made in relation to the executive members, lay members and non-GP clinicians of the governing body: AO, CFO, secondary care clinician and so on. Typically, a process of open competition and advertisement is completed. This may be undertaken by the members' council or governing body dependent upon the constitution. These appointments are usually only made on a permanent basis for executive members, with fixed-term appointments for the other roles.

Elections usually take place in relation to GP members and the chair, with nominations being made by the member practices. An election will then take place if there is more than one candidate. The election may be overseen and administered by the members' council or by the local medical committee.

If a CCG has localities, then votes can only be cast for one of the GPs standing in their own locality area. Depending upon the CCG's constitution, votes may be available to all GPs providing primary medical services to a registered list of patients (based on a general medical services, personal medical services or alternative provider medical services contract) and practicing within the geographical area of the CCG (one person, one vote). Alternatively, votes may be allocated to each member practice based on the population it serves.

Some CCG member councils have established members' council advisory panels, which are small panels comprising three council members and an independent HR adviser. It oversees the process of appointing members to the governing body – including the chair – by assessing prospective candidates to determine their suitability for the role, then inviting suitable candidates to stand for election. The panel then makes recommendations to the members' council on those appointments.

The 'fit and proper' persons test described in earlier chapters also applies to CCG appointments.

Tenure

Terms of office for all elections and appointments to the governing body are as set out in each CCG's constitution. With the exception of executive appointments, which are made on a permanent basis, there is little consistency as to the terms that are offered – some are for two or three years, while others are for five years. There is no mandated limit set on the maximum term of office. The guidance given elsewhere in this handbook may be considered but is only advisory. Even so, it is critical that CCGs consider how to find a balance between continuity of knowledge and renewal of thinking in the governing body.

Disqualification

The NHS Commissioning Board and Clinical Commissioning Group (Responsibilities and Standing Rules) Regulations 2012 set out the standing rules regulations that detail those people who are disqualified from being a chair or member of a CCG governing body. These include:

- an MP, Member of the European Parliament or London Assembly Member;
- a member of a local authority in England, Wales, Scotland or Northern Ireland;

CLINICAL COMMISSIONING GROUPS

- an employee, member, shareholder or partner of an organisation providing commissioning support;
- anyone convicted in the prior five years of any UK offence; or offence outside of the UK if deemed illegal at home and convicted to a sentence of three months or more;
- anyone subject to (interim) bankruptcy restrictions under insolvency legislation;
- anyone dismissed from paid employment (not including redundancy) in the previous five years from any NHS organisation (including Wales, Scotland and Northern Ireland);
- a healthcare professional subject to an investigation or proceedings by a regulatory body resulting in suspension or removal from the register, prevention or conditions on practising from those not removed from the register;
- someone subject to an order or undertaking from company directors' disqualification legislation; and
- a person removed from being a trustee by charities legislation.

The ICSA specimen code of conduct for NHS CCG governing body members

This guidance reflects current best practice from across economic sectors and the requirements of NHSE. It is available to ICSA members at www.icsa.org.uk. It should be read in conjunction with the Professional Standards Authority's standards for NHS boards and governing bodies. It sets out a specimen code, which suggests that governing body members must:

- adhere to the CCG's rules and policies, including the constitution, standing orders and prime financial policies, and support its objectives, in particular those relating to NHS CCG status and developing a successful CCG;
- act in the best interests of the CCG at all times;
- contribute to the working of the governing body in order for it to fulfil its role and functions as defined in the constitution;
- recognise that their role is a collective one;
- support and assist the chief officer, and the accountable officer, in his/her responsibility to answer to NHS England and the group's local community;
- value fellow governing body members, even when there are differences in opinion;
- adhere to the CCG's meeting etiquette policy;
- be mindful of conduct which could be deemed to be unfair or discriminatory;
- conduct themselves in a manner which reflects positively on the CCG when attending external meetings or any other events; and
- seek to ensure that the membership of the CCG, and of its patients, their carers and other interested parties, are properly informed and that their views are fed back to the CCG.

Committees

Like FTs and NHS trusts, the governing body is required by statute to have audit and remuneration committees as a minimum. The extent of each party's authority to act depends on the powers delegated to them by the CCG as expressed through its scheme of reservation and delegation (or terms of reference for committees). However, CCGs are not able to form joint committees (see below) for their remuneration or audit committees, as these are non-delegable functions.

CCGs did not originally have the power to establish joint committees with other CCGs but this was remedied in October 2014. In the interim period, CCGs established committees (known as 'committees-in-common') that could make decisions on behalf of two or more of them. Such committees are now being used to achieve a largescale service reconfiguration within the health economy within the 5YFV (see Chapter 3).

It is important to note that CCGs can now amend their constitutions (with NHSE approval) to also enable their governing bodies to set up joint committees as well and some are doing so in order to jointly enact some key commissioning functions.

Many CCGs have local GP groups, which are often known as 'localities'. The model constitution requires CCGs that wish to delegate authority to their localities (as a committee of the group) to include in their constitution details of the role of the locality and to whom they are accountable. The locality committee must account to the governing body when it undertakes work that falls within the scope of the functions of the governing body. The CCG is free to determine the scope of the responsibilities delegated to locality committees and to include in the terms of reference for each committee how it will be held to account for its work. Reference should also be made as how the locality committee will relate to the broader membership and the governing body in discharging its functions.

In addition, CCGs that have taken on delegated responsibility for primary care commissioning are required to establish a Primary Care Commissioning Committee (PCC Committee). Because the functions being exercised by the PCC Committee are actually NHSE functions, exercised on behalf of NHSE by the CCG, these functions cannot be further delegated. This means that they cannot be delegated to a joint committee. The PCC Committee reports to both NHSE and the governing body. It is chaired by a lay member, has a lay vice chair and GP members are in the minority.

Where CCGs decide not to list their non-statutory committees within the constitution, NHSE require the CCG to maintain and publish a committees' handbook. This should include the full list of committees established and their terms of reference.

The remuneration committee

The NHSE guidance *Remuneration Guidance for Chief Officers (where the senior manager also undertakes the accountable officer role) and chief finance officers* makes it clear that CCGs must have a remuneration committee drawn from its governing body, of whom one member should act as its chair.

Section 15 of The National Health Service (Clinical Commissioning Groups) Regulations 2012 stipulates that the committee chair must be appointed by the CCG for a term to be determined. It also states that all members of the governing body other than lay persons are disqualified from being the chair.

The committee should not include full-time employees or individuals who claim a significant proportion of their income from the CCG, nor should member practices be in the majority. The committee will make recommendations to the CCG governing body as to the determination of remuneration, fees, pension and allowances payable to its employees. No governing body member or senior manager should be present for discussions about their own remuneration (although it is reasonable for the chief officer, the human resources (HR) lead and other senior managers where appropriate, to attend meetings of the committee during which the remuneration of other staff is discussed). In addition, some CCGs have conferred on or delegated to the remuneration committee the authority to make recommendations on remuneration and terms of service for elected governing body members.

CCGs are now subject to the same controls on senior remuneration as NHS providers (see Chapter 11). Consequently, when a CCG is seeking to appoint a clinical chief officer or chief officer who will hold the AO role, early consideration has to be given to the level of remuneration proposed for the post and approval obtained from the DHSC where necessary before the role can be advertised.

Annex 2 of the NHSE guidance *Clinical Commissioning Group Governing Body Members: Role outlines, attributes and skills* recommends that all payments should be evidently in line with the individual's current earnings, commensurate with the average rate for their current employment or the specific role or demonstrably required to provide backfill. The guidance goes on to set out what these principles mean for GPs, other practice staff, lay members, the nurse and the secondary care clinician on the governing body. Good practice would also suggest that robust benchmarking information be available to support the remuneration committee in this decision-making process – for example, remuneration could be in line with NED payments in other NHS organisations or at a rate commensurate with their salary.

National guidance has been published with a set fee for the lay members, secondary care doctor and nurse roles but, where the NHS currently employs these postholders, the guidance recommends their fee is based on their existing NHS salary instead of the set fee. Guidance on salary ranges for executive members based on NHS trust executive pay is provided by NHSE and follows the principles set out in the Hutton Fair Pay Review.

A survey by NHS Clinical Commissioners (January 2016) outlined the variation across CCGs in terms of lay member contract hours, actual hours worked and allowances paid. It revealed that on average CCGs contract with lay members for 3.4 days per month, and the average number of days actually worked is 5.7.

The remuneration committee is required to make a report of its activities in the CCG's annual report and accounts. This is in line with the reports required of FTs and NHS trusts; likewise, the report must also include the relationship between the remuneration of the highest-paid director in their organisation and the median remuneration of the organisation's workforce, in line with the Hutton Fair Pay Review.

The audit committee

Section 15 of The National Health Service (Clinical Commissioning Groups) Regulations 2012 stipulates that the audit committee must have a chair appointed by the CCG (for a term to be determined). The chair must be a lay person with such qualifications, expertise or experience as to enable them to express informed views about financial management and audit matters. The chair of the CCG's governing body and the chief finance officer are disqualified from membership of a CCG's audit committee.

The lay member on the governing body, with a lead role in overseeing key elements of governance, is therefore usually the chair of the audit committee. The committee provides assurance and advice to the governing body, and to the AO, on the proper stewardship of resources and assets, including:

- value for money (VFM);
- financial reporting;
- the effectiveness of audit arrangements (internal and external);
- risk management; and
- control and integrated governance arrangements within the group.

The governing body should approve and keep under review the terms of reference for the audit committee, which include information on the membership of the committee. This should be available upon request to the public. It is recommended that CCGs refer to the Healthcare Financial Management Association (HFMA) NHS Audit Committee Handbook (2014) and this ICSA handbook for further guidance.

Internal audit

Where CCGs have taken on board the delegated powers for primary care commissioning, the *Internal Audit Framework for Delegated Clinical Commissioning Groups (2018)* applies. This framework requires the CCG governing body to evaluate the effectiveness of the arrangements put in place for primary medical care commissioning through an annual internal audit work plan as follows:

- Commissioning and procurement of services
- Contract Oversight and Management Functions

- Primary Care Finance
- Governance (common to each of the above areas).

The outcome of each annual audit will be reported to the CCG Audit Committee and will be reported in the CCG's annual report and AGS.

Duties, rights and powers of the CCG and its governing body

CCGs are accountable to their public and patients, to NHSE (via the regional team) and to their member practices; however, the main functions of the governing body are described in section 14L of the NHS Act 2006 (inserted by section 25 of HSCA 2012). The governing body's principal aim is to ensure that the group has made appropriate arrangements for ensuring that it complies with its obligations to exercise its functions effectively, efficiently, economically and in line with relevant generally accepted principles of good governance.

CCGs need to create their own list of additional functions, which should be cross-referenced with the Scheme of Reservation and Delegation and standing orders where appropriate. The following examples may be useful:

- leading the development of vision and strategy for the CCG;
- overseeing and monitoring quality improvement;
- approving the CCG's Commissioning Plans and its consultation arrangements;
- stimulating innovation and modernisation;
- overseeing and monitoring performance;
- overseeing risk assessment and securing assurance actions to mitigate identified strategic risks;
- promoting a culture of strong engagement with patients, their carers, members, the public and other stakeholders about the activity and progress of the CCG; and
- ensuring good governance and leading a culture of good governance throughout the CCG.

CCGs also have a statutory duty to ensure the effective participation of member practices in the exercise of the CCG's functions as set out in HSCA 2012. This means that practices can challenge the CCG if they feel that it is not fulfilling its statutory duty to ensure effective member participation. For example, the constitution will include electoral procedures and how member practices can remove a CCG governing body member.

Maintaining an effective governing body

The model constitution requires the governing body to have an ongoing role in reviewing the CCG's governance arrangements to ensure that the CCG continues to reflect the principles of good governance.

The research project *Developing CCGs as High Performing Membership Organisations*, in which Calderdale and Greater Huddersfield CCGs worked with Ashridge Business School, established seven areas of competency that demonstrate a high-performing membership organisation. The research was based on the premise that the CCG existed primarily for the benefit of the community, not for the members, but that it was the members who would secure success or otherwise for the CCG. These competencies would make an interesting yardstick for an annual effectiveness review of the governing body and/or members' council. The seven competencies are:

- the membership contract;
- encouraging and promoting best practice;
- information and advice to members;
- the development of member skills;
- promoting the CCG to the membership;
- policy and decision making; and
- engagement with the wider public.

Although there are no mandated requirements to annually assess/evaluate their effectiveness, CCGs would be well advised to consider the guidance on evaluation given elsewhere in this handbook.

The notes for the revised constitution (2018) suggest that the following governance practices should be observed in order to aid effectiveness.

- use of the governance toolkit for CCGs developed in conjunction with the Good Governance Institute;
- undertaking regular governance reviews;
- adoption of standards and procedures that facilitate speaking out and the raising of concerns including a freedom to speak up guardian if one is appointed;
- adopting CCG values that include standards of propriety in relation to the stewardship of public funds, impartiality, integrity and objectivity;
- the Good Governance Standard for Public Services; and
- the standards of behaviour published by the Committee on Standards in Public Life (1995) known as the 'Nolan Principles'.

The chair of the governing body

The chair runs governing body meetings and sets the agenda; they are pivotal in creating the conditions for overall committee and individual effectiveness.

The National Health Service (Clinical Commissioning Groups) Regulations 2012 specify that the chair cannot be the accountable officer or CFO, the mandatory secondary care specialist or nurse, or the lay person with a lead role in overseeing key elements of governance.

If the chair is a GP or other healthcare professional, the deputy chair should be a lay member who should take the chair's role for discussions and decisions involving conflict of interest for the chair.

The chair also plays a key role in managing the relationships between member practices, governing body and committee members and staff. The chair's relationship with the accountable officer is particularly critical to the successful functioning of the CCG, its governing body and other committees. This relationship should be defined clearly in writing.

The chair will also have a key role in overseeing governance, particularly ensuring that the governing body and the wider CCG behaves with the utmost transparency and responsiveness at all times. They will ensure that public and patients' views are heard, their expectations understood and, where appropriate, met. The chair will ensure that the organisation is able to account to its local patients, stakeholders and NHSE, as well as ensuring the CCG builds and maintains effective relationships, particularly with the individuals involved in overview and scrutiny from the relevant local authorities.

The chair of the governing body has specific responsibility for:

- leading the governing body, ensuring it remains continuously able to discharge its duties and responsibilities as set out in the CCG's constitution;
- building and developing the CCG's governing body and its individual members;
- ensuring that the CCG has proper constitutional and governance arrangements in place;
- ensuring that, through the appropriate support, information and evidence, the governing body is able to discharge its duties;
- supporting the accountable officer in discharging the responsibilities of the organisation;
- contributing to the building of a shared vision of the aims, values and culture of the organisation; and
- leading and influencing clinical and organisational change to enable the CCG to deliver commissioning responsibilities.

The accountable officer

The CCG's AO is charged with ensuring that the CCG complies with its statutory duties as set out above. The AO must also ensure that the CCG performs its functions in a way that provides good value for money.

The individual who undertakes the accountable officer role is required to be a member of the CCG's governing body and therefore needs to meet the core requirements for governing body members. Once an individual has been successful in the selection process, to carry out the duties of the accountable officer they may be either:

- an employee of the CCG, or an employee of any member of the CCG;
- a member of the CCG (e.g. a GP); or
- a person specified in the constitution.

Although two or more CCGs may choose to share a single person to undertake their accountable officer roles, it is not possible for a single CCG to appoint two individuals to share this role. The accountable officer may not be the chair of the governing body.

CCGs could decide that their accountable officer role will be held by a clinician supported by an expert manager or undertaken by a manager with expert clinical leadership support. The term chief officer is used to identify senior managers who undertake the accountable officer role, while chief clinical officer is used for senior clinicians who undertake the role. When the accountable officer role is held by a clinician, the CCG's senior manager is called the chief operating officer.

The individual who undertakes the accountable officer role is required to be a member of the governing body. They will therefore need to meet the core requirements as described for governing body members.

The company secretary

While the current legislation does not specify the need for CCGs to appoint a company secretary, good practice from the corporate sector and experience in FTs would suggests that this is also a key role in the governance of an organisation.

ICSA has issued guidance on the role of a CCG head of governance, which encompasses the company secretary role. This role covers three main areas:

- the governing body and CCG committees;
- the CCG itself; and
- the member practices.

In brief, the head of governance would be responsible for ensuring that the CCG complies with relevant legislation and its authorisation (including any conditions attached to it) issued by NHSE. They would establish procedures for the sound governance of the CCG and would advise the governing body, committees and member practices on developments in governance issues. The head of governance would also ensure that meetings of the governing body, committees and member practices run efficiently and effectively, are properly recorded and that all relevant participants receive appropriate support to fulfil their legal duties.

NHS Clinical Commissioners

NHS Clinical Commissioners (NHSCC) is the independent membership organisation of clinical commissioning groups. It provides CCGs with a strong collective voice and represents them in the national debate on the future of healthcare in England. It aims to facilitate shared learning; and deliver networking opportunities for its members so that local clinicians can commission the best possible services for their patients and populations.

NHSCC also leads the engagement function with CCGs, which was previously undertaken by the NHS Commissioning Assembly. The new engagement process aims to ensure that CCGs have every opportunity to be involved in NHSEs work at a national level by creating clearer and more systematic and representative ways of working.

NHSCC is governed by a democratically elected board to provide leadership for the organisation and its six networks. The board is made up of a blend of clinicians, managers and lay people from its membership, through a democratic election process. NHSCC has set up six specialist networks at the request of its members. These provide an opportunity for commissioners involved in these areas to come together and support each other with common challenges as well as share best practice to enhance their work locally.

The Good Governance Institute (GGI)

In 2014, the Good Governance Institute (GGI), with its partner Capsticks, was commissioned by NHSE to carry out a major work programme to assist the ongoing development of CCGs.

In particular, GGI have developed:

- a consistent language to describe governance that is engaging for clinicians and the public;
- a proposed set of outcomes of good governance that can be described and measured; and
- a series of diagnostic tools with which CCGs can measure the outcomes of their governance arrangements supported by a process that CCGs can employ.

Eleven outcomes for good governance were identified by GGI, CCGs and other relevant stakeholders. These are as follows:

1. Clarity of purpose, including setting tone at the top, leading by example, living the values, etc.
2. Leadership and strategic direction, including understanding of market and context, balance between operational demands and strategic goals and creating a pipeline of clinical leaders for the future.
3. Effectiveness of relationships, including co-operative behaviours.
4. Membership and unity, including member ownership of CCG.
5. Public and community engagement, including openness and transparency.
6. Quality and safety structures and systems, including mechanisms to gather patients and carer experience data, adoption of best practice, commitment to research, investment in development, holding each other to account professionally, etc.
7. Focus on outcomes, including understanding what matters to improve health of population, driving quality and safety, co-design with service users, co-ordination of care.
8. Better decision making, including development of key performance indicators (KPIs), use of information, data integrity, ongoing audit, etc. used to support sound decisions, mature management of conflict of interest.

9. Control systems, including clarity of external authority and expectation, risk appetite, internal assurance on resources and quality, effectiveness of governance structures, quality of challenge, etc.
10. Legal and regulatory compliance, including fulfilling statutory and other duties such as the duty of candour.
11. Organisational effectiveness, including resource management, effective procurement, best use of commissioning support, fewer diversions arising from governance failures, etc.

GGI have also now developed a suite of tools that have been tested by more than 40 volunteer CCGs. The tools allow CCGs to self-evaluate the degree to which their governance arrangements deliver on the outcomes of good governance, and include a maturity matrix, a peer review guide, a standards and evidence tool, a board observation guide and a survey that can be administered both online and in hard copy. They are all available for CCGs to use free of charge and can be found at www.ccggovernance.org.

The CCG governance challenge

Non-executive members and independence

The independence of the governing body currently rests on the role of the lay members, of which there must be at least two, with specified roles to oversee elements of governance and to help champion patient and public engagement. This has the potential to be further strengthened with the appointment of the secondary care specialist and the registered nurse member and a third additional lay member in line with the conflicts of interest guidance.

In considering the current makeup of the governing body, the lay members, secondary care specialist and registered nurse member can all be considered non-executive members. They are defined as such in the model CCG Constitution. However, the GP members are also referred to as non-executive members at times.

The Good Governance Standard (following on from the Higgs Report) sets the role of these non-executive members. It says they should:

- contribute to strategy by bringing a range of perspectives to strategy development and decision making;
- make sure that effective management arrangements and an effective team are in place at the top level of the organisation;
- delegate which decisions are reserved for the governing body, and then clearly delegate the rest;
- hold the executive to account, by assessing performance in fulfilling their responsibilities, agreeing levels of remuneration and appointment/removal of executives; and
- be extremely discriminating about getting involved in matters of operational detail.

As a comparison, the UK Code (2018) requires a board and its committees to have the appropriate balance of skills, experience, independence and knowledge to enable them to discharge their duties and responsibilities effectively. This ensures that no individual or group of individuals can dominate the board's decision making. Non-executive members can be either independent or non-independent. Though non-independent non-executives are permissible, the UK Code recommends that the majority of the board should consist of independent non-executives. If there are non-executives who are considered not to be independent, the UK Code suggests that it may be necessary to appoint further independent non-executives to act as a counterbalance. Non-executives are not independent if their opinion is likely to be influenced by the senior executive management of the organisation or by a major stakeholder, or for example, if a person personally stands to gain or otherwise benefit substantially from income from the organisation.

The significant governance issue for CCGs relates to the independence of its non-executive members in carrying out this role of independent scrutiny. The independent non-executives would be identified as the lay members and clinical members. GP members would be classed as non-independent non-executives; good practice would suggest that their number needs to be balanced with an equivalent number of NEDs to ensure good governance.

The boundaries in CCGs can sometimes become further blurred, however. In a number of CCGs, GP members on the governing body take on clinical project leads or operational roles within the CCG. These roles support the CCG in developing robust clinical pathways and models of care in order to deliver the strategic priorities of the CCG. The GPs who undertake these roles will usually have a specific knowledge and expertise in the field in question.

Managing conflicts of interest

As mentioned in the opening remarks of this chapter, managing conflicts of interest is a critical factor in the success of CCGs. Conflicts can arise in the work of CCGs in a variety of ways: for example, if members of the practice became involved in the process of deciding to commission or awarding a service to a GP provider in their locality or to their own practice, they would be potentially conflicted. It would not be clear that they favoured the decision because of the needs of patients rather than their own financial gain.

For a GP or other clinical commissioner, a conflict of interest may also arise when their own judgement as an NHS commissioner could be, or be perceived to be, influenced and impaired by their own concerns and obligations as a healthcare provider; as a member of a particular peer, professional or special interest group; or those of a close family member. Commissioning decisions that are in the overall best interests of taxpayers and the local population may not always be in the best interests of individual patients for whom GPs are required to advocate, or for the companies and partnerships which they own, manage or work for.

Individual behaviour is a major factor in the effectiveness of the governing body, and has an influence on the reputation of the organisation, the confidence and trust members of the public have in it and the working relationships and morale within it. Conflicts, real or perceived, can arise between the organisation's interests and those of individual governors; public trust can then be damaged unless the organisation implements clear procedures to deal with these conflicts.

The guidance *Next Steps Towards Primary Care Co-commissioning* (2014) included a strengthened approach to managing such conflicts in co-commissioning decisions. These requirements related to the make-up of the decision-making committee, where the committee must have a lay and executive majority and have a lay chair. Local Healthwatch and a local authority member of the local HWB will also have the right to serve as observers on the decision-making committee in order to secure the external involvement of local stakeholders.

On 16 June 2017, NHSE published revised statutory guidance on managing conflicts of interest for CCGs. The guidance has been updated to ensure it is fully aligned with the recently published cross-system conflicts of interest guidance: *Managing conflicts of interest in the NHS: Guidance for staff and organisations* (see Chapter 8). A small number of changes have been made, including the following:

- Registers of interest: CCGs are required to have systems in place to satisfy themselves as a minimum on an annual basis that their registers of interest are accurate and up-to-date, and to require that only decision-making staff are included on the published register.
- Gifts from suppliers or contractors: In line with the NHS-wide guidance, gifts of low value (up to £6), such as promotional items, can now be accepted.
- Gifts from other sources: the thresholds for such gifts has been revised to under £50 (rather than £10) and such gifts do not need to be declared. Gifts with a value of over £50 can now be accepted on behalf of an organisation, but not in a personal capacity.
- Hospitality – meals and refreshments: the thresholds have been revised so that hospitality under £25 does not need to be declared. Hospitality between £25 and £75 can be accepted, but must be declared, and hospitality over £75 should be refused unless senior approval is given.
- New care models: a new annex providing further advice on identifying, declaring and managing conflicts of interest in the commissioning of new care models has also been included.

The guidance recognises that conflicts of interest are inevitable in commissioning and it is how they are managed that matters and so it includes a number of strengthened safeguards to mitigate the risk of real and perceived conflicts of interest arising in CCGs:

- CCG employees and practice staff with involvement in CCG business to complete mandatory online conflicts of interest training annually.

- Where a CCG decides not to comply with this statutory guidance, they must include within their next annual self-certification statement the reasons for deciding not to do so.

The general safeguards described in *Towards Establishment: Creating Responsive and Accountable Clinical Commissioning Groups (CCGs)* (2012) included:

- arrangements for declaring interests;
- maintaining a register of interests;
- excluding individuals from decision making where a conflict arises; and
- engagement with a range of potential providers on service design.

The NHSE guidance provides more specific, additional safeguards that CCGs are advised to have in place when commissioning services that could potentially be provided by GP practices. These safeguards are set out in the form of questions which governing bodies are encouraged to ask themselves.

- How does the proposal deliver good or improved outcomes and VFM – what are the estimated costs and the estimated benefits?
- How does it reflect the CCG's proposed commissioning priorities?
- How have the public been involved in the decision to commission this service?
- What range of health professionals have been involved in designing the proposed service?
- What range of potential providers have been involved in considering the proposals?
- How have the HWB(s) been involved?
- How does the proposal support the priorities in the relevant joint health and wellbeing strategy (or strategies)?
- What are the proposals for monitoring the quality of the service?
- What systems will there be to monitor and publish data on referral patterns?
- Have all conflicts and potential conflicts of interests been appropriately declared and entered in registers that are publicly available?
- Why has this procurement route been chosen?
- What additional external involvement will there be in scrutinising the proposed decisions?
- How will the CCG make its final commissioning decision in ways that preserve the integrity of the decision-making process?

Other requirements in the guidance were:

- the strong recommendation for CCGs to have a minimum of three lay members on the governing body;
- the introduction of a conflicts of interest guardian in CCGs undertaken by the audit committee chair as long as they do not have any provider interests;

- the requirement for CCGs to include a robust process for managing any breaches within their conflict of interest policy and for anonymised details of the breach to be published on the CCG's website;
- strengthened provisions around decision making when a member of the governing body, or committee or sub-committee is conflicted;
- strengthened provisions around the management of gifts and hospitality;
- a requirement for CCGs to include an annual audit of conflicts of interest management within their internal audit plans; and
- to include the findings of this audit within their annual end-of-year governance statement.

CCGs will also need to adhere to relevant guidance issued by professional bodies on conflicts of interest (e.g. the British Medical Association (BMA), the Royal College of General Practitioners (RCGP), and to procurement rules such as the Public Contract Regulations 2015 and other legislation such as the Bribery Act 2010 (as discussed in Chapter 5)).

The CCG's public register of conflicts of interest will include information on the nature of the conflict and details of the conflicted parties. The register will form an obligatory part of the annual accounts and be signed off by external auditors. CCGs will also be required to maintain and publish, on a regular basis, a register of all key procurement decisions.

If the governing body is considering a decision in which a member is conflicted, it is good practice for that member to play no part in that decision – normally leaving the room during the discussion of that agenda item. In making the decision as to whether to exclude the member from the discussion, the chair and/or lay member for governance will consider the expertise or insight of the member in relation to the item under discussion. If more than 50% of the members are conflicted, then the chair (or deputy) should have the authority to decide whether the discussion can proceed. Where a quorum cannot be achieved, the chair of the meeting could invite other individuals on a temporary basis to make up the quorum. Such an individual may be a member of a relevant HWB or a member of another CCG.

CCGs are required by *Managing Conflicts of Interest: Statutory Guidance for CCGs* 2017 to appoint a guardian for the management of conflicts of interest. The guidance suggests this should be the chair of the audit committee unless they have a provider interest, as they already have a key role in conflicts of interest management. The guardian should provide oversight of the management of conflicts of interest and provide impartial, unconflicted advice and judgement to the governing body in cases where it is not obvious whether a material conflict exists or how best to manage it. They should define a reasonable balance to avoid conflicts, though enabling the CCG to harness the knowledge of clinicians and other staff for commissioning in order to improve care to patients and value for money to the taxpayer. The deputy chair of the governing body should deputise for the chair of the governing body where the chair has a conflict of interest.

Being a membership organisation

The King's Fund and Nuffield Trust report *Clinical Commissioning Groups: Supporting improvement in general practice?* (2013) states:

'[T]here are significant disparities between the views of those involved in leading CCGs and member GPs, with the latter being less likely to say that their CCG is "owned" by its members, that its decisions reflect their views or that it has had a positive impact to date. There is also significant variation in views from one CCG to another, with levels of member ownership and involvement much higher in some areas than others. Larger CCGs may face a particular challenge in engaging member practices and creating a culture of collective ownership.'

There is a significant challenge here to ensure that the member practices are able to play an influential role in setting the direction of the CCG. The balance of power between the members council and the governing body needs to be handled carefully by the chair and the AO.

Procurement

The National Health Service (Procurement, Patient Choice and Competition) Regulations (No 2) 2013 replace the existing administrative rules governing the procurement of NHS-funded services previously set out in the Principles and rules for cooperation and competition (DH, 2010) and the Procurement guide for commissioners of NHS-funded services (DH, 2010).

The substance of many of these principles and rules is still preserved in the regulations. The regulations require commissioners to ensure good practice in relation to the procurement of NHS healthcare services and to protect patients' rights to make choices regarding their NHS treatment. They also prohibit commissioners from engaging in anti-competitive behaviour unless this is in the interests of health care service users.

It is for commissioners to decide what services to procure and how best to secure them in the interests of healthcare service users. The regulations adopt a principles-based approach that is intended to give commissioners flexibility. NHS Improvement (NHSI)'s role is limited to ensuring that commissioners have operated within the legal framework established by the regulations.

CCGs will need to decide, subject to the National Health Service (Procurement, Patient Choice and Competition) (No 2) Regulations 2013 and current procurement rules set out in the Public Contracts Regulations 2006 where it is appropriate to commission community-based services through competitive tender, through an Any Qualified Provider (AQP) approach or through single tender. In general, commissioning through competitive tender or AQP will introduce greater transparency and help reduce the scope for conflicts.

Governance checklist

- How clear is the vision and aims of the CCG to the member practices and the governing body? Do they understand the constitution and their role as set out there?
- Do the member practices and governing body understand the statutory duties prescribed for a CCG? To what extent does the information that they receive help them to make rigorous decisions in line with those duties?
- What does the size and complexity of the CCG mean for the ways in which they approach each of the main functions of governance set out by the Good Governance Standard for Public Services?
- How clearly defined are the respective roles and responsibilities of the member practices, the governing body and the individual members?
- Do all members of the governing body take collective responsibility for the governing body's decisions?
- How well does the CCG understand the views of the public and service users?
- How does the behaviour of members, both individually and collectively as a governing body, show that their responsibilities to the CCG and its stakeholders are taken very seriously?
- Are there any ways in which member behaviour might weaken the CCG's aims and values?
- Are there formal agreements on the types of decisions that are delegated to the executive and those that are reserved for the governing body and/or the member practices? Is this set out in a clear and up-to-date statement?
- Is there clarity on the election/appointment processes for the members' representatives and the governing body members? What approach will be taken to finding a balance between continuity of knowledge and renewal of thinking in the governing body?
- How well does the role of the lay members support independent scrutiny and challenge? What further measures might be considered to strengthen this if required?
- Is there a process for regularly reviewing the CCG's governance arrangements and practice? Is this independently assessed at any point?

Summary

- The governance of CCGs is maturing, and there are clear signs of consistency developing around the principles, if not around the actual governance processes.
- CCGs were specifically developed as membership organisations; to expect a rigidity of governance more closely aligned to a publicly listed company may not have been appropriate.

- It is clear that there is a requirement for robust governance arrangements within the accountability structure envisaged by NHSE, allowing CCGs the flexibility to develop those arrangements.
- As CCGs seek to integrate and work more closely with their stakeholders, the opportunity to deliver their statutory duties more effectively may present itself. As such, the CCG's role will continue to evolve. As new care models are established, the boundary between what is done by CCGs and by new integrated care providers will shift. However, there will continue to be a need for an effective commissioning function in the NHS. This includes acting as funder, setting local priorities and incentives, oversight of contracts, ensuring best value for the taxpayer, and ensuring the provision of a comprehensive local NHS within the available resources.

16
New models of care

Introduction

According to NHSE, 'one of the original aims of STPs was to develop new care models as blueprints for future care'. The 'vanguard' and 'pioneer' programmes in specific locations initially introduced these new care models and the ongoing commitment to the work of the STPs is not intended to replace new care models; instead, STPs are intended to create the environment in which the success of the vanguards and pioneer programmes is able to evolve and spread. A small number of the STPs are also now evolving into integrated or 'accountable' care systems (ACSs). In these areas, providers and commissioners are coming together, with a combined budget and fully shared resources, to serve a defined population.

Many of the new models of care promoted by the 5YFV are underpinned by different legal structures, which would qualify as a significant transaction (e.g. acquisitions, mergers, foundation groups, hospital chain, accountable care organisations). Given that the Healthcare Commission (now CQC) had already identified back in 2008 that 'it is clear that, in relation to service failure, problems often occur at the borders between one organisation or team and another' (Learning from Investigations (2008)), the good governance of these new models and the relationships that they create is essential. This chapter seeks not only to establish the governance structures for the various models but also explores the key themes that underpin the success of these models.

'It is just as important to have good governance between organisations as within organisations. A service that stops at the doors of the hospital or when a partner fails to deliver is not really a service, it's a broken link in the chain of care. In an increasingly complex and interconnected world organisations can no longer operate in isolation. Boards must seek assurances from partners that they have identified the risks to overall strategic objectives and put adequate controls in place.'

(Integrated Governance II: Governance Between Organisations
(Institute of Healthcare Management, June 2008))

Five Year Forward View (5YFV)

Chapter 3 sets out the main implications of this guidance, but all of the new models of care covered there have their origins in the direction of travel set out in this guidance. The challenge for all boards or governing bodies is to recognise that the drivers within the guidance for transformation and sustainability do not necessarily mean large-scale transactions and structural change. Networks and collaboration may be the better option; perhaps lessons learned from earlier major restructures have demonstrated that changing the structural form does not readily lead to the scale of transformation required for sustainable services.

'The higher the degree of organisational change, the higher the risk that the benefits will not be delivered (the evidence on mergers and acquisitions is pretty unequivocal that the risks from full-scale organisational change are high).'

(*Future organisational models for the NHS. Perspectives for the Dalton review* (The King's Fund and Foundation Trust Network (FTN), July 2014))

What is clear is that, in order to be successful, these new models of care will require a greater clarity of purpose, objective setting and lines of accountability than seen before in the NHS sector. The key principles, then, for any form or structure have to be as follows:

- Ensure each partner to the new structure has the capability to lead and control the agreed objectives.
- Explore the culture of the partner organisations to determine cultural alignment and purpose.
- Ensure that the founders of the new structure can exert control over the vehicle they have collectively created.
- Consider creating a memorandum of understanding between the partners as an indication of the intended direction of travel.
- Be clear about how the new structure will relate to its key stakeholders, particularly the regulators (e.g. will a new CQC registration or provider licence be required).
- Consider the ability of the partners to be able to integrate technology so that information can easily be shared.
- Take the appropriate advice, both legal and financial, to ensure compliance with competition laws.

To be clear then, there are various models of care and their associated organisation forms presented within the Dalton Review, however, these are not necessarily clearly defined legal forms. The STPs, which were developed initially under the 5YFV, will need to consider the best legal form for each aspect of its collaborative work. When considering any of the new models of care, each board and/or governing body within the STP must consider whether a new corporate legal form is required or whether a contractual legal arrangement would be sufficient.

This distinction is helpful as the corporate or contractual form clearly establishes the degree of integration the partner organisations in the new form are trying to create. Where the STP is evolving into an ICS or ACS, clarity on the legal form and/or arrangement being proposed will be important.

The remainder of this chapter will seek to set out the various models that are currently being considered. It will then attempt to define the legal forms that may underpin the model.

Integrated Care

One of the challenges of understanding the governance issues at play in the development of integrated care is the plethora of terms that are used. For clarity, this chapter will follow the definitions set out in the King's Fund Report *Making sense of integrated care systems, integrated care partnerships and accountable care organisations in the NHS in England* (February 2018). These are as follows.

Integrated care systems (ICSs)

These have evolved from STPs and take the lead in planning and commissioning care for their populations and providing system leadership. They bring together NHS providers and commissioners and local authorities to work in partnership in improving health and care in their area. Examples include Great Manchester's and Surrey Heartlands devolution programmes. These systems currently have no statutory basis and rest on the willingness of NHS organisations to work together to plan how to improve health and care. As such, they require fluidity and flexibility in their governance arrangements.

Integrated care partnerships (ICPs)

These are alliances of NHS providers that work together to deliver care by agreeing to collaborate rather than compete. These providers include hospitals, community services, mental health services and GPs. Social care and independent and third-sector providers may also be involved. They are currently being established in ten areas, including South Yorkshire and Bassetlaw.

Accountable care organisations (ACOs)

These are established when commissioners award a long-term contract to a single organisation to provide a range of health and care services to a defined population following a competitive procurement. This organisation may subcontract with other providers to deliver the contract. In contrast to the fluid governance nature of an integrated care system, an ACO will have a formal governance and organisation structure behind it. NHSE has been attempting to develop a new contract to be used by commissioners to establish an ACO on which the DHSC has consulted. This consultation has given rise to two separate legal challenges in the High Court with claims of illegality, increasing privatisation and lack of transparency being alleged. Both challenges failed in 2018.

This model challenges the provider/commissioner split and anti-competition rules established by the HSCA 2012 and set aside earlier government policy to deliver a competitive market in healthcare services as the providers work together to both provide and commission services (e.g. when the ACO subcontracts to other providers for certain services).

Models of care

Many of these new models of care that were adopted by the vanguards required some form of pooling budgets and integration of services, but most of them proceeded on the basis of informal partnerships. Where more formal governance arrangements were sought, then a number of different legal forms were considered (see below). Whatever the form, the models continue to challenge regulators on how to:

- contract for the new systems of care;
- work together with emerging partnerships;
- allocate funding;
- engage with patients and the wider community; and
- share risk and rewards.

Interestingly it is now the scaling-up of these models that is crucial and with funding for the new care models programme coming to an end, it is not clear where the support for this will come from.

Buddying, federations and learning and clinical networks

Buddying is one of the least formal approaches to collaborative working and can start as an informal arrangement to share best practice, experience and learning across organisations. It stems from the buddying arrangements introduced for trusts in 'special measures' and the Dalton recommendation was that this should be expanded in a more formal setting to allow organisations in difficulty to benefit from support and improvement that can be offered by successful trusts. His review recommended that those organisations able to demonstrate a track record of high performance should be encouraged to consider managing an organisation in persistent difficulty through a long-term management contract.

A federation is a group of practices and primary care teams working together, sharing responsibility for developing and delivering high-quality, patient focused services for their local communities, which may include developing, providing or commissioning services, training and education, back office functions, safety and clinical governance. The size and legal entity involved will depend on the purpose for which the federation has been developed. For example, for running out of hours or other urgent care services, a larger organisation with sophisticated risk sharing arrangements is likely to make sense, whereas a joint provider of extended primary care services or a clinical governance group might be smaller and operate as a network.

Learning and clinical networks are also an informal arrangement and can be organised horizontally (e.g. across providers) or vertically (e.g. between GP practices and providers). They may have terms of reference or a memorandum of understanding, but are unlikely to have more substantial contractual arrangements. Learning networks aim to share best practice and may align policies between institutions, but they do not create new integrated delivery structures.

Multi-speciality Community Providers (MCPs)
This is where primary care (e.g. GP federations) and community care are combined. These can be 'virtual', 'partially integrated' or 'fully integrated', depending upon the level of integration envisaged.

Primary and Acute Care Systems (PACSs)
This is where secondary care providers pull the entire health and care system together. These, too, can be 'virtual', 'partially integrated' or 'fully integrated', depending upon the level of integration envisaged.

Acute Care Collaborations (ACCs)
This is where hospital chains, clinical networks, specialty franchises, multi-provider hospital groups or foundation groups combine together to provide secondary care.

Enhanced health in care homes (EHCH)
This is where care homes provide joined up primary, community, secondary and social care to residents of care and nursing homes, with staff from across health and social care organisations working together as part of multidisciplinary teams.

Urgent and Emergency Care Networks (UECNs)
These networks aim to simplify the urgent and emergency care system to provide better integration between A&E departments and other services that provide and support urgent treatments. Such networks include the development of hospital networks with access to specialist centres, new partnership options for smaller hospitals and greater use of pharmacists and out-of-hours GP services.

Foundation groups
A foundation group is the joining together of providers, and at present can present in a variety of different forms. The groups use a mixed economy of membership models, ranging from buddying through to full acquisition. Foundation groups may, for example, involve trusts joining together under the umbrella of a successful NHS provider and sharing management skills, clinical expertise and

back-office functions. There are, however, common themes principally relating to the governance and management of acute services at different locations.

In October 2016, NHSI published *Acute care collaborations – guidance on options for structuring foundation groups*, outlining the current statutory framework for such a foundation group, namely, corporate joint ventures (CJVs) or committees in common (CICs). These are covered in more detail below.

Accountable Clinical Networks (ACNs)

ACNs cover a range of acute services, including maternity and paediatrics, cancer, mental health and radiology services. The network aims to deliver rapid and sustained improvements in the systematic delivery of care by optimising patient pathways for the services covered by the network, and by identifying and implementing best practice at each stage along those pathways. The networks bring groups of providers together to consider how best to serve a defined population rather than just focusing on the services provided by their own individual organisations.

Clinical networks have existed for some time across the NHS, sometimes underpinned by contract, but often based on loose collaborative agreements. However, those arrangements have been quite fragile at times and have not been resilient enough to make the relevant services sustainable. The arrangements for an ACN will involve stricter accountability, which in most cases, means a single provider taking on a single capitated budget for the population and services covered by the network, in a similar fashion to that of MCPs and PACSs.

Specialty franchises

A good example of a speciality franchise would be the model developed by Moorfields Eye Hospital NHS Foundation Trust, one of the world's leading eye hospitals, under which they offer a range of specialist and routine ophthalmology services through satellite clinics in hospitals across London and elsewhere.

Corporate forms

Corporate joint ventures (CJV)

A joint venture (JV) is a strategic alliance where two or more parties, usually businesses, form a partnership to share markets, intellectual property, assets, knowledge, and, of course, profits. It differs from a merger in the sense that there is no transfer of ownership in the deal. In a CJV, the companies start and invest in a new company that is jointly owned by both of the parent companies thus creating a new corporate body. By comparison, a strategic alliance is a legal agreement between two or more companies to share access to their technology, trademarks or other assets. A strategic alliance does not create a new corporate body, which a CJV does.

As CJVs create a separate corporate body, they are only available to FTs, as NHS trusts do not have the power to set up or participate in corporate bodies except for income generation. FTs have the power to invest money 'for the purposes of, or in connection with, their functions', so they are able to make investments, which includes forming bodies corporate or otherwise acquiring membership of bodies corporate.

A CJV can be established by either forming a company (whether established by shares or by guarantee) or an LLP. Regardless of the legal structure used, the most important document is the joint venture agreement, which sets out all of the partners' rights and obligations as well as the objectives of the joint venture, the contributions of the partners and the rights to the profits (and losses).

A CJV between FTs could also be described as a public–public CJV as seen in a foundation group that uses the CJV form. Other CJVs could also be created, such as between an FT and a private sector organisation (public–private CJV).

There are a number of issues that a board would need to consider in establishing a successful CJV, all of which would have to be discussed with commissioners, NHSI and NHSE. These issues include:

- how the financial, operational and other risks are shared between the contracting parties, since a CJV is always a separate legal entity;
- legal and financial advice on the advantages and disadvantages of using a corporate vehicle – for example, how these vehicles are treated for tax purposes;
- whether the investment meets the definition of control or joint control under accounting standards;
- the issues of accounting consolidation within the DHSC's group accounts;
- the cultural fit and responsiveness of the chosen partner since these are as important as any considerations about commerciality;
- the appropriate governance structure, beyond just the shareholding, which balances taking sufficient control to ensure the FT's requirements are met and allowing the partner the necessary freedom to act to achieve them; and
- how to work in a partnership rather than solely enforcing a contractual model.

Interestingly, research by Grant Thornton (*Better together: Building a successful joint venture company (2016)*) demonstrates that public–public CJVs can be more successful as they combine common cultures and all profits are returned to the public sector. The research, although focused on local government, recommends the following relevant considerations, which have been adapted here for NHS joint ventures:

- clear objectives for the CJV (e.g. income growth, costs savings, etc.);
- readiness to work in partnership as well as contractually;
- robust understanding of own services and opportunities for growth;
- access to professional advice and support;
- effective procurement process to test partnering arrangements;
- effective sharing of profit and risk;

- anticipation of future changes, building in flexibility to contracts, performance monitoring, etc.;
- creating a culture of trust and strong working relationship;
- ongoing scrutiny of key outcomes (not inputs or activity);
- allowing the CJV to operate independently not as a division of the FT;
- appropriate corporate structure and governance arrangements – CJV is commercial in its relationship with non-partners and a partnership manner with CJV partners; and
- appropriate plans for an exit if and when it will be required.

Committees in common

The NHSI guidance on foundation groups also offers committees in common as a possible vehicle for a new model of care. The key features of committees in common are as follows:

- They are accountable to their respective boards.
- Although each organisation appoints its own committee, they can meet at the same time and with the same remit.
- Co-ordinated decision making is improved by each committee having, wherever possible, the same membership.
- Commissioning contracts remain with the respective partners.
- Assets remain in each organisation's ownership but committees in common can be given responsibility for managing them.
- Establishing committees in common does not affect the regulatory framework.

Tim Winn, in his article 'Operating Effective Committees in Common' (July 2018), describes two types of committee in common: the advisory committee and the decision-making committee.

> 'An **advisory committee** makes recommendations or gives advice to the member organisations, who then decide what to do. This type of committee may be constituted by the boards of the member organisations, but its membership is entirely flexible because while it is important that its purpose is clear, the committee does not need to fit into the governance structure of its member organisations. What it does, and who sits on it, really is up to [the member organisations], because there are no legal requirements for discussion groups, however formally or informally they might be constituted.
>
> A **decision-making committee** takes decisions for the member organisations. Therefore, each organisation's decision is taken by its own representatives. The appointment of the organisation's representatives – and the way in which the representatives take decisions – must comply with that organisation's internal governance structure and the terms on which they have delegated authority to those who represent them at the committee's meetings. This category includes committees that take decisions, including those that take

irreversible decisions or those that take decisions that can be overturned by the member organisations, or those committees whose decisions have to be "ratified" by the member organisations.'

For NHS Trusts, under the usual NHS Trust Standing Orders, the board can delegate its authority to a committee, to an ED or an employee of the Trust. For FTs, the board can only delegate its authority to a committee of directors or an individual ED.

'This means that legally, individual FT NEDs operating at system-level are doing so as individuals and have no powers to bind their organisation. This problem may be overcome by two or more NEDs representing a FT as a committee with delegations from the board.'

(Collaborative Working – Tackling Governance Challenges in Practice – Hempsons/NHS Providers re (November 2018))

In CCGs, depending upon their constitution the CCG can delegate its authority to a member of the CCG (a member GP), to the Governing Body, to a committee of the CCG or to an employee of the CCG. Those new models that involve local authorities have different rules again.

Tim Winn goes on to outline a number of practical consequences:

- The delegate actually has to have the authority to take the decisions required.
- Quoracy is key and for a committee in common to be quorate and able to take decisions it will need all of the organisations to be represented at the necessary level.
- Provision for substitutes should be considered at authorisation level, as well as at committee level. The committee in common's terms of reference need to say that organisations can send substitutes, but so does the donor organisation.
- Unanimous decisions. No organisation can be outvoted on a committee in common as each represented organisation takes its decisions, separately – so decisions have to be made unanimously.
- Abstentions – if an organisation's delegate abstains, then that organisation has not taken any decision at all.
- Responsibility for the decisions taken by each organisation lies with its delegates. This suggests that organisations should choose their delegates with care.

The committees can be supported by a legally binding contractual joint venture between the participating partners (see below).

Committees in common may be useful where three or more providers, including an NHS trust, wish to form a foundation group. Some provider boards have appointed a joint CEO and/or a chair as a practical first step in setting up these arrangements. If a foundation group comprises a single FT and a single NHS trust, the NHS trust could appoint a committee whose membership consists of all the directors of the NHS FT.

Mergers and acquisitions

Ultimately, however, the legal forms above are limited in that accountability remains with each organisation's board. Consequently, some boards may conclude that the real value of the structural change is to develop clinical and management integration as the first step towards a full merger or acquisition. A word of caution does need to be mentioned here since the King's Fund's review found that, although reconfigurations are sometimes undertaken to produce financial savings, the evidence that these savings are delivered is almost entirely lacking (see Imison, Sonola, Honeyman and Ross, King's Fund, 2014). Trust mergers are often seen as enabling change to services by removing organisational barriers. Again, a parallel study of 20 mergers between 2010 and 2015 by the King's Fund found a cost to the DH (now DHSC) of approximately £2 billion to support 12 of these mergers. This funding was used for various purposes, including paying off legacy debt, tackling underlying deficits, and investing in new buildings and upgraded facilities to enable clinical services to be reconfigured (see Collins, King's Fund, 2015). There was no clear evidence that these mergers had produced commensurate financial benefits through changes to clinical care or through cutting back on management costs.

Nevertheless, this is still a regularly used vehicle for improving sustainability and delivering transformation, particularly in relation to dealing with poorly performing organisations. The NHS Act 2006 governs NHS mergers and acquisitions with different provisions (and implications) depending on whether the transaction is structured as a merger or an acquisition. The Single Operating Framework sets out that NHSI is responsible for reviewing mergers and acquisitions to understand their potential impact on both the risk profile of the acquiring FT and its ability to continue to meet its provider licence conditions. NHSI has a role in approving mergers and acquisitions (see Chapter 14). Both the NHS organisations involved in the transaction, as well as commissioners of their services, are also required to consider their obligations under the Public Contracts Regulations 2015, as such obligations may be triggered as a result of the merger or acquisition. Finally, each NHS trust and/or FT must comply with its own internal governance arrangements when making a decision to merge or acquire another organisation.

Contractual forms

Contractual joint ventures

Both NHS FTs and NHS trusts can enter into contractual joint ventures that are legally binding. Such ventures do not establish new bodies but can create legally binding rights and responsibilities (e.g. establishing a contractual joint venture for pathology services). In principle, contractual joint ventures could be used to establish prime contractor/subcontractor arrangements to address changes to commissioning arrangements/proposals for service reconfiguration and financial adjustments/risk share arrangements.

Alliance Agreement

Alliance contracting for delivering projects has grown rapidly since it was first adopted with outstanding results in the early 1990s for the development of the BP Andrew oil field in the North Sea. An alliance contract creates a collaborative environment without the need for new organisational forms. By having one alliance contract, all parties are working to the same outcomes and are signed up to the same success measures. There is a strong sense of 'your problem is my problem, your success is my success'. The parties share risk, collectively own opportunities and are all responsible for the delivery of a contract. Unlike a contract co-ordinated by a prime contractor, there are no sub-contractual arrangements. All organisations within the alliance are equal partners and organise their own internal governance to manage the delivery of care.

The Alliance Agreement is a contractual arrangement being consulted upon by NHSE for use by virtual MCPs/PACSs and does not replace or override existing services contracts (i.e. contracts between the commissioner and the provider for delivery of care). Instead, it is intended to bring providers together around a common aspiration for joint working across the system by setting out a number of shared objectives and a set of shared governance arrangements. The governance arrangements establish an alliance leadership team, an alliance management team and an alliance programme manager. The alliance leadership team is a forum, in which the representatives of each provider and commissioner have been given delegated decision-making authority. This allows them to make decisions on behalf of each alliance member. The need for unanimity in decision making to make such an arrangement effective is set out in the terms of reference for the alliance leadership team.

Integration Agreement

The NHSE Integration Agreement is a contractual arrangement for use in partially integrated MCPs/PACSs. It will ensure that the GPs involved have the necessary commitment to integration for the MCP/PACS to succeed. The Agreement will perform two main functions:

1. to create a framework for shared governance and decision making between practices and the MCP/PACS; and
2. to set out how the integration of services will be affected, setting out the primary care contribution to the MCP/PACS care model.

MCP/PACS Contract

The MCP/PACS Contract is a contractual arrangement being consulted upon by NHSE to make sure that the contracting and financial environment supports integration and delivery of the MCP/PACS care model. By awarding an MCP/

PACS Contract, commissioners can ensure that the integrated working and aligned incentives that providers have built through the model are sustainable and that organisational siloes are truly dissolved. The MCP Contract will be awarded for up to 15 years, and NHS bodies (e.g. FTs) and non-NHS bodies (e.g. a GP LLP) can bid for the contract. The PACS Contract will be of longer duration than those that are typically offered to NHS providers at present but with an initial early breakpoint (e.g. after the first two or three years of the contract term).

Bidders will need to demonstrate to commissioners, NHSI and NHSE through the procurement process and the Integrated Support and Assurance Process (see below), that they are capable of holding and delivering the contract. Any bidder for the MCP Contract (fully or partially integrated) will be required to demonstrate how they will work with GPs.

The PACS contract could be held by a new entity, formed (e.g. through a joint venture between a group of GPs, an acute trust, and other local health and care providers, or held by an existing NHS provider).

Formal agreement

Implementing the EHCH care model does not involve the creation of a single lead provider; nor are care home providers expected to merge with an MCP or a PACS in a new organisational form. Consequently, a formal agreement is the contractual arrangement whereby care home providers may, if they wish, enter into an agreement with an MCP or PACS, or existing commissioners and providers, to formalise their commitment to whole-system, partnership working.

Section 75 agreements

Section 75 is an agreement made under section 75 of the National Health Services Act 2006 between a local authority and an NHS body in England. They have been used extensively prior to the 5YFV and are now being used in conjunction with other contractual forms as they can include arrangements for pooling resources and delegating certain NHS and local authority health-related functions to the other partner(s) if it would lead to an improvement in the way those functions are exercised. Section 75 agreements are not a contract nor an operational model or a transfer of functions. It is a partnership of equal control whereby one partner can act as a 'host' to manage the delegated functions, including statutory functions of both partners who remain equally responsible and accountable for those functions being carried out in a suitable manner.

Regulation of new models of care

NHSI worked with NHSE to develop and implement the ISAP. *The Integrated Support and Assurance Process: An introduction to assuring novel and complex contracts* was published in November 2016, and was designed to be a consistent, streamlined NHSE and NHSI process for supporting and assuring novel procurements. Commissioners wishing to make use of the ACO contract will have to go through the ISAP and demonstrate that their plans are robust. The alternative is to use existing contracts underpinned by agreements among providers to work in partnership as is happening in the new models of care and ICPs.

In addition, NHSI has indicated that it must be consulted when new care models involve transactions, mergers or raise other oversight considerations. NHSI must also be involved if NHS trusts or FTs are entering into new or novel contracts with their commissioners to deliver a new care model.

For FTs, NHSI will also continue to review transactions that are material, significant or statutory (see Chapter 14). For NHS trusts, NHSI also has a role, on behalf of the SoS, in overseeing and assuring transactions.

NHSI has issued guidance called *Transactions guidance – for trusts undertaking transactions, including mergers and acquisitions* (2017) to advise and support NHS trusts and FTs through the process.

Governance implications

The challenges for governance going forward will relate to clear accountability structures and the identification and management of the risks that are created by these new configurations with a range of partners.

New models of care such as integrated care systems, integrated care partnerships and accountable care organisations can consider corporate or contractual forms such as joint ventures, mergers & acquisitions to help formalise their governance as they have governance frameworks in existence elsewhere outside of the NHS sector. The idea of the Dalton Review was to borrow these models and adapt them to the NHS sector.

Many STPs are underpinned by some form of shared governance arrangements to take forward their planned changes and to support joint decision making and accountability.

Most of the published STPs set out a delivery structure which, with variations, typically includes a strategic board and delivery board supported by a programme management office (PMO). These boards are generally fed by either workstream groups, sector groups or local area groups. The extent to which the key enablers of workforce, estates and IT are included is largely consistent, although the resource allocated to the PMO is mixed (ranging from some full-time teams to those working on it in addition to their day jobs). Some plans explicitly distinguish groups as decision making, operational or advisory. However, they do not generally include details about how the governance structures will work in practice and how they will need to evolve as the STP progresses.

Many STPs have developed or are developing a memorandum of understanding (MOU), which is signed up to by individual boards and provides a clear model for accountability. *Governing for Transformation: STPs and governance* (NHS

Providers and Hempsons, November 2016) provides a template MOU covering: scope and clarity of purpose; agreed principles; governance for decision making; disagreements and disputes; opting out; risk and assurance; and resources.

Accountability

Who will be accountable for the delivery of STPs? Most STPs have been organised by consensus and collaboration, wholly appropriate for developing plans, but not for implementation. At present, NHSE and NHSI are clear that each board or governing body retains authority over the decision for each individual organisation that is part of the STP and that each board or governing body has a responsibility to the wider health economy, not just the performance of their individual part. This raises interesting questions when financial and performance targets are still set for each individual organisation not pooled for the STP. STPs also require full engagement with local authorities whose governance arrangements are completely different to that within the NHS.

In addition, there is an inherent tension at the heart of each individual organisation involved in these collaborative new forms, with the benefits for 'the corporation' and for 'the public' not necessarily being the same thing. The King's Fund (2017) reports that 'some places are beginning to consider ways of bringing NEDs into the governance structures of their integrated care system, for example by having a NEDs, lay members and elected members group. NEDs of the future may well be judged not by how much time they spend in meetings but by their contribution to the ecology of system relationships.'

The HFMA Handbook (2018) recognises the increasing need for joint and partnership working raises some interesting governance issues. Chapter 6 of the HFMA Handbook (2018) explores the role of the audit committee in supporting good governance and establishing clear assurance processes for partnerships working at scale. It acknowledges that risks tend to arise at the borders between organisations and recommends that the audit committee consider assurance and accountability in the following areas:

- any pooled budget arrangements
- aligned board reporting,
- shared financial control totals
- shared performance goals
- clear procurement arrangements for complex transactions
- steps to address the key lines of enquiries for all novel contracts

In some instances, audit committees may end working together under a committee in common arrangement. The HFMA Handbook (2018) offers good practice for such collaborative arrangements, these include separate chairs, separate terms of reference, separate agenda and minutes, separate attendance records, separate reports to their respective governing bodies and a robust process for managing conflicts of interest.

Patient and public engagement

How are the needs of patients and the public kept at the heart of STPs? Involvement with clinicians, CCG lay members, NEDs, FT governors, patient forums and by having wider engagement with local politicians and the public will be essential. Early involvement in STP planning and delivery will bring long-term benefits and there is evidence that already plans have progressed too far without this engagement and the reputation of the STPs and their leadership risk being damaged, perhaps fatally.

Local government

How are the right relationships being built within STPs? STPs are about integration – social care and health integration, closer collaboration of CCGs, and bringing together responsibility for the commissioning and provision of services within innovative arrangements. As such, building relationships across the NHS and local government within each footprint is paramount for STP delivery. This integration will require careful thought and open debate, as it will combine different forms of governance (e.g. unitary board and cabinet decision making).

Balancing the tension between making decisions quickly and openly and transparently

There is an inherent tension between making decisions quickly to speed up transformation and making the right decisions openly and transparently, with the support of the main stakeholders in the system. Governance structures will need to be streamlined, but absolutely require good communication channels that support feedback gathering and information dissemination.

The clinical voice

How can STPs preserve the clinical voice? It is essential for implementation that clinical input and the clinical voice sits equally alongside the managerial input and voice to drive service transformation and improvement.

Independent scrutiny

What role will lay members, NEDs and FT governors have in delivering STPs? Each STP footprint has been left to determine its governance form and despite this flexibility it will be essential to ensure that independent challenge should be represented throughout the decision-making process to ensure that scrutiny, transparency and decision making remains firmly in the interest of the public and patients.

The Art of the Possible by Hempsons and NHS Providers (2017) suggests that 'over-reliance on delegations can mean that decisions are not subjected to rigorous challenge that is the standard way of working at trust board level and constitutes best practice'. The appointment of associate NEDS is being considered to resolve this.

Audit and assurance

What assurance processes will be available to support that independent scrutiny? Effective assurance systems that include risk management and internal controls will need to be developed for the STPs. Where new models of care are being used that are recognised forms of organisational structure, such as joint venture, then using their existing governance may be sufficient. However, there may also be a need for different central government policy and/or legislation to enable these new forms to develop.

Scale and complexity

As ACOs and ICSs develop the resulting organisations may be very large, which may make it very difficult for a single board to direct and control. Outside of the NHS, such large corporate organisations establish group structures to provide the necessary corporate governance; these examples may be of use to NHS in exploring governance frameworks. *The Art of the Possible* (2017) suggests that the greatest risk lies in the period of transition 'where multiple health and care body corporates are working together'.

The King's Fund (2017) makes the following observation, which sets out clearly the challenges that may lie ahead for STPs and illustrates the consequences where there are poor governance arrangements:

> 'STPs are a conscious "workaround" by national bodies of the complex and fragmented organisational arrangements that are the legacy of the Health and Social Care Act 2012. They rely on the willingness of NHS leaders at a local level to collaborate with their peers in the best interests of the populations they serve. STPs have no basis in statute, and their proposals need to be endorsed and supported by the boards of the NHS organisations involved as they move from planning to implementation.
>
> There is an ever-present risk that these proposals will be challenged by those who oppose them through judicial review and other means. This would introduce further delays to the implementation of planned changes and so it is important therefore that the governance and decision-making processes are formalised to align the ambition to collaborate in STPs with the sovereignty, accountability and legal duties of the boards of NHS organisations and local authorities.'

A way forward

Legislative change

The King's Fund (2017) recommends that the HSCA 2012 be revisited to amend those sections that are not aligned to the 5YFV and STPs, in particular the aspects of anti-competitive rules and to acknowledge the formal role of STPs.

Whilst this is not likely in the short term, in June 2018, prime minister Theresa May said, 'As our NHS evolves, and delivers more joined-up care across different services, we should make sure the regulatory framework keeps in step and does not become a barrier to progress.' This was echoed by Simon Stevens, CEO of NHSE, who recently called for 'pragmatic changes' to be made. In particular, he called for:

- 'the ability for local NHS organisations to function in a way that is more consistent with the move towards systems working [and population health]';
- 'impediments [to local organisations working as systems] which exist [in] procurement and competition legislation' to be removed; and
- the 'streamlining of some of the national accountability arrangements', thus building on NHSE and NHSIs joint working.

Regulatory change

The increasing focus on working with partners across health and social care required by STPs, integrated care systems, integrated care partnerships and accountable care organisations creates a tension for providers and commissioners alike; as they continue to work on organisational performance as part of wider system performance. This is increasingly being recognised in the guidance being published. The Well-Led Framework (June 2017) maintains its focus on organisations because this is the statutory basis for service provision, but it has increased the emphasis on working proactively with partners. It recommends that many of the principles of good governance at organisational level are also applicable at system level and the guidance encourages local system partners to use the framework for development opportunities within STPs if it is appropriate. The CQC is also now beginning to assess commitment to system working as part of its well-led assessment.

Integrating the work of NHSE and NHSI is also a step towards supporting an integrated system of care. The joint working arrangements between NHSE and NHSI offer the opportunity for a 'single financial and operating planning process for the NHS, a single performance management process and the alignment of regulatory interventions'. As such, it might begin to remove the mixed and conflicting messages that providers and commissioners receive. In addition, it should reduce the regulatory burden of reporting.

In *The Future Shape Of The NHS*, John Coutts of NHS Providers (November 2018) suggests that a 'slimmed down NHSE/NHSI could act as an institutional shareholder on behalf of the public taking a strategic oversight, acting as a conduit for political input – intervening in extremis but largely abstaining from interference in operational business'. He goes onto suggest that the regional functions of NHSI and NHSE would be integrated into the responsibilities of the system itself.

As John Deffenbaugh states in his article *Accountable Care is the New Paradigm of Healthcare* (British Journal of Healthcare Management 2018), 'stakeholders in accountable care will face a tension between legal duties and partnership working, so they will need to give up sovereignty to take these collective risks.'

Practical change

NHS Providers in its briefing for governors, No Trust is an Island (2018), recommends that where significant changes for FTs are proposed, governors are consulted, especially if this falls within the FT's definition of a significant transaction. It also notes that governors can be a key avenue to facilitate the FT's engagement with the public around STPs and ICSs, as they act on behalf of the interests of the trust's members and the public, and have experience in engaging with communities that are traditionally hard to reach, or groups with certain protected characteristics.

There is a role too for NEDs as John Deffenbaugh in his article 'Becoming an Integrated (Accountable) Care System' (*British Journal of Healthcare Management* 2018) recognises 'the emerging governance structure at ICS level will need to incorporate a role for NEDs. They will be as valuable, if not more so, in shaping the effectiveness of the ICS as they will be in the partner organisations that comprise the ICS.'

In *The Future Shape of the NHS* (November 2018), John Coutts comments that 'non-statutory partnerships are usually more difficult environments in which to make binding decisions, and to control, than single organisations. They often have differing cultures and rely on good relationships, relationships that are bound to change as personnel change. Non-statutory partnerships provide a short-term solution to collaborative working but are unlikely to be sustainable in the longer term.'

He goes on to suggest another view which would retain the advantages of the FT unitary board leadership and autonomy which is to use existing trusts as 'one key building block for system working'. In his words, 'this could mean four or five quite large vertically and horizontally integrated trusts, alliances of trusts and GP federations using a lead contractor model or a locally agreed variation.' To achieve this, he suggests that some mergers/acquisitions might be required but using a lead contractor model may also be viable. In due course, the system itself (the ICS) would need to be created as a corporate body with a board of directors that reflected the system. He suggests that forming special health authorities under the 2012 Act, might be a feasible option.

The viability of the special authorities option is rejected by Nicholas Timmins in *Amending the 2012 Act: can it be done?* (Kings Fund October 2018) as he argues that:

- they would not meet the criteria for special authorities and could be open to legal challenge
- they would be subject to a shelf life of three years as prescribed by the legislation and would always be preparing their own demise; and
- NHSI and NHDSE would have no regulatory powers over them as a special health authority as such bodies are answerable to the SoS.

He argues that 'a more likely route for an integrated care system within the existing Act is for CCGs to merge or form joint committees'.

In order to address the issues of accountability *The Future Shape* recommends a local accountability which could be achieved through 'bringing together health and wellbeing boards across regions, widening membership to include a broader range of stakeholders and changing their role to patient/service user champion with limited/defined powers to hold trust boards and regions to account'. Currently they have limited formal powers and it is possible that further legislation would be needed to enable this.

Tackling governance challenges

The Hempsons/NHS Providers report *Collaborative Working – Tackling Governance Challenges in Practice* (November 2018) sets out some common principles that boards could adopt to ensure that the risk inherent in system-wide working are identified and managed for the benefit of their populations.

- **Directors and boards need to prioritise the best interests of patients and the public across the system's catchment area,** rather than thinking about the interests of the system infrastructure or the narrower interests of their trust.
- **The envelope for delegations needs to be carefully defined.** It should include the right to make decisions that accord with trust strategy, policy and culture, accord with the agreed system strategy, will not destabilise the trust financially and will not bring the trust into disrepute.
- **Boards need to consider what classes of decision they will continue to reserve for themselves.** If boards across the system can reach an agreement on decisions they choose not to delegate, but reserve to themselves, all the better, but it is not essential.
- **Boards need to work within the system with colleagues to reconcile top-down decision making with staff engagement programmes from the frontline.** This is particularly important in managing change involving job and organisation design. It should not be an insurmountable process, since strategy development needs to be simultaneously top down and bottom up so the staff are brought along with strategy as it emerges, can shape its development, and own and deliver any change.
- **Boards should be clear with one another that while they will endeavour not to overturn decisions made under delegation at system levels, they reserve the right to do so.** However, they will inform partner organisations at the earliest opportunity if this seems likely to happen.
- **Boards should extend their risk management systems to incorporate system-wide risk.** The system itself should also develop a risk management system that allows individual boards to escalate and de-escalate risk within the system.
- **Boards should re-examine how they will obtain assurance on system-wide risk** and decide what actions they will take in the absence of such assurance or if there are concerns about the quality of assurance.

NEW MODELS OF CARE

- **Boards should introduce a process of informal call overs (meetings on an informal basis) between NEDs/chairs and EDs** so that potential decisions can be challenged on an ad hoc basis prior to being taken.
- **Boards should consider retrospectively decisions taken under delegation, examine the risk and look for assurance that it is being mitigated,** and if necessary take steps
- **The guiding principle for everyone should be: doubt is your friend, if in doubt, don't suppress it, act on it for the good of the trust, patients and the wider system.**

Governance checklist

- What systems or processes are available to help clarify the different levels at which decisions will be made within the STP?
- Given that STPs have no legal accountabilities, how will collective decisions be reached (eg formal schemes of delegation, committees in common, terms of reference, etc)?
- How are provider NEDs, CCG lay members, and councillors represented throughout the STP decision-making process, and what role do they play in scrutiny and assurance?
- What needs to be in place to ensure that individual statutory responsibilities can still be delivered?
- How involved have local authority health and overview scrutiny committees and health and wellbeing boards been in developing and scrutinising STPs? What are the plans for involving them during implementation?

(Taken from the STP checklist by NHS Clinical Commissioners.)

Summary

- There is much technical and legal guidance in this area and it is clear from the wealth of resources being made available that there is still more clarity to be gained on how to implement the new models of care and how to address their implications in terms of the statutory and regulatory frameworks.
- Interestingly though, the key to success in all of these structural forms is related to clear governance processes which foster trust and collaboration.
- Such processes require a new type of leadership, which is set out in the NHSI's new national framework, *Developing People – Improving Care. A National Framework for action on improvement and leadership development in NHS-funded services* (2016). High-performing health systems show that compassionate and inclusive leadership behaviours create cultures where people can deliver sustainable quality and efficiency improvements quickly.

- '[A]ny of the arrangements under consideration could bring benefits but it is not the organisational form that will determine the outcome, it is the quality of leadership alongside a culture of excellence in performance and accountability for results' ('New organisational models for the NHS won't be built in a day', *King's Fund, Blog*, 1 July 2014).
- Despite the uncertainty of the future success of STPs and whether they can deliver the widespread transformation required to deliver ongoing sustainability, there are key health service governance principles that need to be enshrined to guide the governance structures going forward for the STPs and their new models of care.
- Without any change to the legislative framework likely in the short term, STPs and new models of care are being required to develop workarounds that may be unstable and the Kings Fund (2017) makes it clear 'their effectiveness hinges on the willingness of local leaders to work in this way and if necessary to give up some of their own sovereignty for the greater good of the populations they serve'.

17
Risk management

Introduction

The responsibility of boards for effective risk management came under close scrutiny following the 2007–09 banking crisis. Banks were criticised for getting into financial difficulty because of reckless business strategies and failing to recognise the business risks that they were taking.

From a more positive aspect, research by Ernst & Young (2015), *Turning Risk into Results*, has found that companies with more mature risk management practices generate three times the level of earnings before interest, tax and depreciation as those with the least mature risk management practices.

Within NHS organisations, the scrutiny of risk management is also the responsibility of the board; however, there tends to be rigorous external scrutiny as well. The leaders of NHS organisations are responsible for deciding risk strategies and risk policies, and for ensuring that the systems to support the management of those risks are effective.

There are some similarities between a risk management system and an internal control system, but each has a different purpose. It is important to distinguish between them: in essence, the risk management system is the overarching system that is then underpinned and supported by the internal control system.

The boards of publicly quoted companies faced a step change in their approach to risk management with the introduction of the FRC Guidance on *Risk Management, Internal Control and Related Financial and Business Reporting* (2014) (FRC Risk Guide). This guidance revised, integrated and replaced the previous editions of the FRC risk guidance *Internal Control: Revised Guidance for Directors on the Combined Code* (formerly known as the Turnbull Guidance) and the *Going Concern and Liquidity Risk: Guidance for Directors of UK Companies*. The FRC Board Guide now also references the 2014 guidance and recommends that board directors familiarise themselves with it.

The FRC Risk Guide sets out its aims as 'bring[ing] together elements of best practice for risk management; prompt[ing] boards to consider how to discharge their responsibilities in relation to the existing and emerging principal risks faced by the company; reflect[ing] sound business practice, whereby risk management and internal control are embedded in the business process by which a company pursues its objectives; and highlight[ing] related reporting responsibilities'.

The FRC Risk Guide states that board responsibilities for risk include 'financial, operational, reputational, behavioural, organisational, third party, or external risks, such as market or regulatory risk, over which the board may have little or no direct control'.

Consequently, the challenge is to include behavioural and organisational risk into their risk management systems. The FRC's rationale behind this has been the recognition that the root causes of most crises lie in human behaviour and in the way that organisations are led, structured and managed. The FRC Risk Guide recommends that boards should evaluate their skills as to understanding risk as part of the annual board evaluation process so ignorance of risk will cease to be an excuse. Boards therefore need to understand:

- the nature of their principal risks;
- the responsibility of the board to decide how much risk the organisation should be prepared to accept in order to achieve hoped-for financial or performance returns; and
- how much risk the organisation should be able to tolerate.

Exposures to business risk should not exceed the levels determined by the board. The business risk management system should be effective in ensuring that board strategies and policies are implemented and reviewed.

Risk has a higher profile within NHS organisations with the active involvement of the audit committee in the board assurance framework (BAF) and the regular scrutiny of principal risks, or the existence of specific committees, which consider risk as part of the quality and/or governance agenda. Even so, the FRC Risk Guide provides a benchmark for consideration.

The regulatory framework for risk management and internal control

Though not required to follow the UK Code or the FRC guidance, NHS organisations and health service governance can benchmark best practice against the provisions in recognition of the connection between good corporate governance and risk management. It is therefore worth setting out these provisions in more detail.

The Turnbull Guidance on internal control

When principles and provisions relating to internal control and risk management were first introduced under the Combined Code in 1998, a working party known as the Turnbull Committee published guidelines to listed companies on how to apply them. This was referred to as the Turnbull Guidance, and was the responsibility of the FRC.

This guidance has now been replaced by the FRC Risk Guide, which links the traditional Turnbull Guidance on internal control with emerging good practice for risk management. However, the Turnbull Guidance still offers helpful insights on the effective working of an internal controls system.

The Turnbull Guidance applied to the entire system of internal control, including operational and compliance controls as well as financial controls. It defined an internal control system as 'the policies, processes, tasks, behaviours and other aspects of an organisation' that, taken together:

- help it to operate effectively and efficiently so that the organisation can respond in an appropriate way to principal risks to achieving the organisation's objectives;
- help it to ensure the quality of external and internal reporting; and
- help to ensure compliance with applicable laws and regulations, and also with internal policies for the conduct of business.

According to Turnbull, internal control should be embedded in the business and its operating systems. Controls should not be applied occasionally or from an external source, and they should be applied regularly and automatically as part of established procedures. Controls also have to remain relevant over time. As circumstances change, controls should be altered or adapted to meet the new requirements, as controls that are appropriate to an organisation should take account of its particular circumstances.

The Turnbull Guidance also suggested that a system of internal control includes control activities, information and communications processes and process for monitoring the effectiveness of the system. The system of internal control should:

- be embedded in the operations of the organisation and form part of its culture;
- be capable of responding quickly to evolving risks to the business arising from factors within the organisation and to changes in the business environment; and
- include procedures for reporting immediately to appropriate levels of management any significant control failings or weaknesses that are identified together with details of corrective action being undertaken.

FRC Guidance on Risk Management, internal Control and Related Financial and business Reporting (The FRC Risk Guide)

The FRC Risk Guide:

- brought together elements of best practice for risk management;
- prompted boards to consider how to discharge their responsibilities in relation to the existing and emerging principal risks faced by the organisation;
- reflected sound business practice, whereby risk management and internal control were embedded in the business process by which an organisation pursued its objectives; and
- highlighted related reporting responsibilities.

The guidance is primarily aimed at companies subject to the UK Code, but provides useful best practice benchmarking for NHS organisations and will be referenced throughout this chapter.

UK Code

A core principle of the UK Code is that: 'the board should establish procedures to manage risk, oversee the internal control framework, and determine the nature and extent of the principal risks the company is willing to take in order to achieve its long-term strategic objectives.'

The UK Code also includes the following principle: 'the board should establish formal and transparent policies and procedures to ensure the independence and effectiveness of internal and external audit functions and satisfy itself on the integrity of financial and narrative statements.'

In other words, the board's responsibility for reviewing internal controls (and risk management) extends beyond financial matters to business operations and regulatory compliance. Indeed the FRC Board Guide also recognises that risks can emerge and crystallise rapidly, so the systems in place to monitor risks should include procedures to elevate any concerns to the board's attention as quickly as possible. 'Processes for doing this and agreed triggers should be clear and be implemented quickly.'

The UK Code recommends that principal risks should include those risks that could result in events or circumstances that might threaten the company's business model, future performance, solvency or liquidity and reputation. In deciding which risks are principal risks companies should consider the potential impact and probability of the related events or circumstances, and the timescale over which they may occur.

The nature of risk

Risk refers to the possibility that something unexpected or unplanned for will happen. In many cases, risk is seen as the possibility that something bad might happen. In everyday life, there is a risk of becoming seriously ill, being involved in a road accident, having a house burgled or flooded, having a motorcar breakdown, and so on. This can be described as downside risk, because it is a risk that something will happen that would not normally be expected.

There is also upside risk – the possibility that events might turn out better than expected. In a health service context, an example is the possibility that activity levels will be higher than planned or that working days lost through industrial action will be lower than anticipated. Another example is investment decisions. Every investment is risky, and actual returns could be lower or higher than expected. In deciding whether to undertake an investment, the risks as well as the potential returns should be considered. Some risks are easy to recognise because they are always present and an NHS organisation may have had many years of experience in dealing with them. For example, financial risks include the risk that tariff will be set at a substantially lower level or that the costs of pharmaceutical supplies will increase. Other risks, however, are more difficult to identify and anticipate.

RISK MANAGEMENT

The FRC Risk Guide describes the board's responsibilities for an organisation's overall approach to risk management and internal control as follows:

- ensuring the design and implementation of appropriate risk management and internal control systems that identify the risks facing the company and enable the board to make a robust assessment of the principal risks;
- determining the nature and extent of the principal risks faced and those risks which the organisation is willing to take in achieving its strategic objectives (determining its 'risk appetite');
- ensuring that appropriate culture and reward systems have been embedded throughout the organisation;
- agreeing how the principal risks should be managed or mitigated to reduce the likelihood of their incidence or their impact;
- monitoring and reviewing the risk management and internal control systems, and the management's process of monitoring and reviewing, and satisfying itself that they are functioning effectively and that corrective action is being taken where necessary; and
- ensuring sound internal and external information and communication processes and taking responsibility for external communication on risk management and internal control.

That said, it is still management's role to implement and take day-to-day responsibility for board policies on risk management and internal control. The board needs to satisfy itself that management has understood the risks, implemented and monitored appropriate policies and controls, and are providing the board with timely information so that it can discharge its own responsibilities.

Risk appetite and risk tolerance

The board has overall responsibility for risk management and for deciding the organisation's risk appetite. Risk appetite is the level of risk that an organisation is willing to take in the pursuit of its objectives and can be defined as the combination of the desire to take on risk to obtain a specific return (financial or quality), risk capacity and risk tolerance. The 'desire to take on risk' refers to the amount and type of risk that the board of directors would like the organisation to have exposure to. Risk capacity is the maximum risk exposures that the organisation can accept without threatening its financial stability. Risk tolerance is the amount of risk that the organisation is prepared to accept to achieve its financial objectives. Risk tolerance is therefore the amount of risk that an organisation's board of directors allows the organisation to accept.

Risk appetite and risk tolerance are closely related. One is the amount of business risk (and types of business risk) the board would like the organisation to have and the other is the amount of risk that the board is prepared to tolerate.

The FRC Risk Guide confirms that the board has ultimate responsibility determining its risk appetite. The board should review risk appetite regularly, and decisions should be taken about the scale of risk that is desired or acceptable. Risk tolerance could be expressed in numerical terms, such as the maximum loss that the board would be willing to accept on a particular venture if events turn out adversely or in terms of the quality of the service that is provided. Alternatively, risk tolerance could be expressed in terms of a total ban on certain types of business activity or behaviour.

The relevance of risk for health service governance

NHS organisations must take risks in order to deliver healthcare. How much risk should they be prepared to tolerate, and would they be able to withstand 'shocks' in the business environment if an unexpected event or development were to occur? The board has the responsibility for strategic decisions on risk, and an important aspect of health service governance is for the board to recognise its responsibilities and ensure that the risk management system in the organisation is effective. The board has a responsibility to govern the organisation in the interests of the stakeholders. A part of this responsibility is to decide the objectives and strategic direction for the organisation, to approve detailed strategic plans put forward by management, and to monitor and review the implementation of those plans. An important objective of NHS organisations is to make economic, efficient and effective use of public resources in its provision of healthcare, and the organisation's strategies should be directed towards this. However, any business strategy involves taking risks and actual results may be better or worse than expected.

Bad health service governance can result in the collapse of an organisation, and excessive risk-taking is one aspect of poor governance. The board should consider risk when it makes strategic business decisions. It should choose policies that are expected to deliver the key objectives but should limit the risks to a level that it considers acceptable. For example, when the board takes major investment decisions or decides on a new corporate strategy such as a clinical services strategy, risks as well as expected returns must be properly assessed. The board should also be satisfied that managers take risk as well as expected outcomes into account in their decision making. The Cadbury Report (1992) described risk management as:

> 'the process by which executive management, under board supervision, identifies the risk arising from business ... and establishes the priorities for control and particular objectives.'

The significance of risk management for corporate governance was demonstrated forcibly by the global banking crisis in 2007–2009. In the UK, the government initiated the Walker Report to look into the failures in the banking industry commented that while there were failures in the regulation of the banking industry, much of the blame for the crisis was attributable to poor governance, and in particular inadequate attention to risk management.

RISK MANAGEMENT

Types of risks

A distinction can be made between business risk and internal control risk (sometimes called governance risk). Business risks are risks that occur and arise in the business environment in which an organisation operates. Business risks may also be referred to as strategic risks, as they are determined by the strategies that the organisation pursues. Risks will differ between organisations but may include financial, operational, reputational, behavioural, third party, or external risks, such as market or regulatory risk, over which the board may have little or no direct control. In the NHS, business risks could be risks to patient safety and financial security that arise from factors in their external environment, including competition or government policy, over which management has no direct control.

Categories of business risk

The nature and severity of business risks varies from one organisation to another. Risks change over time: some become less significant, and new risks emerge. Business risks are risks that the actual performance of the business could be much worse (or better) than expected due to unexpected developments in the business environment. For example, when an organisation develops a new service, it will have an expectation of the likely activity level. Actual levels could be higher or lower than expected. With some new services, the risk that activity levels will differ from expectation could be much more severe than with other new services. There are various reasons why activity levels may be less than expected or may fall unexpectedly. Competitors may take away some of the organisation's market share; an organisation may suffer from bad publicity; there may be new regulations making the provision of a particular service more difficult.

Business risks can be categorised or identified in different ways, but it may help to understand the variety of risks by considering the following sources of risk.

- **Financial risk:** these are risks that financial conditions may change, with adverse changes in tariff or interest rates, higher losses from bad debts or changes in prices from major suppliers.
- **Operational risk:** the risk of losses resulting from inadequate or failed internal processes, people and systems, or external events.
- **Reputational risk:** the risk of loss in customer loyalty or customer support following an event that damages the organisation's reputation.
- **Behavioural risk:** these are risks connected with the workplace and lifestyle behaviours of employees and organisations that have a negative impact on its productivity.
- **Third-party or competition risk:** the risk that business performance will differ from expected performance because of actions taken (or not taken) by other organisations.

- **External risks:** these are risks of significant changes in the business environment from political and regulatory factors, economic factors, social and environmental factors and technology factors (the so-called 'PEST' factors). For example, business performance may be affected by the introduction of new regulations, a change of government, economic decline or growth, environmental issues, unexpected changes in social habits or technological change.

Each industry and each organisation within an industry faces different risks. The questions that management should ask are 'What risks does this organisation face?' and 'How can these risks be measured?' It has to be possible to assess the risk in a business, even one with unpredictable variations in key factors such as activity levels or market prices. High volatility is associated with high business risk.

Though all manner of principal risks in the business environment may cause an organisation to fail to achieve its objectives, further principal risks are failures or weaknesses within its own internal systems and operating procedures or human error. These failures and weaknesses could be avoided, or the consequences of failures could be limited, by means of internal controls. Internal controls are measures or arrangements that are intended to prevent failures from happening, limiting their potential effect, or identifying when a failure has occurred so that corrective measures can be taken. The failure or weakness of these controls is classified as an internal control risk.

Internal control is also an aspect of governance, because the board of directors has a responsibility to ensure that the assets of the organisation are not threatened, and that the interests of the stakeholders are not damaged, by making sure that an effective system of internal control is in place.

Internal control risks

An internal control system is the system that an organisation has for identifying internal control risks, applying controls to reduce the risk of losses from these risks and taking corrective action when losses occur. There should be controls to ensure that the organisation, its systems and procedures operate in the way that is intended, without disruption or disturbance. In addition, there should be controls to ensure that assets are safeguarded, such as controls to ensure that money received is banked and is not stolen, and that operating assets such as items of equipment and computers are not damaged or lost. Such controls should include measures to reduce the risk of fraud and financial controls that should ensure the completeness and accuracy of accounting records, and the timely preparation of financial information. Controls should also be in place to ensure compliance with key regulations, such as CQC regulations, NHSI regulations or health and safety regulations.

However, just like risk management, the board needs to be clear on its strategy and corporate objectives in order to assess what internal risks exist and therefore what controls are needed. The Auditing Practices Board says:

> 'Clear business objectives need to be identified before an effective system of internal control can be established. Without clear objectives, management will be unable to identify and evaluate the risks that threaten the achievement of their objectives and design and operate a system of internal control to manage those risks.'

Internal control risks are risks that arise within an organisation because of weaknesses in its systems, procedures, management or personnel. Unless there are controls to deal with them, internal control risks can lead to losses because of operational failures, errors or fraud. The controls for these risks are 'internal controls' and internal controls are applied within an internal control system. It is the responsibility of the board of directors of an organisation to ensure that the internal control system (and the internal controls within this system) is effective in preventing losses from internal control risks, or identifying losses and taking corrective action when they occur.

Categories of internal control risks

A useful definition of internal control was given by the US Committee of Sponsoring Organizations of the Treadway Commission (COSO). The COSO Framework defines internal control as 'a process, effected by an entity's board of directors, management and other personnel, designed to provide reasonable assurance regarding the achievement of objectives' in the areas of effectiveness and efficiency of operations (through operational controls), the reliability of financial reporting (through financial controls) and compliance with relevant laws and regulations (through compliance controls).

It follows then that internal control risks can be categorised into three broad types, namely: financial, operational and compliance.

- **Financial risks:** these are risks of errors or fraud in accounting systems and accounting and finance activities. Errors or fraud could lead to losses for the organisation, or to incorrect financial statements. Weak controls may also mean that financial assets are not properly protected. Examples of financial risks include the risk of failure to record transactions in the bookkeeping system, failure to collect money owed by customers, failure to protect cash and misreporting (deliberate or unintentional) in the financial statements.
- **Operational risks:** this is the risk of losses resulting from inadequate or failed internal processes, people and systems, or external events. Operational risks include the risks of a breakdown in a system due to machine failures or software errors, the risk of losing information from computer files or having confidential information stolen, the risk of a terrorist attack, and losses arising from mistakes or omissions by staff.

- **Compliance risks:** these are risks that important laws or regulations will not be complied with properly. Failure to comply with the law could result in legal action against the organisation and/or fines.

Responsibilities for risk management and internal control

The organisation's risk management strategy should set out how the authority, responsibility and accountability for risk management and internal control is defined, co-ordinated and documented throughout the organisation from individual employees through to board members. This strategy should be reviewed and approved by the board.

The board

The board is responsible for risk at a high level, but responsibilities for the management of risk are delegated to executive management. The board should decide the level of risks that are acceptable at a strategic level and should ensure that the management team consider risk in the decisions that they make.

The FRC Risk Guide explains:

'The board should define the processes to be adopted for its on-going monitoring and review [of risk management and internal control systems], including specifying the requirements, scope and frequency for reporting and assurance. Regular reports to the board should provide a balanced assessment of the risks and the effectiveness of the systems of risk management and internal control in managing those risks. The board should form its own view on effectiveness, based on the evidence it obtains, exercising the standard of care generally applicable to directors in the exercise of their duties.'

It also goes on to recommend questions that the board should consider throughout the year.

- How effectively have the risks been assessed and the principal risks determined?
- How have they been managed or mitigated?
- Have the necessary actions been taken promptly to remedy any significant failings or weaknesses?
- Do the causes of the failing or weakness indicate poor decision-taking, a need for more extensive monitoring or a reassessment of the effectiveness of management's on-going processes?

In addition to the board's ongoing monitoring and review role, the FRC Risk Guide recommends that it should undertake an annual review of the effectiveness of the systems to ensure that it has considered all significant aspects of risk management and internal control for the year under review, up to the date of approval of the annual report and accounts. An effectiveness review of should consider:

- the organisation's willingness to take on risk (its risk appetite), the desired culture within the organisation and whether this culture has been embedded;
- the operation of the risk management and internal control systems, covering the design, implementation, monitoring and review and identification of risks and determination of those which are principal to the organisation;
- the integration of risk management and internal controls with considerations of strategy and business model, and with business planning processes;
- the changes in the nature, likelihood and impact of principal risks, and the organisation's ability to respond to changes in its business and the external environment;
- the extent, frequency and quality of the communication of the results of management's monitoring to the board which enables it to build up a cumulative assessment of the state of control in the organisation and the effectiveness with which risk is being managed or mitigated;
- issues dealt with in reports reviewed by the board during the year, in particular the incidence of significant control failings or weaknesses that have been identified at any time during the period and the extent to which they have, or could have, resulted in unforeseen impact; and
- the effectiveness of the organisation's public reporting processes.

At board level, responsibility for reviewing the effectiveness of the risk management system may be delegated by the board to the audit committee, which is also likely to have responsibility for reviewing the internal control system. Alternatively, the board may prefer to establish a separate risk committee. Where delegation does occur, the FRC Risk Guide makes it clear that:

> 'The board should be satisfied that the arrangements for the work carried out, for the co-ordination of their work (if more than one committee is involved), and for reporting to the board are appropriate and operating effectively. The board retains ultimate responsibility for the risk management and internal control systems and should reach its own conclusions regarding the recommendations it receives.'

The board should also ensure that the remuneration committee takes appropriate account of risk when determining remuneration policies and awards, and should ensure that the links between the remuneration committee and the risk and/or audit committee are operating effectively.

Risk committees

The advantages of having a separate risk committee are as follows.

- It can focus on risk issues and reviewing the organisation's risk management system, without having to concern itself with other issues (such as the external auditors). It would give advice to the board on matters such as risk appetite and risk strategy.

- The composition of the board is not restricted by statutory requirements. A risk committee should ideally consist mainly of NEDs but should also have the finance director as a member. If the audit committee had responsibility for the oversight of risk management, the finance director could not be a committee member (although they could be invited to meetings of the audit committee to give their views).

The Walker Report recommended that a risk committee could be established, consisting of senior executives and chaired by the CEO. This committee would be responsible for risk management at an operational level. The responsibilities of this committee and the board risk committee would be very different as:

'The role of the board risk committee is to advise the board on all high-level risk matters and should not extend into operational matters which are for the executive within the overall risk framework determined by the board. The NEDs on the committee cannot be expected to be able to replicate the industry expertise of the executive team nor will their capacity to contribute be enhanced by information overload. The materials presented to them should be in succinct format, highlighting major issues.'

This provides an interesting consideration for larger NHS organisations, where a similar structure may be helpful.

Risk management systems and procedures

To enable the board of directors to carry out its responsibilities for risk management effectively, there are two essential requirements. Firstly, board members should have an understanding of risks and risk management. Secondly, there should be a risk management system in place that the board as a whole or the appropriate board committee can review.

Risk registers

An organisation might use a risk register for recording identified risks, the evaluation of the risks, and the measures that have been taken to deal with them. Executive management maintains the risk register, but it can be used by the risk committee of the board (or the audit committee) as a way of reviewing the effectiveness of the risk management system. At board level, there should be regular programmed scrutiny of the register of principal risks, including:

- the risk score;
- mitigation/action being taken; and
- escalation or de-escalation of risks.

Individual areas or divisions within the organisations should have processes in which the same risk management system operates with the responsibility of escalating risks, which are outside of their resources or authority to manage.

RISK MANAGEMENT

Interestingly, the King III Code is much more explicit about risk management than the FT Code and UK Code. Provisions in the King III Code relating to risk management include the following.

- The board's risk strategy should be executed by management by means of risk management systems and processes.
- The board should ensure that effective and ongoing risk assessments are performed by management.
- Risks should be prioritised and ranked, in order to focus on areas where action is most needed.
- The board should regularly receive and review a register of the organisation's key risks.
- Key risks should be quantified where practicable (e.g. in terms of maximum potential loss or expected loss).
- The board should ensure that processes are in place for anticipating unpredictable risks.
- Management should identify and note in the risk register the responses that have been decided upon and taken.
- Management should provide assurances to the board that the risk management plan is integrated into the daily activities of the business.

Stress testing

'Stress testing' is widely used by major organisations to assess their ability to withstand extreme 'shocks' or unexpected events in the business environment. This can be done by taking the normal business planning or forecasting model used by the organisation and altering a key variable, such as the rate of growth (or decline) in economic growth, a very large increase in a major resource such as staff costs, loss of access to a key market for service provision, and so on. The purpose of stress testing is to assess whether the organisation could survive the shock. If there are doubts about this ability, the organisation should consider measures to reduce the risk, perhaps by developing contingency plans, or taking measures to improve their capital or liquidity.

Elements of the risk assessment process

The FRC Risk Guide does not set out in detail the procedure by which a company designs and implements its risk management and internal control systems. Defining a single approach to achieving best practice would be misguided, as it would lead boards to underestimate the crucial importance to high-quality risk management of the culture and behaviour they promote. However, it is still possible to identify some basic elements to a risk management system. These elements are:

- risk identification;
- risk evaluation;

- risk management measures; and
- risk control and review.

A further element that might be considered is that of risk training. Risk identification involves an organisation having a procedure in place for reviewing and identifying the risks it faces. Risks change over time, and risk reviews should therefore be undertaken regularly.

Risk evaluation calls for procedures to assess the potential size of the risk. The expected losses that could occur from adverse events or developments depend on the probability that an adverse outcome will occur and size of the loss in the event of an adverse outcome. Where a risk is unlikely to materialise into an adverse outcome, and the loss would in any case be small, no management action might be necessary. Where the risk is higher, measures should be taken to protect the organisation so that the remaining exposure to risk is within the organisation's tolerance level and consistent with its risk appetite.

The 2008 NHS National Patient Safety Agency publication *A Risk Matrix for Risk Managers* was developed to assist NHS risk managers in implementing an integrated system of risk assessment. The guidance sets out a matrix for NHS organisations to score both the probability and the size of the loss. The matrix covers risks associated with:

- adverse publicity/reputation;
- business objectives/projects;
- environmental impact;
- finance, including claims;
- human resources/organisational development/staffing/competence;
- impact on the safety of patients, staff or public (physical/psychological harm);
- quality/complaints/audit;
- service/business interruption; and
- statutory duty/inspections.

Management should decide the measures taken to deal with each risk and is accountable to the board for these measures. In broad terms, risks can be dealt with by avoiding them or by taking steps to limit the exposure. Some risks can be avoided but many risks have to be accepted as an inevitable feature of business.

For principal risks, an organisation should decide what measures might be necessary to reduce the risk to acceptable proportions. Risks may be reduced through measures such as stakeholder management and collaborative ventures. From a health service governance perspective, it should be a responsibility of the board to make sure that risks are reviewed regularly, and that management takes suitable measures to deal with them.

Executive management should establish control systems to monitor risks that include identifying situations that are getting out of control, or where significant events have developed or are developing.

A further consideration for NHS organisations is the requirement of the FRC Risk Guide that:

> 'the board should consider whether it, and any committee or management group to which it delegates activities, has the necessary skills, knowledge, experience, authority and support to enable it to assess the risks the organisation faces and exercise its responsibilities effectively. Boards should consider specifically assessing this as part of their regular evaluations of their effectiveness.'

This should ensure that they are capable of contributing proactively to board discussions on risk strategy. Training in risk management should be particularly important for members of the board committee (audit committee or risk committee) with responsibility for reviewing the risk management system.

Internal control systems and procedures

The board of directors is responsible for maintaining a sound system of risk management and internal control, as shown earlier in the UK Code and FRC Risk Guide. They require the board of directors to set appropriate policies on internal control, to seek regular assurance to satisfy itself that the system is operating effectively and to ensure that the system of internal control is effective in managing risks in the way that it has approved.

In deciding its policies for internal control and assessing what constitutes an effective system of internal control, the board should consider:

- the nature and extent of the risks facing the organisation;
- the amount of risk and types of risk that it regards as acceptable for the organisation to bear;
- the likelihood that the risks will materialise;
- the organisation's ability to reduce the impact on the business of the risks that do materialise; and
- the costs of operating particular controls relative to the benefits to be obtained from managing the risks they control. Controls are not worth having if they cost more than the expected benefits or savings they will provide.

Having identified the responsibilities of the board for maintaining a sound system of internal control, the FRC Risk Guide adds that it is the job of management to implement the board's policies on control. Management must have procedures for identifying and evaluating the risks faced by the organisation, as well as designing, implementing and monitoring a control system to deal with these risks in a way that is consistent with the board's policies. In addition, all employees have some responsibility for internal control – for example, to avoid making mistakes in their work, and also to ensure that the control procedures for which they are responsible are properly performed.

The board needs to have assurance that there is a robust and resilient internal control system for managing internal control risks that feeds into and underpins the risk management system. Having established the internal control risks to the organisation's strategic objectives, management needs to identify the internal controls to limit or manage those risks. The controls are an essential part of an internal control system; their nature and extent will depend largely on the organisation's size, what controls it can afford and whether the benefits obtained from any particular control measure are sufficient to justify its cost. The internal control system should be sufficiently robust and effective to minimise the risk of serious losses through error or fraud. In a large organisation, there would be thousands of different financial operational and compliance controls, each designed to prevent particular financial, operational or compliance failures, or to detect them if they occur.

An important aspect of health service governance is to ensure that the system of internal control (and the internal controls within that system) is adequate and effective in preventing or detecting failures in the system. For example, if the system is ineffective, an organisation may be exposed to a high risk of fraud and to a high risk that its annual financial statements will not be accurate or reliable.

A sound system of internal control should be embedded in the operations of the organisation and form part of its culture. It should be capable of responding quickly to risks to the business as they emerge and develop, should include procedures for reporting immediately to the management responsible and control failings that have been identified and any corrective action that has been undertaken. The Turnbull Guidance emphasised that a sound system of internal control cannot provide certain protection against an organisation suffering losses or breaches of laws or regulations or failing to meet its business objectives. The possibility will always exist of 'poor judgement in decision making, human error, control processes being deliberately circumvented by employees and others, management overriding controls and the occurrence of unforeseen circumstances'. A sound system of internal control provides reasonable assurance that risks will be suitably controlled, but cannot provide absolute assurance that there will not be any material losses, fraud, errors or breaches of laws and regulations.

In addition to the internal controls themselves, an internal control system should also have other elements to be effective and achieve its objectives. The COSO Framework identifies five elements to a system of internal control (also recognised in the Turnbull Report).

- A control environment that describes the awareness of (and attitude to) internal controls in the organisation, shown by the directors, management and employees generally. It therefore encompasses corporate culture, management style and employee attitudes to control procedures.
- There should be a system or procedures for identifying the risks facing the organisation (and how these are changing) and assessing their significance.

- Controls or management initiatives should be devised to deal with significant risks.
- Controls should be devised and implemented to eliminate, reduce or control risks.
- All employees who are responsible for the management of risks should receive information that enables them to fulfil this task.
- The effectiveness of internal controls and the internal control system generally should be monitored regularly. Internal audit is one method of monitoring the internal control system. Internal controls are also monitored by executive management and (as part of their annual audit) by the external auditors. The board of directors also has a responsibility to review the effectiveness of the system.

Types of internal controls

Financial controls

Financial controls are internal accounting controls that are sufficient to provide reasonable assurance that:

- transactions are made only according to the general or specific authorisation of management;
- transactions are recorded so that financial statements can be prepared according to accounting standards and generally accepted accounting principles;
- transactions are recorded so that assets can be accounted for;
- access to assets is only allowed according to the general or specific authorisation of management;
- the accounting records for assets are compared with actual assets at reasonable intervals of time; and
- appropriate action is taken whenever there are found to be differences.

The maintenance of proper accounting records is an important element of internal control. Effective financial controls should ensure the quality of external and internal financial reporting, so that there are no material errors in the accounting records and financial statements. They should ensure that no fraud is committed (or that fraud is detected when it occurs) and that the financial assets of the organisation are not stolen, lost or needlessly damaged, or that these risks are reduced.

A useful method of categorising internal financial controls was used in an old guideline issued by the UK Auditing Practices Board, using the mnemonic SPAMSOAP. In this guideline (no longer in issue) internal financial controls are categorised as follows.

- **S: Segregation of duties**: where possible, duties should be split between two or more people, so that the work done by one person acts as a check on the work done by another. With segregation of duties, it is more difficult for fraud to

take place, because several individuals would have to collude in the fraud. It is also more difficult for accidental errors to occur, because when several people are involved in a task, they act as a check on each other.
- **P: Physical controls**: measures to ensure the physical safety of assets, such as putting cash in a safe, banking cash receipts immediately, and preventing unauthorised access to computer systems through the use of passwords and internet firewalls.
- **A: Authorisation and approval**: all financial transactions should require the authorisation or approval of an appropriate responsible person, and there should be an authorisation limit to how much spending each responsible person can approve.
- **M: Management controls**: management should exercise control over financial systems, for example by preparing a budget and then monitoring actual performance by comparing it with the budget. Management controls can also be exercised by reviewing other financial statements, such as a balance sheet, profit and loss account and cash flow statement.
- **S: Supervision**: the day-to-day work of employees should be properly supervised. Good supervision will reduce the likelihood of errors or fraud.
- **O: Organisation**: everyone should be fully aware of their responsibilities, and lines of authority, lines of reporting and levels of responsibility should be clear. Errors and fraud are much more likely where it is uncertain who is responsible for what and who should be reporting to whom.
- **A: Arithmetical and accounting controls**: these are procedures in an accounts office to check the accuracy of the records and the numbers. They include the use of control totals and reconciliations.
- **P: Personnel**: the quality of internal controls is dependent on the quality of the individuals working in the organisation. Personnel selected to do a job should have the right personal qualities and be properly trained and/or qualified.

This list of different types of control is provided as a guide to the nature of financial controls. Health service governance is concerned with the adequacy of internal controls and the effectiveness of the internal control system; designing and implementing controls is a responsibility of management.

Operational controls

Operational controls are controls that help to reduce operational risks or identify failures in operational systems when these occur. They are designed to prevent failures in operational procedures, or to detect and correct operational failures if they do occur. Operational failures may be caused by machine breakdowns, human error, failures in the performance of systems (possibly due to human error), weaknesses in procedures and poor management. Operational controls are measures designed to prevent these failures from happening or identifying and correcting problems that do occur. Regular equipment maintenance, better training of staff, automation of standard procedures, and reporting systems that make managers accountable for their actions are all examples of operational controls.

Compliance controls
Compliance controls are concerned with making sure that an entity complies with all the requirements of relevant legislation and regulations. It can be difficult to understand the nature of internal control risks and internal controls to deal with them. There are many different risks and many controls that are applied. The following are simple examples.

Reviewing the effectiveness of risk management and internal control

The UK Code states that the board of directors (or the audit committee) should carry out a review of the effectiveness of the system of risk management and internal control at least annually. NHS bodies, as part of the Department of Health and Social Care (DHSC)'s NHS Controls Assurance project, were required to include a statement on internal controls (SIC) in its annual report and accounts. This has now been replaced by the AGS (see Chapter 18).

In order to review the effectiveness of the system, there must be procedures for monitoring and review. The board or audit committee needs to form its own view about the effectiveness of the system, based on the information and assurances it receives. The sources of information about risk management and internal control are management, the internal auditors (if the organisation has an internal audit function) and the external auditors, who notify management and the audit committee about weaknesses in internal controls that they have discovered in their audit. Their roles are set out in more detail in Chapter 19.

In its Guidance on Audit Committees (revised 2010), the FRC states that except where the responsibility is retained by the entire board, or delegated to a risk committee:

> 'The audit committee should receive reports from management on the effectiveness of the systems they have established and the conclusions of any testing carried out by internal and external auditors.'

Emergency preparedness and business continuity

Emergency preparedness is a plan of what to do if a disaster that is unconnected with the organisation's business and outside the control of management occurs. Disaster recovery planning goes beyond procedures that should be taken in an emergency, such as a fire or explosion in a building. It is intended to establish what should be done if an extreme disaster threatens the ability of the organisation to maintain its operations. Examples of disasters are natural disasters (such as major fires or flooding or storm damage to key installations or offices), major terrorist attacks and pandemics.

The NHS needs to be able to plan for and respond to a wide range of incidents and emergencies that could affect health or patient care. These could be anything from extreme weather conditions to an infectious disease outbreak or a major transport accident or a terrorist act. This work is referred to in the health service as 'emergency preparedness, resilience and response' (EPRR), and is underpinned by legislation contained in the Civil Contingencies Act 2004 (CCA 2004) and the NHS Act 2006 (as amended).

Emergency preparedness plans are vital for NHS organisations, as lengthy or widespread overwhelming demand or shutdown of operations could be catastrophic. While the training of appropriate NHS staff regarding such arrangements in the UK is the responsibility of NHS organisations, the DHSC funds an extensive training programme delivered by the Health Protection Agency to support the NHS in England in planning and preparing for major incidents.

The NHSE Emergency Preparedness, Resilience and Response Framework (2015) is a strategic national framework containing principles for health emergency preparedness, resilience and response for the NHS in England at all levels including NHS provider organisations, providers of NHS-funded care, CCGs, GPs and other primary and community care organisations.

Further guidance is given in NHSE Core Standards for Emergency Preparedness, Resilience and Response (EPRR) guidance (2018) which enable health agencies across the country to share a common approach to EPRR, allow coordination of EPRR activities according to the organisation's size and scope, provide a consistent and cohesive framework for EPRR activities and inform the organisation's annual EPRR work programme. The CCA 2004 and the NHS Act 2006 (as amended) underpin EPRR within health. Both Acts place EPRR duties on NHSE and the NHS in England.

The NHSE Core Standards for EPRR are split into ten domains:

1. Governance
2. Duty to risk assess
3. Duty to maintain plans
4. Command and control
5. Training and exercising
6. Response
7. Warning and informing
8. Cooperation
9. Business continuity
10. Chemical Biological Radiological Nuclear (CBRN) and Hazardous Material (HAZMAT).

The CCA 2004 defines an emergency as:

> 'An event or a situation which threatens serious damage to human welfare in a place in the UK, the environment of a place in the UK, or war or terrorism which threatens serious damage to the security of the UK.'

The definition is concerned with consequences rather than the cause or source. For the NHS, incidents are classed as either:

- Business Continuity Incident;
- Critical Incident; or
- Major Incident.

Each will impact upon service delivery within the NHS, may undermine public confidence and require contingency plans to be implemented. NHS organisations should be confident of the severity of any incident that may warrant a major incident declaration, particularly where this may be due to internal capacity pressures, if a critical incident has not been raised previously through the appropriate local escalation procedure.

Business Continuity incident

A business continuity incident is an event or occurrence that disrupts, or might disrupt, an organisation's normal service delivery, below acceptable predefined levels, where special arrangements are required to be implemented until services can return to an acceptable level. (This could be a surge in demand, requiring resources to be temporarily redeployed.)

Critical incident

A critical incident is any localised incident where the level of disruption results in the organisation temporarily or permanently losing its ability to deliver critical services, patients may have been harmed or the environment is not safe requiring special measures and support from other agencies, to restore normal operating functions.

Major incident

A major incident is any occurrence that presents serious threat to the health of the community or causes such numbers or types of casualties, as to require special arrangements to be implemented. For the NHS, this will include any event defined as an emergency as above.

Although not formally described, there may be events occurring on a national scale, such as fuel strikes, pandemics or multiple events that require the collective capability of the NHS nationally. In each NHS organisation, the CEO is responsible for ensuring that their organisation has a Major Incident Plan in place that will be built on the principles of risk assessment, cooperation with partners, emergency planning, communicating with the public and information sharing.

The plan will link into the organisation's arrangements for ensuring business continuity as required by the CCA 2004.

The CEO will ensure that the board receives regular reports, at least annually, regarding emergency preparedness, including reports on exercises, training and testing undertaken by the organisation, and that adequate resources are made available to allow discharge of these responsibilities. As a minimum requirement, NHS organisations will be required to undertake a live exercise every three years, a tabletop exercise every year and a test of communications cascades every six months. A review of emergency preparedness plans may therefore be a part of the annual review of the effectiveness of internal control by the board or audit committee.

NHS organisations and providers of NHS funded care must:

- nominate a director level accountable emergency officer who will be responsible for EPRR; and
- contribute to area planning for EPRR through local health resilience partnerships (LHRPs) and other relevant groups.

Business continuity management also forms an important part of risk management arrangements and is a further requirement of the CCA 2004. The aim of business continuity management is to ensure that NHS organisations are able to maintain the highest level of service possible whatever might happen to the infrastructure. There is a range of problems that might affect NHS organisations and services at any time, for example, loss of water or power, flooding, or criminal action. The aim of business continuity planning is to enable planning and reaction in a coordinated manner. While business continuity and major incident planning are usually separate processes within an organisation, a major incident may occur at the same time as a business continuity issue, or be triggered by it.

Business continuity management, including processes for recovery and restoration, should be considered by NHS organisations as part of its everyday business processes. Business continuity should be seen as embedded in the culture of the NHS as principles of health and safety, and there must be demonstrable commitment to the process from the boards of NHS organisations. The skills to develop business continuity plans are complementary to those involved in emergency planning and may therefore need to be undertaken by separate officers. It is critical though that both plans are integrated and complementary to each other.

High reliability organisations

There has been some interesting work carried out in recent years with regard to major hazard organisations such as airlines and oil refineries, which have been attempting to influence the organisational and safety culture at their sites to transform them into high reliability organisations (HROs) with a positive safety culture. These are organisations that are able to manage and sustain almost error-free performance despite operating in hazardous conditions where the consequences of errors could be catastrophic.

Descriptions of HROs usually include organisations where failure may have far-reaching, potentially catastrophic consequences. Such organisations will be typically characterised by a high level of interactive complexity: for example, interaction among system components is unpredictable and/or invisible, and there is a high level of interdependence amongst a system's component parts (including people, equipment and procedures). Much like many HROs, the healthcare industry does complex, high-stakes work where mistakes can equal great harm.

A review of the literature published by the Health and Safety Executive in 2011 identified key features and characteristics that could be adopted by organisations to achieve ongoing high reliability and safety objectives.

Successful containment of unexpected events by:

- having in place back-up systems in the event of failures and cross-checking of important decisions (redundancy);
- allowing people with expertise, irrespective of rank, to make important safety-related decisions in emergencies, though maintaining a clear hierarchical structure and an understanding of who is responsible for what during routine operations (deference to expertise in emergencies; oscillation between hierarchical and flat organisational structures), investment in training and technical competence; and
- well-defined procedures for all possible unexpected events.

Effective anticipation of potential failures through:

- engagement with front-line staff in order to obtain 'the bigger picture' of operations (sensitivity to operations);
- attentiveness to minor, or what may appear as trivial, signals that may indicate potential problem areas within the organisation; using incidents and near misses as indicators of a system's 'health' (preoccupation with failure); and
- systematic collection and analysis of all warning signals, no matter how trivial they may appear to be, and avoiding assumptions regarding the nature of failures. Explanations regarding the causes of incidents tend to be systemic rather than focusing on individual, 'blame the operator' justifications (reluctance to simplify).

Just culture, characterised by:

- open reporting systems for near misses and accidents without fear of punishment;
- follow-up of accident investigation outcomes by implementing corrective actions;

- empowering staff to abandon work on safety grounds; and
- fostering a sense of personal accountability for safety.

Learning orientation, characterised by:

- continuous technical training;
- systematic analysis of incidents to identify their root causes and accident types or trends within the organisation;
- open communication of accident investigation outcomes; and
- updating procedures in line with the organisational knowledge base.

Mindful leadership, characterised by:

- proactive commissions of audits to identify problems in the system (often in response to incidents that occur in other similar industries);
- 'bottom-up' communication of 'bad news';
- engagement with front-line staff through site visits; and
- investment of resources in safety management and the ability to balance profits with safety.

In addition to this review, further research into the applicability of the characteristics and systems of HROs for the healthcare sector has been carried out to further the safety culture in healthcare services. The most commonly applied resulting principles include:

- attempts to improve safety culture;
- checklists and other tools;
- initiatives to build teamwork using crew resource management and human factors approaches; and
- standardised processes using care bundles.

It will be interesting to see how developments in this area can be built into NHS risk management processes.

Governance Checklist

- How is the risk management strategy communicated throughout the organisation? How does the board determine whether this is clear, appropriate and effective?
- How effectively is the organisation able to withstand risks, and risk combinations, which do materialise? How effective is the board's approach to risks with 'low probability' but a very severe impact if they materialise? 3 What are the channels of communication that enable individuals, including third parties, to report concerns, suspected breaches of law or regulations, other improprieties or challenging perspectives?

RISK MANAGEMENT

- What are the responsibilities of the board and senior management for crisis management? How effectively have the organisation's crisis management planning and systems been tested?
- To what extent has the organisation identified risks from joint ventures, third parties and from the way in which the organisation's business is organised?
- How are these managed?
- How effectively does the organisation capture new and emerging risks and opportunities? How and when does the board consider risk when discussing changes in strategy or approving new transactions, projects, products or other significant commitments?
- To what extent has the board considered the cost-benefit aspects of different control options?
- How does the board ensure it understands the organisation's exposure to each principal risk before and after the application of mitigations and controls, what those mitigations and controls are and whether they are operating as expected?
- What are the processes by which senior management monitor the effective application of the systems of risk management and internal control?
- In what way do the monitoring and review processes take into account the organisation's ability to re-evaluate the risks and adjust controls effectively in response to changes in its objectives, its business, and its external environment?
- How are processes or controls adjusted to reflect new or changing risks, or operational deficiencies? To what extent does the board engage in horizon scanning for emerging risks?
- How has the board satisfied itself that the disclosures on risk management and internal control contribute to the annual report being fair, balanced and understandable, and provide shareholders with the information they need?
- How has the board satisfied itself that its reporting on going concern and the longer-term viability statement gives a fair, balanced and understandable overview of the organisation's position and prospects?

(Adapted from Appendix C of the FRC Risk Guide.)

Summary

- The FRC Risk Guide is very clear that good stewardship by the board should not inhibit the sensible risk-taking that is critical to growth.
- The assessment of risks as part of the normal business planning process should support better decision making, ensure that the board and management respond promptly to risks when they arise, and ensure that stakeholders are well informed about the principal risks and prospects of the organisation.

- The addition of behavioural and organisational risk into the risk management system highlights the challenge that is embedding risk management processes into an organisation.
- This seems to be a critical area for boards to consider as part of their ongoing training and development.

18
Assurance

Introduction

In corporate governance, the annual report and accounts is seen as the most important communication between a company and its stakeholders. This is not the case in health service governance. Although significant, the annual report and accounts is not the sole means of communication for NHS organisations; instead, there are a wide variety of reporting and disclosure requirements. These complex requirements seek to provide assurance to the board and its stakeholders.

One of the major stakeholders for any board or a governing body within the NHS will be the regulators applicable to their context. The reporting requirements of these regulators have created an industry in itself and to understand the scale of those mechanisms is beyond the scope of this Handbook. The intention here is to provide an introduction to the main reporting frameworks. The chapter will explore the reporting requirement of NHSE, NHSI and the CQC, as these are the main regulators that most boards will have to engage with. Whilst the intention of reporting to regulators is to provide assurance to the regulators; at the same time, it provides assurance to a board on the effectiveness of their executive team and at times their own effectiveness as a board.

Assurance can be understood as the provision of accurate and current information about the efficiency and effectiveness of an organisation's policies and operations, and the status of its compliance with statutory obligations. Assurance is the process of establishing the integrity and validity of disclosures, including statements and reports. Good assurance is confidence backed by sufficient evidence: the board should obtain assurance that performance and quality are as they should be, that risks are properly controlled and that strategy is being implemented successfully and sustainably. Board members, regulators and others need to have information from more than one source in order to be able to validate this evidence.

Trustworthy reporting and auditing is probably the most significant issue for health service governance. Good health service governance should ensure that performance, quality and financial reporting is reliable and honest, and that the opinion of the external auditors is objective and unbiased.

Regulatory reporting

Frameworks for the NHS in England are published each year. They describe the national priorities, system levers and enablers needed for NHS organisations to maintain and improve the quality of services provided, while delivering transformational change and maintaining financial stability.

Currently, NHSI monitors and assures the performance of individual NHS trusts and foundation trusts through the Single Oversight Framework (SOF), while NHSE carries out this role for individual CCGs using the CCG Improvement and Assessment Framework (CCG IAF). CQC monitors and assures the quality performance of individual health and social care providers through an intelligence driven and risk-based inspection scheme.

All of this performance information is publicly available through publications from the regulators and on the UK's biggest health website NHS Choices, which provides a comprehensive health information service.

NHSI's Single Oversight Framework

NHSI's Single Oversight Framework describes in detail how each provider trust's compliance with its licence is monitored. It sets out NHSI's approach to overseeing provider trust compliance with the governance and continuity of services requirements of their provider licence. The objective of the Framework is to help NHSI support 'providers to attain and maintain Care Quality Commission ratings of "Good" or "Outstanding", meet the NHS constitution standards and manage their resources effectively, working alongside their local partners'.

The information collected and reviewed under the SOF includes annual plans and reports, regular financial and operational information and other exceptional or significant data, including relevant third-party material. A summary of this is shown in Figure 18.1.

Based on this information, NHSI identifies where a provider trust may need support across its five themes of quality of care, finance and use of resources, operational performance, strategic change, and leadership and improvement capability. NHSI then uses a segmentation approach, in which the level of support is tailored to the needs of the provider as dictated by their segmentation as follows:

1. No potential concerns identified across the five themes – lowest level of oversight.
2. Triggering criteria of concern in one or more of the five themes – but not in breach of licence (or equivalent for NHS trusts) and/or formal licence action not needed.
3. Serious issues – the provider is in actual/suspected breach of the licence (or equivalent for NHS trusts).
4. Critical issues – the provider is in actual/suspected breach of its licence (or equivalent for NHS trusts) with very serious/complex issues (e.g. including

ASSURANCE **393**

	In-year	Annual/less frequently	By exception[1]
Quality of care	In-year quality information to identify any areas for improvement (see Appendix 1)	Annual quality information	Results of CQC inspections CQC warning notices, fines, civil or criminal actions and information on other relevant matters
Finance and use of resources	Monthly returns	Annual operational plans Information relating to Use of Resources (UoR) assessments	One-off financial events (eg sudden drops in income/ increases in costs) Transactions/mergers
Operational performance	Quarterly/monthly/weekly operational performance information (see Appendix 3)		Any sudden and unforeseen factors driving a significant failure to deliver
Strategic change	Delivery of sustainability and transformation plans Progress of any new care models, devolution plans	Sustainability and transformation plans	Any sudden and unforeseen factors driving a significant failure to deliver
Leadership and improvement capability	Third-party information with governance implications[2] Organisational health indicators - staff absenteeism - staff churn - board vacancies	Staff and patient surveys Third-party information with governance implications[2]	Findings of well-led reviews and developmental well-led reviews Third-party information with governance implications[2]

[1] Providers are also expected to notify NHS Improvement of any other material changes in performance or risks that fall outside routine monitoring
[2] eg reports from quality surveillance groups (QSGs), General Medical council, ombudsman, CCGs, Healthwatch England, NHS Digital, auditors, Health and Safety Executive, patient groups, complaints, whistleblowers; medical Royal Colleges

Figure 18.1: Summary of information requirements for monitoring

providers requiring major intervention on multiple issues to return to sustainable performance).

Support may be universal, targeted or mandated. Universal support would be associated with a segment 1 classification and targeted support segment 2. Where a provider is at risk of a suspected breach of its licence then this would require mandated support (i.e. a segment 3 classification). Where the trust is in breach of its licence and is in special measures (see later), then the classification would be segment 4.

Key triggers for NHSI as areas of concern include:

- CQC rating of 'inadequate' or 'requires improvement' in overall rating, or against any of the safe, effective, caring or responsive key questions;
- CQC warning notices;
- failure to agree a control total for finance;
- use of Resources rating of 'inadequate' or 'requires improvement';
- failure to meet any operational performance standard for at least two consecutive months;
- material concerns about a provider's delivery against the local transformation agenda, including (where relevant) new care models and devolution; and
- CQC 'inadequate' or 'requires improvement' assessment against the 'well-led' domain.

The SOF has included oversight of NHS-controlled providers since February 2018 as the advent of new care models meant that joint ventures and subsidiaries were becoming more common as providers deliver more integrated care. Plans for new subsidiaries were put on hold in September 2018 as NHSI launched a new consultation on the regulatory approach for such structures.

NHSE's Improvement and Assessment Framework

NHSE introduced the CCG Improvement and Assessment Framework in 2017/18 and it identifies how local health and care systems and communities can assess their own progress. In addition, the CCG IAF fulfils the NHSE's statutory assessment function, by aligning the NHSE's Mandate and planning guidance to unlock change and improvement in four key areas of better health, better care, sustainability and leadership.

The IAF is designed to assess an individual CCGs' fitness to operate successfully in the changing environment envisaged by the 5YFV. It therefore considers a CCG's individual performance indicators as well as wider indicators that demonstrate its influence and relevance as a local system leader.

NHSE has a statutory duty to conduct an annual performance assessment of each CCG and the IAF covers 58 indicators across 29 areas such as financial stability, leadership and care quality in services such as maternity and A&E; these ratings are available to patients on the myNHS website. These ratings follow the same structure as the CQC rating structure of:

ASSURANCE

- Outstanding
- Good
- Requires Improvement
- Inadequate.

The methodology to apply a year-end assessment is agreed during the year; it also requires regional and national moderation to ensure assessments have been applied consistently across all CCGs. The framework allows a tailored place-based support package to be created around each CCG. NHSE has also introduced special measures interventions (see later) for CCGs so that tailored intensive support can be provided where NHSE has grave concerns about a CCG's performance.

New models of care

This individualised approach by NHSI and NHSE to monitoring and assurance runs counter to the movement towards system-level planning and delivery and so, the planning guidance in 2018–19 (NHSE, NHSI, 2018) has begun to describe how the regulatory system will align with system collaboration by focussing on the assurance of system plans, rather than organisation-level plans. This will only be the case, however, where the ICSs are judged mature enough to become operational. Such ICSs will enjoy a more autonomous regulatory relationship with NHSE and NHSI, who intend to utilise their powers of intervention in conjunction with the ICS's leadership.

For example, the ICS's leadership will have a key role in deciding on the remedial action to be taken if regulatory intervention in a trust or CCG is required. In addition to this, NHSE in 2017 awarded each STP with an overall rating based on performance across nine domains and signalled a move towards the performance assessment of local health systems. A further important step towards collaboration in regulation is the alignment in approach by CQC and NHSI with regard to the well-led framework and the use of resources assessments.

In due course, the regulatory system will be informed by a new integrated oversight framework that will form a key part of the regular performance discussions between NHSE, NHSI and STPs/ICSs. Alongside this, NHSE, NHSI and STPs/ICSs will continue to review trust-level data – and CCG-level data – to help agree when individual organisations need support or intervention and who should provide that support or intervention. Development of this new framework will be aligned to The NHS Long Term Plan, due for publication in early 2019.

CQC inspections

Having completed inspections of all the services, CQC has developed a baseline understanding of the quality of care in England. On the basis of this, the CQC has gone on to conduct focused inspections on core services where there were concerns about the quality and safety of a service provided or where there have been perceived improvements in the quality of the service. These inspections have consistently asked the same five questions of every service:

- Is it safe?
- Is it effective?
- Is it caring?
- Is it responsive?
- Is it well-led?

Since March 2018, Use of Resources assessments carried out by NHSI have been considered by the CQC as a sixth question. The CQC's trust-level quality ratings are then combined with the Use of Resources rating to produce an overall trust-level rating. The Use of Resources assessment is intended to assess how effectively and efficiently trusts are using their resources – including their finances, workforce, estates and facilities, technology and procurement – to provide high quality, efficient and sustainable care for patients.

In addition to the core services that the CQC selects to inspect (at least one core service will be inspected annually), the CQC will also assess the overall leadership of the provider. This will include an assessment of how well the board assures itself that basic systems underpinning safe care are in place (e.g. learning from incidents).

Comprehensive inspections have also continued. They happen at different times and are mostly unannounced. Such inspections are only carried out for newly registered providers or where there are significant concerns. The well-led focused inspection is announced to ensure the appropriate interviews can be scheduled for designated trust employees.

Following each inspection, the CQC publish an independent assessment of how the organisation performed. It rates services on a four-point scale of:

- Outstanding
- Good
- Requires Improvement
- Inadequate.

The CQC also has a range of interventions and sanctions at its disposal. These include:

- using requirement notices or warning notices to set out what improvements the provider must make and by when;
- making changes to a provider's registration to limit what they may do – for example by imposing conditions for a given time;
- placing a provider in special measures, where CQC closely supervises the quality of care while working with other organisations to help them improve within set timescales; and
- holding the provider to account for their failings by:
  - issuing simple cautions
  - issuing fines
  - prosecuting cases where people are harmed or placed in danger of harm.

For planning purposes, previous ratings are then used as a guide to setting maximum intervals for re-inspecting core services as follows:

- one year for ratings of Inadequate;
- two years for ratings of Requires Improvement;
- three-and-a-half years for ratings of Good; and
- five years for ratings of Outstanding.

The CQC will normally recommend that a trust is placed in special measures (see later) when an NHS trust or foundation trust is rated as inadequate in the well-led key question (for example, there are concerns that the organisation's leadership is unable to make sufficient improvements in a reasonable timeframe without extra support) and inadequate in one or more of the other key questions (safe, effective, caring and responsive).

Failure regimes/special measures

Failure regimes and special measures apply when NHS trusts and FTs have serious problems and there are concerns that the existing leadership cannot make the necessary improvements without support. They consist of a set of interventions designed to remedy problems within a reasonable timeframe. Trusts may be placed in special measures as a result of serious failures in quality of care and/or serious financial problems. NHSE also uses special measures as an intervention when it has grave concerns about the performance of a CCG.

In the worst-case scenarios, the failure regime, or 'trust special administrator regime', is the process by which 'unsustainable' or 'failed' trusts may be placed into administration. The failure regime is imposed upon trusts which are deemed to be failing financially or in terms of governance, or quality of care. The failure regime was designed to be used as a last resort and so far has only been used twice since its creation.

NHSE's special measures

Previous assurance frameworks have linked a CCG's assurance status with intervention actions. A CCG assessment moving down to limited assurance or not assured in a particular component would signal the need for an improvement plan. An improvement plan could form part of the application of special measures or legal directions. The CCG IAF does not make in-year assessments to provide these triggers. However, the process remains the same. If the data, or wider sources of insight, raise concerns that initiate a discussion between NHSE and a CCG, the outcome could be an improvement plan. If the circumstances match the description of special measures or the statutory definition of directions, these actions may also be taken.

NHSE is supported by legislation in exercising formal powers of direction if it is satisfied that a CCG is (a) failing or (b) is at risk of failing to discharge its functions. Formal intervention action would be proposed, as laid out in section 14Z21 of the NHS Act 2006 (as amended). These interventions include:

- directing the CCG as to how it discharges its functions;
- directing the CCG or the AO to stop carrying out any functions for a defined period;
- terminating the AO's appointment and appointing a new AO;
- varying the CCG's constitution;
- carrying out certain functions on behalf of a CCG or arranging for another CCG to do so; and
- dissolving the CCG.

Since the use of such formal direction affects CCG autonomy, careful consideration is required before this course of action can be implemented

NHSI's special measures

NHSI has assumed all of NHS TDA's and Monitor's powers to intervene in a provider trust in the event of failings in its healthcare standards, as judged by the CQC, or other aspects of its leadership that result in a significant breach of its licence conditions.

NHSI assesses a breach or a potential breach of the governance and continuity of service licence conditions through a risk-based system of regulation. This determines the intensity of the monitoring undertaken at each provider trust. Its intervention powers are broad, ranging from closing a specific service – if there are serious concerns about it – and requiring a board either to take or not take a specific action(s), to requiring a board to obtain external advice on a particular issue or – in extreme cases – removing any or all of the directors (or governors in the case of an FT) and appointing replacements.

In the most serious cases, where intervention by NHSI cannot resolve the breach, a provider trust could be dissolved after consultation. If this were to happen, the NHS Act 2006 provides mechanisms to ensure that NHS patients and users continue to receive high-quality treatment.

Quality of care

A special measures intervention for quality of care failings is usually instigated by the CQC Chief Inspector of Hospitals, when an NHS trust or FT is rated 'Inadequate' in the well-led domain and 'Inadequate' in one or more of the other domains (safe, caring, responsive and effective).

When the NHSI receives a recommendation from the Chief Inspector to place an NHS trust or FT in special measures, the NHSI will consider the evidence that CQC provides to them alongside other relevant evidence. Based on the full range of information, the NHSI will make a decision whether the trust or FT will be placed in special measures.

The NHSI may also place a trust or FT into special measures without receiving a recommendation from the Chief Inspector, based on its own evidence. In these circumstances, the NHSI will always seek advice from CQC. An NHS trust or FT will not enter special measures until the NHSI formally makes that decision. The NHSI will communicate its decision to the trust and then make a formal public announcement through a press release. The period of special measures begins when the NHSI formally and publicly announces that a trust is in special measures. It is intended that the usual period of time a trust remains in special measures will be a maximum of 12 months, although this may be extended in some circumstances.

The CQC will focus on identifying failures in the quality of care and judging whether improvements have been made. The NHSI will use their respective powers to support improvement in the quality of care provided. Typically, providers will be subject to the following interventions, although their detailed application will vary according to the specific circumstances of the organisation.

- The NHSI will appoint an improvement director who will act on their behalf to provide assurance of the trust's approach to improving performance.
- In most cases, the NHSI will also appoint one or more appropriate partner organisations to provide support in improvement. Partner organisations are selected for their strength in the areas of weakness at the trust in special measures. Arrangements for this appointment will be set out in a memorandum of understanding between the NHSI and the partner ('buddy') organisation. Partner organisations will be reimbursed by NHSI for reasonable expenses and may receive an incentive payment.
- The NHSI will review the capability of the trust's leadership. If needed, this may lead to changes to the management of the organisation to make sure that the board and executive team can make the required improvements.
- The NHSI will require trusts in special measures to publish their progress against action plans every month on the NHS Choices and their own website, and to participate as required in national and local press conferences.

A provider will only come out of special measures if it has made the required improvements. This is usually expected to take place within one year; however, as can be seen by Medway and North Cumbria, for some providers it can take a number of years. It is for the relevant Chief Inspector to inspect the provider and judge whether improvements have been made and if it is delivering good enough care to exit special measures. The NHSI will only take a provider out of special measures after it has been re-inspected, is no longer rated as 'inadequate' in the 'well-led' domain and has improved to at least 'requires improvement' across the other four CQC domains.

Whilst a trust will be looking to exit from special measures, the Chief Inspector of Hospitals can recommend a variety of outcomes, namely:

- exiting from special measures;
- exiting from special measures with some continued support in place;
- remaining in special measures until the end of an extension period;
- remaining in special measures while NHS Improvement addresses financial concerns; and
- remaining in special measures while urgent support is provided or a long-term solution is found.

The NHSI must also be confident that improvements will be sustained in order to accept the removal of the special measures intervention.

Financial special measures

The financial context for the NHS has also led to a growing number of commissioners and providers being placed in 'financial' special measures. NHSI, in partnership with NHS England, is using a suite of measures for providers and commissioners to restore financial discipline and help ensure ongoing financial sustainability for the NHS. NHSI and NHSE placed several challenged NHS providers and commissioners in financial special measures in order to bring about swift improvement in their finances. As part of this, each organisation undergoes a rapid financial review and agrees a financial recovery plan. Specialist teams, led by a financial improvement director, oversee intensive, accelerated action to bring about financial improvement, including support from peer organisations where appropriate. Each organisation receives a package of support designed to achieve rapid financial improvement, whilst maintaining or improving quality. The support can include:

- ensuring that financial systems and controls operate effectively, so that money isn't being spent without proper checks and controls – including, for example, in the authorisation of agency and locum spend;
- improving efficiency and productivity, including learning lessons from higher performing organisations;
- improving the way workforce is managed and rotas planned to use permanent staff most effectively; and
- ensuring commissioners and providers charge and get paid appropriately for the work carried out.

NHSI will place a trust into special measures for financial reasons if:

1. The trust has not agreed a control total and is planning or forecasting a deficit (or has recently delivered a significant year-end deficit).
   or:
2. The trust has agreed a control total but:
   - has a significant negative variance year to date against the control total plan and
   - is forecasting (or has recently delivered at year-end) a significant deficit.
   or:

3. The trust has an exceptional financial governance failure (e.g. significant fraud or irregularity).

NHSI will consider exceptional mitigating circumstances or existing robust recovery plans as evidence not to intervene through special measures. However, if NHSI are satisfied that the FT is in breach of its licence conditions (or the equivalent conditions applicable to an NHS trust) or it has reasonable grounds to suspect a breach, in relation to financial governance, then it will place the trust into special measures.

NHSI will then support the trust with the following interventions:

- Financial Improvement Notice issued.
- NHSI ED sponsor appointed.
- Regular formal progress and challenge meetings with ED sponsor, typically every one to two months.
- A financial improvement director, appointed by NHS Improvement.
- Appointment of turnaround/recovery support, including an NHSI team and possibly wider support (e.g. peer support).
- Board vacancies filled on the direction of NHSI.
- Trust required to publish on its website home page that it is in special measures for financial reasons.
- Any FT in special measures for financial reasons is required to notify its Council of Governors, and give the reasons for it and the planned response.

In order to leave financial special measures, organisations have to demonstrate rapidly that they are returning to financial discipline, which includes developing a robust financial recovery plan and any governance failures have been addressed. NHSI must also be confident that there has been no deterioration in the quality of care as a result of the financial improvement.

New models of care and failure regimes

The creation of STPs, ICSs and ACOs along with other new models of care raised questions around regulation and oversight for NHSE, NHSI and the CQC. The main issues to be addressed are as follows:

- Any collaboration that does not create a new legal entity cannot hold a provider licence and as such cannot be held to account by NHSI and thus placed in special measures if they are in difficulty.
- Where organisations merge or acquire another, a legal entity is created and will require a licence.
- NHSI is currently considering whether reporting and monitoring of finance, leadership and strategic change could be done at board level, and reporting on quality and operational performance at trust level.

- The setting up of subsidiaries and joint ventures which deliver healthcare (e.g. MCPOs or PACS care models were previously classed an independent provider and as such received a lighter touch of regulation).
- NSHI has confirmed that independent providers (now termed 'NHS controlled providers') will, for the purposes of oversight, be classified as NHS providers and overseen as such. Since April 2018 'NHS-controlled providers' have been required to hold a new provider licence which is inclusive of a licence condition imposing requirements around good governance. Consequently, NHS controlled providers will be subject to the SOF by NHSI and where they breached their licence conditions due to serious failures in quality of care or financial problems, they will be placed in segment 4, and placed in either the special measures regime or the financial special measures regime.

Quality governance

The growing political agenda for assurance on the delivery of quality services, as well as quality outcomes for patients, has led to the growth of quality governance as a specialised area of governance for provider trusts. While not strictly part of health service governance, many NHS company secretaries or governance practitioners will find themselves involved in the quality agenda purely because the board is required by its regulators to give regular and specific assurance on the delivery of quality within their organisation.

Quality has been part of government strategy for modernising the NHS for many years. A First Class Service: Quality in the new NHS, published in July 1998, set out the agenda for quality improvement in the NHS. The publication of Lord Darzi's 2008 report Quality Care for All revived and reinforced this strategy. He highlighted four key areas that would demonstrate improving quality of care, which were:

- patient safety;
- effectiveness, including clinical outcomes and patient reported outcome measures (PROMs);
- user experience; and
- innovation.

The Darzi Report resulted in greater clarity on quality standards; the development of quality metrics; publication of Quality Accounts; the creation of Commissioning for Quality Improvement (CQUINs) incentives and the National Quality Board.

Since, ultimately, the board of a healthcare provider organisation is responsible for the quality of care delivered across all services that it provides, this has to be achieved through governance arrangements which delegate responsibility down to the operating levels in the organisation. In the case of quality, this means that, although individuals and clinical teams are at the frontline and responsible for delivering quality care, it is the responsibility of the board to create a culture within the organisation that enables clinicians and clinical teams to work at their best.

In addition, the board must have in place arrangements for measuring and monitoring quality and for escalating issues, including, where needed, to the board. Boards should encourage a culture where services are improved by learning from mistakes, where staff and patients are encouraged to identify areas for improvement, and where they are not afraid to speak out.

The term 'quality governance' is used to refer to the values and behaviours and the structures and processes that need to be in place to enable the board to discharge its responsibilities for quality.

The arrangements for quality governance should complement and be fully integrated with the governance arrangements for other aspects of the board's responsibilities, such as finance governance and research governance. The National Quality Board (NQB) framework *Shared Commitment to Quality* (2016) promotes improved quality criteria across all national health organisations for the first time and provides a nationally agreed definition of quality and guide for clinical and managerial leaders wanting to improve quality.

The approach has been agreed across NHS and social care organisations to provide more consistency and to enable the system to work together more effectively. The 5YFV confirms a national commitment to high-quality, person-centred care for all; the framework describes the changes that are needed to deliver a sustainable health and care system in key areas which matter most to the users of the service:

- **Safety:** people are protected from avoidable harm and abuse. When mistakes occur lessons will be learned.
- **Effectiveness:** people's care and treatment achieves good outcomes, promotes a good quality of life, and is based on the best available evidence.
- **Positive experience:** Caring, responsive and person-centred.

The framework goes on to describe the standards required for those providing services as high performing providers and commissioners working together and in partnership with, and for, local people and communities, that:

- are well-led: they are open and collaborate internally and externally and are committed to learning and improvement;
- use resources sustainably: they use their resources responsibly and efficiently, providing fair access to all, according to need, and promote an open and fair culture; and
- are equitable for all: they ensure inequalities in health outcomes are a focus for quality improvement, making sure care quality does not vary due to characteristics such as gender, race, disability, age, sexual orientation, religion, belief, gender reassignment, pregnancy and maternity or marital or civil partnership status.

Quality accounts

The significant report relating to quality is the annual quality account, which reports on the quality of services provided by an NHS healthcare service. Quality accounts are not intended as marketing documents, but as an opportunity for NHS providers to enter into an open and honest dialogue with the public regarding the quality of care in the organisation. All providers of NHS services are required to produce a quality account as set out in the Health Act 2009 and supporting regulations. The Quality Account must be presented to the SoS and published on the NHS Choices website each June.

NHS trusts and FTs are required to report on a prescribed set of quality indicators in their Quality Accounts. The Health and Social Care Information Centre (HSCIC) Indicator Portal provides the latest data reported for each of the indicators. As trusts use the same data sources, they can easily be compared with each other. Trusts are asked to report the result for each quality indicator by following a prescribed statement, including what actions they have taken, or will take, to improve the results and therefore the quality of care they provide. There are 15 quality indicators; however, trusts only have to report on those that are relevant to the services they provide. For example, an ambulance trust will include different indicators to those of a mental health trust as they provide different services.

Organisations must decide on at least three areas where they are planning to improve the quality of their services. They should also provide details about how they prioritise improvements and why and how they are planning to report back on progress to their patients and the public. Patients' views should be taken into account when organisations decide on the priorities for improvement. The Quality Account also reports on the organisation's participation in national, local and clinical audits as well as clinical research.

The Quality Account must also make two statements to the CQC. The first statement gives information on a provider's registration status (either without any conditions, with conditions, or not registered). The CQC can also apply specific conditions in response to serious risks that it finds. For example, it can demand a ward or service is closed until the provider meets safety requirements or that it is suspended or taken off the register if absolutely necessary. Such action must be disclosed in the Quality Account. The second statement provides information on what reviews and/or investigations the provider has taken part in and what the CQC said about the provider.

More recently, the National Quality Board published its National Guidance on Learning from Deaths (March 2017) which sets out a framework for providers on identifying, reporting, investigating and learning from deaths in care. As a result of this publication, all providers are required to report on their learning from deaths in the Quality Accounts.

The accuracy of data is key in being able to measure and compare quality improvements. The Quality Account requires organisations to make statements, which give an indication of the quality and accuracy of the information an organisation collects.

To ensure that the information presented in the Quality Account is accurate and interpreted fairly, and that the range of services described and priorities for improvement are representative of the services delivered, assurance is required to ensure accuracy. Commissioners have a legal obligation to review and comment on the Quality Accounts, while the council of governors, local Healthwatch organisations and OSCs will be offered the opportunity to comment on a voluntary basis.

NHS trusts and FTs are required to gain external audit assurance on their quality accounts and two of their quality indicators. The auditors will issue a limited assurance report on whether anything has come to their attention that leads them to believe that:

- the quality account has not been prepared in line with the requirements set out in the Regulations;
- the quality account is not consistent with specified documentation detailed in section 3 of the annual guidance; and
- one or both quality indicators are misstated.

Quality report

In addition to the Quality Accounts, FTs must also include a report on the quality of care they provide (the quality report) within their overall annual report as set out by FT Annual Reporting Manual (ARM) for the year under review. The quality report specifically aims to improve public accountability for the quality of care.

The quality report incorporates all the requirements of the quality account regulations as well as a number of additional reporting requirements set by NHSI. The additional NHSI requirements are as follows:

- A statement which gives a monetary total for the amount of income in the year under review conditional upon achieving quality improvement and innovation goals, and a monetary total for the associated payment in the previous year.
- An explanatory note for clinical coding stating that the results should not be extrapolated further than the actual sample audited and which services were reviewed within the sample.
- An overview of the quality of care offered by the FT based on performance in the year under review against indicators selected by the board in consultation with stakeholders, with an explanation of the underlying reason(s) for selection. The indicator set selected must include at least three indicators each for patient safety, clinical effectiveness and patient experience. Where the quality indicators are the same as those used in the previous year's report, the data reported should be consistent.
- Performance against the relevant indicators and performance thresholds set out in the oversight documents issued by NHSI.

The FT board is also required to make a statement of directors' responsibilities that the quality report meets the requirements set out in FT Annual Reporting Manual (FT ARM) for the year under review. FTs are also required to obtain a limited assurance report from their external auditors on the content of the quality report and to include it in the annual report. The limited assurance report has reported on whether anything has come to the attention of the auditor that leads them to believe that the content of the quality report has not been prepared in line with the requirements set out in FT ARM. The auditors must also undertake substantive sample testing on two mandated performance indicators and one local indicator selected by the governors of the FT. The auditors must then provide a report to the FT's council of governors and board of directors of their findings and recommendations for improvement on the content of the quality report, mandated indicators and a locally selected indicator.

Financial reporting

The annual report and accounts is an important document for governance because it is a means by which the directors are made accountable to the stakeholders, and it provides a channel of communication from directors to stakeholders. The report and accounts enable the stakeholders to assess how well the organisation has been governed and managed. It should therefore be clear and understandable to a reader with reasonable financial awareness, and reliable and 'believable'.

If financial statements are produced in a way that is intended deliberately to mislead stakeholders, the persons responsible would be guilty of fraud, which is a crime. Misleading financial statements, however, could only be issued if the audit committee is satisfied with their preparation, external auditors provide a 'clean' audit report, and the board of directors approves the financial statements. In most organisations, this would require deception by a small group of EDs, such as the CEO and finance director.

NHS trusts are obliged to comply with the determination and directions given by the SoS in the preparation of their annual report and annual accounts. These directions are set out in the NHS Finance Manual, published by the DH. In addition, the government publishes the Financial Reporting Manual (FReM), which is the technical accounting guide to the preparation of financial statements. Foundation trusts are required to follow the guidance given by NHSI in the FT ARM; CCGs should follow the guidance in the CCG Annual Reporting Manual (CCG ARM).

The UK Code states as a main principle that: 'the board should present a balanced and understandable assessment of the company's position and prospects' in its report and accounts, as well as in its interim reports and other public statements. This principle applies to narrative reporting in the annual report as well as to the financial statements. These principles are mirrored in the FReM, the FT ARM and the CCG ARM.

The FReM, FT ARM and CCG ARM have adopted these changes, and the previous directors' report (including an operating and financial review) has now been split into a strategic report and a directors' report.

As previously mentioned, regular financial reporting to the regulators is part of the oversight approach of the NHSI and NHSE, however, the other key financial reporting tool for NHS organisations is the annual report and accounts.

NHS organisations must publish an annual report and (full) audited accounts as one document and present it at a public meeting, whether or not summary financial statements are also produced. Where an NHS body has dissolved, or taken FT status, an annual report and audited accounts for its final accounting period must still be published and presented at a public meeting by a successor organisation. NHS organisations still have the option to prepare and distribute an annual report and summary financial statements; however, this is additional to the annual report and accounts described above which must be available if requested.

The year-end for all NHS organisations is 31 March and the timetable for the production of the annual accounts is quite constrained. For 2018/19, the deadline for submitting audited accounts to DH was 29 May 2019. FTs are required to lay their annual report and accounts, with any report of the auditor on them (including the limited assurance opinion on the Quality Report), before Parliament in July each year. The annual accounts of each NHS organisation are then summarised as part of the NHS Annual Accounts, which are also laid before Parliament in July of each year

The guidance sets out the minimum content of the annual report. Beyond this, however, the entity must take ownership of the annual report. It should ensure that additional information is included where necessary to reflect the position of the NHS body within the community and give sufficient information to meet the requirements of public accountability.

The financial statements report on the financial performance of the organisation over the previous financial year and the financial position of the organisation as at the end of that year. The directors' report and other statements published in the same document provide supporting information, much of it in narrative rather than in numerical form. Stakeholders use the information in the annual report and accounts to assess the stewardship of the directors and the financial health of the organisation.

Under the STP process, progress is being made in defining system control figures for financial performance. This raises interesting questions as to the reporting requirements for system control totals, which will be multi-level across the footprint. At present, each individual organisation will continue to report financial performance through its own governance route and in addition as part of the system control group. NHSE and NHSI will continue to monitor and report the financial performance of individual organisations against their agreed plans.

Annual report and accounts – FT

The annual report of NHS FTs must, as a minimum, include:

- the performance report, comprising:
  - overview of performance
  - performance analysis; and
- the accountability report, comprising:
  - directors' report
  - remuneration report
  - staff report
  - the disclosures set out in the FT Code of Governance
  - NHSI's Single Oversight Framework
  - statement of accounting officer's responsibilities
  - annual governance statement
  - a quality report.

The accounts should include:

- the accounting officer's statement of responsibilities;
- the auditor's opinion and certificate;
- a foreword to the accounts;
- four primary financial statements; and
- notes to the accounts.

The annual report may, at the FT's discretion, include additional reporting covering equality, the Modern Slavery Act 2015 and the NHS Constitution. FTs are also required to include progress against their sustainable development plan in their annual report.

Annual report and accounts – CCGs

CCGs also have a statutory obligation to develop and publish an annual report. The annual report and accounts is a single document, which presents the story of the CCG's activities during the previous financial year ending 31 March. The form and content of the annual report and accounts is directed by NHSE and must be in line with the DHSC's manual for accounts. In practice, this is achieved by following NHSE's annual reporting guidance (ARG3). The CCG's annual report and accounts must contain:

- an annual report, including:
  - member practices' introduction;
  - the strategic report;
  - the members' report; and
  - the remuneration report;
- a statement of the accountable officer's responsibilities;
- a governance statement;
- four primary financial statements;

- notes to the accounts; and
- a report and opinion from an independent auditor.

The member practices' introduction is produced collectively by the GP practices that make up the membership of the CCG. It should include:

- reflections on the CCG's progress and performance in relation to the health priorities of the local community as set out in the CCG's strategy and business plan;
- consideration of the impact the council of members and governing body have had in key areas; and
- a statement which sets out how the annual evaluation of effectiveness of the council of members and/or governing body was conducted and how any recommendations are being taken forward.

The strategic report and members' report are based on the requirements of sections 414A, C and D and section 416 of the CA 2006 tailored to be relevant to CCGs. The strategic report should stand alone, but can include summarised information cross-referenced to other parts of the annual report.

It is the responsibility of the CCG's AO to prepare the annual report and accounts. Usually, the governing body approves the annual report and accounts for submission to NHSE and wider publication, but this may vary depending on the CCG's constitution. In approving the annual report and accounts, the members of the governing body confirm that they are satisfied that they present the CCG's year in an appropriate, comprehensive, balanced and coherent way. Before 30 September, each CCG must present its annual report and accounts to stakeholders, including members of the public, at an AGM. The HFMA's Introductory Guide – CCG Annual Report and Accounts (2014) was published to assist members of the CCG and its governing body through the process of reviewing and approving the annual report and accounts. CCGs do not need to present their annual reports and accounts to Parliament.

Responsibilities of the directors for financial reporting

An organisation's directors are responsible for the preparation and content of the financial statements. The UK Code states that the directors should explain in the annual report their responsibility for preparing the annual report and financial statements. There should also be a supporting statement by the auditors (in their report) about their reporting responsibilities. The UK Code also requires that the directors should include in their annual report an explanation of the basis on which the company generates or preserves value over the longer term (its 'business model'), and strategy for delivering the objectives of the company.

There is sometimes confusion and misunderstanding about responsibilities for financial reporting, and a mistaken belief that the external auditors are responsible for the 'true and fair view' in the financial statements. If misleading and incorrect financial statements are produced, it may therefore be supposed that the auditors have been negligent and must be to blame. This view is incorrect. The directors are responsible for the financial statements: they prepare the financial statements and have the primary responsibility for the reliability of the information they provide. Management and the directors are therefore responsible for identifying and correcting any errors or misrepresentations in the financial statements.

The responsibility of the external auditors is to obtain reasonable assurance, in their professional opinion, that the financial statements are free from material error or misstatement. They present a professional opinion to the stakeholders, not to the directors of the organisation, and the directors should not rely on the opinion of the external auditors in reaching their own view.

In UK law, the directors are also potentially liable for any errors or misleading information in the annual report and accounts. Any person (e.g. an investor) suffering a loss because of an error or misstatement in an organisation's report and accounts may sue the organisation, and the organisation may then take legal action against the directors to recover any losses it has occurred from the legal action.

Going concern statement

A key accounting concept is the 'going concern' concept. This is the view that the organisation will continue to trade for the foreseeable future (at least the next 12 months). This is different to an understanding of an organisation's viability.

In the UK Code, the board is required to make an explicit statement in the financial statements about whether the going concern basis of accounting has been adopted and whether there are any material uncertainties about the company's ability to continue to do so in future. It is also required to make a broader statement about the board's reasonable expectation as to the company's viability based on a robust assessment of the company's principal risks and the company's current position. This is developed in the latest FRC Risk Guide which states:

> 'A company that is able to adopt the going concern basis of accounting and does not have related material uncertainties to report, for the purposes of the financial statements, is not necessarily free of risks that would threaten the company's business model, future performance, solvency or liquidity were they to materialise. The board is responsible for ensuring this distinction is understood internally and communicated externally.'

The financial statements are therefore prepared on the going concern basis, and assets are valued differently from what their value might be if the organisation went into liquidation. The statement of going concern should also give reasons why the directors have reached their view, and indicate any doubts there might be. Where there is fundamental uncertainty over the going concern basis (for instance, continuing operational stability depends on finance or income that has not yet been approved), or where the going concern basis is not appropriate, the directors will need to disclose the relevant circumstances and should discuss the basis of accounting and the disclosures to be made with their auditors. Similarly, the UK Listing Rules require the directors to make a statement in the report and accounts that the company is a going concern, together with supporting assumptions and qualifications as necessary. These requirements are mirrored in the NHS Finance Manual, FReM, NHS FT ARM and CCG ARM.

The going concern basis has come under greater scrutiny due to the severe financial circumstances faced by many providers and commissioners. There are continuing significant financial pressures within the sector, with NHS trusts, FTs and CCGs requiring additional financial support.

There is no presumption of going concern status for FTs. Directors must decide each year whether or not it is appropriate for the FT to prepare its accounts on the going concern basis, taking into account best estimates of future activity and cash flows. FTs are required to prepare their accounts in accordance with the relevant international accounting rules as interpreted by the FT ARM, which sets out that:

> 'An entity should prepare its financial statements on a going concern basis, unless:
> (a) The entity is being liquidated or has ceased trading; or
> (b) The directors have no realistic alternative but to liquidate the entity or to cease trading, in which circumstances the entity may, if appropriate, prepare its financial statements on a basis other than going concern.'

In recent years, NHS trusts have been issued letters from their regulator, where required, confirming that the DHSC would continue to make funding available to the trust. On this basis, such NHS trusts in financial deficit have been able to declare themselves as a going concern. Such letters were not issued for 2016/17, which created additional challenges for boards of any NHS trust that could not meet the definition of a going concern as set out in the DHSC's Group Accounting Manual (GAM) 2016/17. This specifies that unless an NHS trust expects its services to cease to be provided in the public sector the going concern basis should be assumed. If an NHS trust is dependent upon financing which is not confirmed, this would ordinarily be an uncertainty for the going concern basis and the DHSC GAM requires that these be disclosed in the annual report and accounts. However, while this uncertainty is being disclosed it does not affect the going concern basis itself. The NHS trust should consider preparing a paper for its board and/or audit committee if necessary. If the NHS trust's auditor considers this disclosure to be of sufficient importance, they may enter an 'emphasis of matter' as part of their annual report. This does not constitute a 'qualified opinion', and would not cause a concern for NHSI as long as the NHSI was already aware of the matters being disclosed.

The auditor's responsibility is to consider the appropriateness of the use of the going concern assumption in preparing the financial statements. They should also consider if there are material uncertainties about the organisation's ability to continue as a going concern that need to be disclosed in the financial statements.

A typical going concern statement within an annual report might be as follows:

> 'After making enquiries, the directors have a reasonable expectation that the NHS foundation trust has adequate resources to continue in operational existence for the foreseeable future. For this reason, they continue to adopt the going concern basis in preparing the accounts.'

In the UK, disclosures about the assumptions or qualifications about going concern status are becoming more extensive. The directors may be personally liable if they make a statement that the organisation is a going concern without giving the matter careful consideration. Liability could arise if the organisation subsequently goes into liquidation within the next 12 months and stakeholders claim that they relied on the going concern statement when making their investment decisions.

In the strict accounting sense, NHS bodies cannot prepare accounts on any other basis than as a going concern. Various Acts of Parliament prevent NHS organisations from becoming insolvent in the strict accounting sense, as the DH bears the ultimate liability for any debts. Even so, NHS annual reporting requirements still require NHS organisations to include a statement on whether or not the financial statements have been prepared on a going concern basis and the reasons for this decision, with supporting assumptions or qualifications as necessary. The distinction between going concern and viability make for interesting audit committee discussions, particularly in the current financial climate and in the context of shared financial controls across STPs.

The corporate governance statement

In 2006, the European Union (EU) adopted a Company Reporting Directive that required quoted companies to produce a corporate governance statement in their annual reports. The statement must refer to the corporate governance code applied by the company (e.g. the UK Code) and explain whether, and to what extent, the company complies with that code. The statement must also include a description of the main features of the company's internal control and risk management systems in relation to the financial reporting process, and provide a description of the composition and operation of the board and its committees.

In the UK, listed companies were already required to report much of the corporate governance information required by the Company Reporting Directive. The UK Listing Rules require companies to include in their annual report a statement of how they have applied the principles of the UK Code, for example disclosures about the composition of board committees and their work.

However, the Company Reporting Directive required the information to be presented in a separate 'corporate governance statement' and that the statement should include a description of the main features of the company's internal control and risk management systems relating to the financial reporting process, neither of which were contained in the UK Code.

The parallel arrangement for FTs is that they are required to include a statement of compliance with the FT Code in their annual report.

The annual governance statement

A model statement of the FT annual governance statement is set out in FT ARM. It is a backwards-looking statement that captures information on risk management and internal control, and includes some specific requirements on quality governance. It replaced and expanded upon the former requirement for a statement on internal control and is signed by the FT's chief executive officer (CEO).

This requirement is in line with the UK Code, which states that the board should report to shareholders each year that it has conducted the annual review of the effectiveness of the systems of internal control and risk management. The Financial Services Authority (FSA)'s Disclosure and Transparency Rules for listed companies also requires companies to report on the main features of their internal control and risk management systems in relation to financial reporting.

All public bodies (including NHS organisations) must provide assurance that they are appropriately managing and controlling the resources for which they are responsible. The requirement for an AGS has now been rolled out across all NHS organisations and a template for guidance issued for NHS trusts, FTs and CCGs. The annual guidance from the DHSC continues to set out the key elements that need to be considered when producing the AGS. While NHS organisations will have risk management, control and review processes in place, the detail of these processes vary from one organisation to another depending on circumstances such as size and the complexity of the risks faced. The annual guidance, therefore, offers a summary of characteristics under six high-level elements to help with consideration of the completeness of the processes that have been put in place in a particular body.

This requirement is in line with the UK Code, which states that the board should report to shareholders each year that it has conducted the annual review of the effectiveness of the systems of internal control and risk management. The Financial Services Authority's Disclosure and Transparency Rules for listed companies also requires companies to report on the main features of their internal control and risk management systems in relation to financial reporting.

NHS organisations are required to ensure that they have sufficient evidence to demonstrate that they have implemented processes appropriate to their circumstances under the following high-level elements:

1. scope of responsibility;
2. the purpose of the system of internal control;
3. capacity to handle risk;

4. review of economy, efficiency and effectiveness of the use of resources;
5. information governance;
6. annual quality account;
7. review of effectiveness; and
8. conclusion.

The conclusion must either:

- clearly state that no significant internal control issues have been identified (as supported by the HOIA opinion); or
- specifically list the significant internal control issues which have been identified in the body of the AGS.

A single definition of a significant internal control issue is not possible and NHS organisations are required to exercise their judgement in deciding whether or not a particular issue should be regarded as falling into this category. The guidance sets out factors that may be helpful in exercising that judgement, including the following:

- Might the issue prejudice achievement of priorities?
- Could the issue undermine the integrity or reputation of the NHS?
- What view does the audit committee take on this point?
- What advice has the internal or external audit given?
- Could delivery of the standards expected of the accountable officer (AO) be at risk?
- Has the issue made it harder to resist fraud or other misuse of resources?
- Did the issue divert resources from another significant aspect of the business?
- Could the issue have a material impact on the accounts?
- Might national or data security or integrity be put at risk?

The audit committee plays a key role in the production of the AGS. It supports the board and AO by reviewing the comprehensiveness of assurances in meeting the board and AO's assurance needs and reviewing the reliability and integrity of the assurances. The audit committee also advises the board and AO of any control issues that could be considered significant and are therefore appropriate for disclosure in the AGS.

The board assurance framework

In order to sign off the AGS, NHS boards need to be assured that the systems, policies and people they have put in place are operating in a way that is effective, focused on key risks and driving the delivery of objectives. There is, however, the potential for a lack of clarity within the board (and beyond) to what is meant by the term 'assurance'. This can extend to uncertainty over the level of assurance required, where that assurance comes from and how the reporting of assurance is managed in a co-ordinated manner.

Although the process of securing assurance has always been a fundamental principle of good management and accountability, the requirement for all NHS AOs to sign the AGS has focused attention on the level of assurance that boards receive. To provide this statement, boards need to be able to demonstrate that they have been properly informed through assurances about the totality of their risks, not just financial, and have arrived at their conclusions based on all the evidence presented to them. Assurance is the foundation of evidence that gives confidence that risk is being controlled effectively, or conversely, highlights that certain controls are ineffective or there are gaps that need to be addressed.

The HM Treasury Guidance on Assurance Frameworks (2012) defines an 'assurance framework' as:

> 'A structured means of identifying and mapping the main sources of assurance in an organisation, and co-ordinating them to best effect.'

The board assurance framework (BAF) is a framework that NHS organisations are required to put in place to identify the key risks to the trust's achievement of its strategic objectives and how these risks are being managed. It provides an organisation with a method for the effective and focused management of the principal risks to meeting its objectives. It also provides a structure for the evidence to support the AGS. It identifies which of the organisation's objectives are at risk because of inadequacies in the operation of controls or where the organisation has insufficient assurance about them. At the same time, it provides structured assurances about where risks are being managed effectively and objectives are being delivered. This allows the board to determine where to make efficient use of resources and to address the issues identified to improve the quality and safety of care. As a natural extension of risk management, it is reasonable to incorporate the board assurance arrangements into the risk management documentation, therefore ensuring that risk, control and assurance identification and monitoring processes are considered as one and not disparate activities.

It is also a key tool for a well-led organisation and if used as a live and dynamic tool offers significant evidence in the well-led assessment (see Chapter 6).

Baker Tilly and NHS Providers issued a toolkit, *Board Assurance: A toolkit for health sector organisations – Do we really know what we think we know?*, in 2015. This explains:

> '[A]ssurance mapping as a key part of developing and maintaining board assurance arrangements and producing a BAF. Mapping provides an organisation with an improved ability to understand and confirm that they have assurance over key controls or where control gaps exist and whether actions are in place to address these gaps. The assurance mapping process and the way of illustrating the results using a BAF can give confidence to management and the board that they "really know what they think they know".'

In documented form, a BAF would include:

- the trust's strategic objectives;
- the key risks to achieving the objectives;
- the controls in place to manage the risks;
- the assurances that the trust used to provide evidence that the controls were operating effectively;
- any gaps in the assurances; and
- an action plan to address the gaps.

Three types of assurance can be sought: verbal, written and empirical. All can be of use depending on the circumstances. Each will be valued differently depending on other factors. The governing body has defined the overarching levels of assurance as noted below:

- Level 1 – Operational (Management)
- Level 2 – Oversight functions (Committees)
- Level 3 – Independent (Audits/Reviews/Inspections etc.).

The evidence supporting assurance should be sufficient in scope and weight to support the conclusion and be:

- relevant;
- reliable;
- understandable;
- free from material misstatement;
- neutral/free from bias; and
- such that another person would reasonably come to the same conclusion.

All evidence does not carry the same weight, and should be weighted in accordance to independence and relevance. Evidence may be flawed in terms of both quality and quantity, leading to limitations in the assurance that can be provided. Every NHS organisation must design its own framework, which will relate to the delivery of its own objectives within the context of an understanding of the principal risks that the organisation faces. The BAF should enable the board to:

- establish principal objectives (strategic and directorate);
- identify the principal risks that may threaten the achievement of these objectives – typically in the range of 75–200 depending on the complexity of the organisation;
- identify and evaluate the design of key controls intended to manage these principal risks, underpinned by core controls assurance standards;
- set out the arrangements for obtaining assurance on the effectiveness of key controls across all areas of principal risk;
- evaluate the assurance across all areas of principal risk;
- identify positive assurances and areas where there are gaps in controls and/or assurances;

- put in place plans to take corrective action where gaps have been identified in relation to principal risks; and
- maintain dynamic risk management arrangements including, crucially, a well-founded risk register.

The audit committee should not be responsible for creating the BAF; instead, it should satisfy itself that line management is carrying it out appropriately and that the processes and format are valid, relevant and effective. The committee needs to be satisfied that it contains the high-risk areas pertinent to the organisation.

Governance checklist

- Does the board have a good understanding of the requirements imposed by the relevant framework for performance reporting? Is the board clear about how this aligns to its overall strategy and corporate objectives for the organisation?
- Is the board confident that the performance and quality dashboard it reviews is supported by robust and viable data?
- Is the board confident that the annual report and accounts present a balanced and understandable assessment of the organisation's position and prospects?
- Does the annual report meet the appropriate reporting requirements, including the addition of a strategic report?
- Is the board clear about the its compliance with the relevant codes of governance?
- Does the board regularly review the board assurance framework and what actions does it take to address the issues it raises?

Summary

- Boards need to be confident that the systems, policies and people they have put in place are operating in a way that is effective, is focused on key risks and is driving the delivery of objectives.
- The concept of assurance can be a source of misunderstanding and mismatched expectations. Potentially, there can be a lack of clarity within, and beyond the board, as to what is meant exactly by the term 'assurance'. This can extend to uncertainty over the level of assurance required, where that assurance comes from and how the reporting of assurance is managed in a coordinated manner.
- Assurance can also sometimes be hard to find in the NHS, not because of the lack of information but because there is so much information. In addition, the validity and robustness of some of the information can also create difficulties, such as problems with coding.
- There is clearly a large and complex reporting structure for NHS organisations with NHSE, the NHSI and the CQC responsible for the design of much of its content.

- Since the publication of the Francis Inquiry findings and 5YFV, there has been a growing commitment for these agencies to work together and align their reporting requirements. This alignment can already be seen; for example, in the use of a Single Oversight Framework, and the commitment to develop the Well-Led Framework.
- There is, however, a significant amount of information in the public domain, allowing key stakeholders and the general public to assess whether, indeed, the board is fulfilling its statutory duties.
- In the context of this highly regulated sector, the work of internal and external audit and the role of the audit committee is a significant contribution to the assurance evidence required by the NHS board to fulfil its statutory duties.

19
Audit

Introduction

The role of audit is important in ensuring accurate reporting, which is one of the foundations for health service governance. Given the range and diversity of reporting requirements that are imposed on NHS organisations, the role of audit clearly becomes a crucial tool in the reliability and robustness of those reports and provides vital independent assurance to NHS boards.

All stakeholders rely on the quality, performance and financial information that is published by the organisation. It is important, therefore, that the information is objective and robust. As a result, the work of both internal and external audit is vital in making sure that, as far as is reasonably possible, the information is objective and can be relied on. Within NHS organisations, the remit of internal and external audit includes the review of quality, performance and financial information. Part of the audit committee's role is to monitor the work of both internal and external auditors and to ensure that the external auditors can place full reliance on the work of internal audit in these three areas of information.

The role of internal audit

According to the Chartered Institute of Management Accountants (CIMA) official terminology, internal audit is the:

> 'independent appraisal activity established within an organisation as a service to it. It is a control which functions by examining and evaluating the adequacy and effectiveness of other controls'.

Internal audit is intended to provide independent assurance that an organisation's risk management, governance and internal control processes are operating effectively. The work done by any internal audit unit is not prescribed by regulation, but is decided by management or by the board (or audit committee). The possible tasks of internal audit include the following:

- **Reviewing the internal control system:** traditionally, an internal audit department has carried out independent checks on the financial controls in an organisation; however, this has now extended to include quality and performance controls as well. The checks would be to establish whether suitable quality, performance and financial controls exist and if so, whether they are applied properly and are effective. It is not the function of internal auditors to manage risks, only to monitor and report them, and to check that risk controls are efficient and cost-effective.

- **Special investigations:** internal auditors might conduct special investigations into particular aspects of the organisation's operations (systems and procedures), to check the effectiveness of operational controls.
- **Examination of financial and operating information:** internal auditors might be asked to investigate the timeliness of reporting and the accuracy of the information in reports.
- **VFM audits:** this is an investigation into an operation or activity to establish whether it is economical, efficient and effective.
- **Reviewing compliance by the organisation with particular laws or regulations:** this is an investigation into the effectiveness of compliance controls.
- **Risk assessment:** internal auditors might be asked to investigate aspects of risk management, and in particular the adequacy of the mechanisms for identifying, assessing and controlling significant risks to the organisation, from both internal and external sources.

Function and scope of internal audit

Unlike external auditors, internal auditors look beyond financial risks and statements to consider wider issues such as the organisation's reputation, growth, its impact on the environment and the way it treats its employees.

An organisation might have an internal audit unit or section, which carries out investigative work. An internal audit function should act independently of ED managers, but normally reports to an ED such as the finance director. The NHS Accounting Officer Memorandum requires all NHS trusts to have an internal audit function. The NHS Internal Audit Standards (or Government Internal Audit standards for FTs) set out the requirements for internal audit and how to assess the service that is delivered. The FT Code requires the FT audit committee to monitor and review the effectiveness of the FT's internal audit function.

In the corporate sector, the FRC Guidance on Audit Committees (FRC Audit Guide) suggests that the audit committee should ensure that the internal auditor has direct access to the board chair and the audit committee, and is responsible to the audit committee. This means that the internal auditors maybe in an unusual position within the organisation. For operational reasons they may have a line reporting responsibility to an ED such as the finance director. EDs may also ask the internal auditors to carry out audits or reviews of the systems or procedures (and internal controls) for which they are responsible. However, the senior internal auditor should have some control over deciding what aspects of the organisation's systems should be investigated or audited, and has a responsibility for reporting to the audit committee and the chair of the board.

Investigation of internal financial controls
Internal auditors are commonly required to check the soundness of internal financial controls. In assessing the effectiveness of individual controls, and of an internal control system generally, the following factors should be considered.

- Whether the controls are manual or automated: automated controls are by no means error- proof or fraud- proof, but may be more reliable than similar manual controls.
- Whether controls are discretionary or non-discretionary: non-discretionary controls are checks and procedures that must be carried out. Discretionary controls are those that do not have to be applied, either because they are voluntary or because an individual can choose to dis-apply them. Risks can infiltrate a system, for example, when senior management chooses to dis-apply controls and allow unauthorised or unchecked procedures to occur.
- Whether the control can be circumvented easily: an activity can be carried out in a different way where similar controls do not apply.
- Whether the controls are effective in achieving their purpose: are they extensive enough or carried out frequently enough? Are the controls applied rigorously? For example, is a supervisor doing their job properly?

Reports by internal auditors can provide reassurance that internal controls are sound and effective or might recommend changes and improvements where weaknesses are uncovered.

The objectivity and independence of internal auditors
The manager of a directorate or department should monitor the internal controls within the operation and try to identify and correct weaknesses. However, a line manager cannot be properly objective, because they could face 'blame' for control failures in the system or operation for which they are responsible.

In contrast, internal auditors ought to be objective, because they investigate the control systems of other directorates and departments. However, they are also employees within the organisation and report to someone on the organisation structure. If the internal auditors report to the finance director, they will find it difficult to be critical of the finance director. Similarly, if the internal auditors report to the CEO, they will be reluctant to criticise the CEO. In this respect, their independence could be compromised.

In its Guidance for Audit Committees, the Institute of Chartered Accountants in England and Wales (ICAEW) comments that the internal auditors should be separate and independent from line management, but that 'independence' for internal auditors does not have the same meaning as independence for external auditors. To protect the independence of the internal audit function, the FRC's

Guidance on Audit Committees suggests that the audit committee should have the responsibility for the appointment of the head of internal audit, and the head's removal from office.

Review of the effectiveness of the internal audit function

The board or audit committee should review the effectiveness of the internal audit function each year. As part of this review, the 2014 HFMA NHS Audit Committee Handbook (HFMA Handbook) suggests that the audit committee should make sure that the head of internal audit has direct access to the chair of the board and the audit committee and is accountable to the audit committee.

There should also be a review and assessment of the annual internal audit work plan along with regular reports on the results of work done by the internal auditors. The review should consider and monitor the responses of management to the recommendations made to them by the internal auditors. The audit committee should also meet with the head of internal audit at least once a year without EDs being present. The HFMA Handbook states that the audit committee should actively review the plans of both internal and external audit and assess the quality of the services that are provided.

The role of external audit

External audit traditionally has been the process by which the annual accounts of public and private sector bodies are subject to external scrutiny to provide independent assurance that they have been prepared in accordance with relevant legal and professional standards and give a 'true and fair' view of the financial performance and financial position of the audited body. More recently, however, external audit has comprised a wider brief including quality and performance audits as well. According to the Public Audit Forum:

> 'It is one of the basic principles of audit in the public sector, that the scope of the audit should be understood to go beyond giving assurance on the accounts, to include examination of aspects of corporate governance and the use of resources.'

External audit in the public sector is characterised by three distinct features:

- Auditors are appointed independently from the bodies being audited.
- The scope of auditors' work is extended to cover not only the financial statements, but also aspects of corporate governance and arrangements to secure the economic, efficient and effective use of resources.
- Auditors may report aspects of their work to the public and other key stakeholders.

Function and scope of external audit

The statutory responsibilities and powers of appointed auditors for public bodies including NHS organisations are set out in the Local Audit and Accountability Act 2014. In discharging these specific statutory responsibilities and powers, auditors will be required to carry out their work according to the NAO's Code of Audit Practice. Auditors are required to have regard to this guidance under the Act.

Schedule 7 to the National Health Act 2006 (NHS Act 2006) provides the Comptroller and Auditor General (C&AG) with access rights to FTs that allow National Audit Office (NAO) representatives to inspect the accounts and any records relating to them, including the auditor's report. Although the C&AG is not the appointed auditor of individual FTs, NAO may wish to examine financial aspects of one or more FTs in the context of its wider role in providing assurance to Parliament over the proper use of public monies.

After completing their annual audit, auditors are required to prepare a report to the stakeholders of the organisation, which is included in the published report and accounts. The audit report has two main purposes:

- to give an expert and independent opinion on whether the financial statements give a true and fair view of the financial position of the organisation as at the end of the financial year covered by the report, and of its financial performance during the year; and
- to give an expert and independent opinion on whether the financial statements comply with the relevant laws.

However, in carrying out their audit, external audit must also pay attention to aspects of the organisation's corporate governance and it's securing of economy, efficiency and effectiveness in the use of resources.

Auditors must be appointed by 31 December of the year prior to the relevant financial year. Any public body that fails to do so must notify the SoS, who will have reserve powers to make, or direct the body to make, an appointment.

Reliance on the work of internal audit

It is expected that the external auditors will liaise with the internal audit function to obtain a sufficient understanding of internal audit activities to assist in planning the audit and developing an effective audit approach. The auditors may also wish to place reliance upon certain aspects of the work of internal audit in satisfying their statutory responsibilities as set out in the NHS Act 2006 and in the NAO Audit Code. In particular, the auditors may wish to consider the work of internal audit when undertaking their procedures in relation to the annual governance statement (AGS).

This demonstrates the key relationship between internal and external audit as it is vital for the external auditors to be able to rely on the work undertaken by internal audit, not just on financial controls but on quality and performance controls as well.

Audit report

The audit report is contained in the organisation's annual report and accounts and is addressed by the auditors to the stakeholders of the organisation. The main purpose of the audit report is to give the users of an organisation's financial statements (and in particular the stakeholders) some assurance that the information in the statements is believable and that the financial statements present a 'true and fair view' of the organisation's financial position and performance. The opinion of the auditors should be the opinion of independent professional experts, based on an investigation of the organisation's control systems, accounting systems and financial/business transactions. The audit report itself provides only limited information to stakeholders, even though stakeholders often assume that an unqualified audit report means that the financial statements of the organisation are accurate and reliable.

An unmodified audit report (sometimes called an 'unqualified opinion') is given when the auditor believes that the accounts give a true and fair view of the organisation's financial position and performance. The wording of an unmodified audit report is usually fairly standard, although reports are longer for public companies (where the auditors might also report on some corporate governance statements) and differ between countries. Such a report may include an 'emphasis of matter' paragraph where, although the audit report is unmodified (i.e. the auditors consider that the financial statements present a true and fair view), there is an item that the auditor wants to bring to the attention of users because it is of some importance for an understanding of the statements (e.g. as specified for NHS organisations, who have to disclose issues with regard to their going concern statement).

Alternately, external auditors may present a modified audit report, although this is unusual. If it happens, there is a potentially serious problem with the financial statements and, by implication, the financial condition of the organisation. It also means that the auditors have been unable to agree with the directors of the organisation about what information the financial statements should contain. There are three types of modified audit opinion, namely, a qualified opinion, an adverse opinion, and a disclaimer of opinion.

A qualified audit opinion is sometimes called an 'except for' opinion. It is given when, in the opinion of the auditor, the financial statements would give a true and fair view except for a particular matter, which the auditor explains.

An adverse opinion is given when the auditor considers that there are material misstatements in the accounts and that these are 'pervasive'. In effect, the auditor is stating that the figures in the accounts are seriously wrong.

A disclaimer of opinion is given in cases where the auditor has been unable to obtain the information that they need to give an audit opinion. The lack of information means that the auditor is unable to state that the financial statements give a true and fair view, and that there may possibly be serious misstatements that the auditor has been unable to check.

Responsibility for detecting errors and fraud

Stakeholders would probably like to assume that if the auditors provide a favourable audit report, the financial statements must be 'correct', and there has not been any fraud or error that has resulted in incorrect use of accounting policies, omissions of fact or misinterpretation of fact. This view is based on the belief that if professional accountants have checked the figures, they must be correct – unless the accountants have been negligent and have failed to do their job properly.

This is not the case. The board of directors is responsible for preventing fraud in their organisation or detecting fraud if it occurs. The organisation's system of internal control, described in Chapter 18, should be designed to limit the risk of fraud and error, and the board is responsible for monitoring the effectiveness of the internal control system. The responsibility of the board (with delegated responsibility of management) for the prevention and detection of fraud and error is a core principle of corporate governance. The directors are fully accountable to the stakeholders and so are fully responsible for the information presented in the annual report and accounts.

It is not the primary responsibility of the external auditors to detect fraud. The auditors will assess the risk or possibility that fraud or error might have caused the financial statements to be materially misleading. The external audit might act as a deterrent to fraud, because the auditors will carry out checks of control procedures, documents and transactions in the course of their audit work. They might discover fraud during the course of their audit work, in which case it would be their responsibility to report the matter to the directors (unless the fraud is carried out by the directors themselves).

An area for dispute, however, is whether the auditors ought to be able to identify fraud or a significant error during the course of their audit work, whenever a fraud or error occurs. Although they are not responsible for the financial statements, it can be argued that a failure by the auditors to discover a major fraud or material error might be the result of professional negligence. If they are negligent, they should be held liable to the organisation and its stakeholders. In the UK, the CA 2006 introduced new rules on auditors' liability for negligence, breach of duty or breach of trust regarding the conduct of the audit.

Shareholders of both public and private companies can vote by ordinary resolution to limit the liability to the company by the auditor in respect of negligence, default, breach of duty or breach of trust occurring in the course of the audit of accounts. The Act states that in considering what is fair and reasonable in the circumstances, the court should have no regard to the possibility or otherwise of recovering compensation from other persons who are jointly or partly responsible for the loss that has been incurred. The CA 2006 Act also introduced two new criminal offences for auditors in connection with the auditors' report: it is a criminal offence, punishable by a fine, to knowingly or recklessly cause an audit report to 'include any matter that is misleading, false or deceptive in any material particular', or knowingly or recklessly cause an audit report to omit a statement that is required by certain specified sections of the Act.

Auditors' liability to third parties

The auditors have a legal duty of care to the organisation and its stakeholders. There is some doubt as to whether they might also have a duty of care to other parties. In the UK, the extent of auditor liability to external parties has been tested in two legal cases: *Caparo Industries plc* v *Dickman* [1990] and *Royal Bank of Scotland* v *Bannerman Johnstone Maclay* [2002]. The latter case, crucially, concluded that the absence of any disclaimer of liability to third parties was a significant contributing factor to the duty of care owed to them. In response to this, auditors have since included a disclaimer of liability to third parties using its audit reports.

No firm decision has yet been reached in the UK as to how to protect auditors from the entire burden of liability where others (e.g. directors, may also to be to blame). The consequence of which is a limited competitive market for audit services that is dominated by the 'Big Four' (Deloitte, PwC, Ernst & Young, KPMG). There are an increasing number of advocates for a 'proportional' system of liability replacing the current 'joint and several' one. Under this proposal, the audit firm would accept their proportion of the blame in a negligence case and would pay that proportion of the compensation. This system, as introduced in Australia in 2004, would ensure a fair outcome for the plaintiff without placing the entire financial burden upon the audit profession.

The Local Audit and Accountability Act 2014 requires that any agreements to limit the liability owed to an NHS organisation by the auditor in respect of negligence, default, breach of duty or breach of trust must comply with regulations made by the SoS. These state that:

- a restriction on the duration of an agreement: it cannot cover more than the financial year or years to which the appointment of the external auditor relates; and
- an agreement for limiting the external auditor's liability cannot be less than such amount as is fair and reasonable given the circumstances.

Independence of external audit

The external auditor should be independent of the client organisation so that the audit opinion will not be influenced by the relationship between the auditor and the organisation. The auditors are expected to give an unbiased and honest professional opinion to the stakeholders about the financial statements.

It could be argued that unless suitable governance measures are in place, a firm of auditors may reach audit opinions and judgements that are heavily influenced by their wish to maintain good relations with the management of a client organisation. If this happens, the auditors are no longer independent, and the stakeholders cannot rely on their opinion. For example, in the corporate sector, an official 2010 report on the collapse of Lehman Brothers in 2008 criticised the external auditors Ernst & Young for allowing the company to account for certain transactions in a way that misleadingly improved the look of the end-of-quarter balance sheets during 2007 and 2008, in the months before the bank eventually collapsed.

The audit profession has identified five categories of potential threats to auditor independence.

- **Self-interest threat:** if the audit firm earns a large proportion of its revenue from a client organisation, it may be unwilling to annoy that client by challenging the figures and assumptions used by management to prepare the organisation's financial statements.
- **Self-review threat:** this can arise when the audit firm does non-audit work for the organisation, and the annual audit involves checking the work done by the firm's own employees. The auditors may not be as critical of the work, or prepared to challenge it, because this would raise questions about the professional competence of the audit firm.
- **Advocacy threat:** this can arise if the audit form is asked to give its formal support to the organisation by providing public statements on particular issues or supporting the organisation in a legal case. Acting as advocate for an organisation means taking sides; this implies a loss of independence.
- **Familiarity threat:** a threat to independence occurs when an auditor is familiar with an organisation or one of its directors or senior managers, or becomes familiar with them through a working association over time. Familiarity leads to trust and a willingness to believe what the other person says. The auditor will also be unwilling to think that the other person is capable of making a serious error or committing fraud. A familiarity threat arises through personal association (e.g. family connections) and through long association with the organisation and its management.
- **Intimidation threat:** an auditor may feel threatened by the directors or senior management of an organisation. Both real and imagined threats can affect the auditor's independence. Intimidation may result from a domineering and bullying personality on the organisation's board of directors (e.g. the CEO). An organisation may also threaten to take away the audit or stop giving the firm non-audit work unless the auditor accepts the opinions of management.

Threats to auditor independence must be identified, and measures should be taken to limit the threat to an acceptable level of risk. Two areas of debate about how to ensure auditor independence have been whether auditors should be prevented from carrying out non-audit work for clients or whether the amount of non-audit work they do should be restricted, and whether there should be a regular rotation of either the audit firm or the audit partner and other senior members of the audit team.

Non-audit work for a client by an audit firm

The codes of conduct of national professional accountancy bodies lack any clear restrictions on the performance of non-audit work for an audit client. Suggestions for regulatory measures to ensure auditor independence have included proposals to restrict the amount of non-audit work, or the type of non-audit work, that the firm of auditors is permitted to carry out for a client organisation. Non-audit work might include:

- consultancy on taxation issues (helping an organisation to minimise tax liabilities);
- investigating targets for a potential takeover bid;
- helping an organisation to construct a bid for a major government contract;
- providing advice and expert assistance on IT systems;
- internal audit services;
- valuation and actuarial services;
- services relating to litigation; and
- services relating to recruitment and remuneration.

The main problem with auditors doing non-audit work is that when the firm audits transactions recommended by its consultancy arm, it is unlikely to take an independent view.

The risk to auditor objectivity and independence from carrying out non-audit work became apparent in the wake of the Enron collapse. Arthur Andersen were the auditors of Enron, and in the financial year before the company's collapse in 2001, Andersen earned more fee income from Enron for non-audit work than from audit work. The audit firm was suspected of failing to carry out a proper audit of the company. It was claimed that the audit firm would have been reluctant to question the accounts of Enron because it would risk losing not just the audit work but also the substantial non-audit fee income. In addition, it was suggested that since the information in the company's financial statements reflected the non-audit consultancy advice given by the audit firm, the firm's auditors would be unlikely to challenge the fairness and accuracy of the statements. In other words, Andersen's auditors would not challenge the opinions of Andersen's consultants.

Audit firms have denied that fees from non-audit work will affect their independence, arguing that the individuals who work as consultants for a client organisation (such as on IT projects) are not the same individuals who work on the audit. Even so, activist shareholder groups continue to challenge this assertion. There are three broad approaches to the regulation of non-audit work by audit firms:

- There should be no restrictions at all on non-audit work by the audit firm.
- There should be a total prohibition on non-audit work for a corporate client by the audit firm.
- There should be a partial prohibition on non-audit work for a corporate client by the audit firm.

A partial restriction could take either of two forms. There could be a prohibition on audit firms from taking on certain types of consultancy work where their independence as auditors could be put at risk, such as tax planning advice work. However, audit firms would be free to carry out other types of non-audit work. The second approach to restricting non-audit work would be to set a limit on the amount of fees an audit firm could earn from non-audit work, expressed perhaps as a proportion of the fees it earns from the audit. For example, a limit might be imposed restricting non-audit fees to, say, 50% of the fees from the audit work.

The difficulty with a partial restriction on non-audit work is that rules have to be devised and agreed as to what permissible and non-permissible non-audit work should be, or what the maximum amount of non-audit fee income should be. In the UK, the audit profession is governed by ethical principles rather than rules and regulations about non-audit work for audit clients. The ICAEW has made the following statements about non-audit work:

> 'The most effective way to ensure the reality of independence is to provide guidance centred around a framework of principles rather than a detailed set of rules that can be complied with to the letter but circumvented in substance.'

> 'A blanket prohibition on the provision of non-audit services to audit clients can be inefficient for the client and is neither necessary to ensure independence, nor helpful in contributing to the knowledge necessary to ensure the quality of the audit.'

The need for auditor independence when the audit firm does non-audit work is recognised in the UK Code. The code includes a provision that 'the annual report should explain to stakeholders how, if the auditor provides non-audit services, auditor objectivity and independence is safeguarded'.

Rotation of audit firm

Another suggestion for protecting auditor independence is that there should be 'rotation' of auditors. There is an important distinction, however, between the rotation of an audit firm, whereby a firm is required to give up the audit for an organisation after a maximum number of years, and the organisation must appoint different auditors, and rotation of audit personnel, whereby the audit engagement partner and other key individuals involved in the annual audit should be removed from the audit after a certain number of years, and new individuals assigned to the work..

Rotation of the audit firm would enhance auditor independence because a firm of auditors would have little to gain by agreeing with the wishes of the client organisation, and carrying out a less than rigorous audit, if it knows that it will soon lose the audit work anyway. The work of outgoing auditors would also be subject to review – and criticism – by the firm of auditors taking their place.

In 2019, the Competition and Markets Authority issued its final summary report on the statutory audit services market. The report made four recommendations to the Government to address concerns raised by cases such as Carillion or BHS and inherent deep-seated problems such as companies selecting their own auditors and a high concentration of statutory services provided by four big audit firms, resulting in limited choice and a market that is not resilient. The four recommendations are:-

1. Robust regulatory oversight of the committees that run the selection process for audited companies, and oversee the audit, to make them more accountable and ensure that they prioritise quality.
2. Mandatory joint audit, to increase the capacity of challenger firms, to increase choice in the market and thereby drive up audit quality. There should be initial limited exceptions to the requirement, based on criteria set by the regulator – mainly the largest and most complex companies. Any company choosing a sole challenger auditor should also be exempt. Audits of exempt companies may be subject to rigorous, real- time peer reviews commissioned by and reporting to the regulator.
3. An operational split between the Big Four's audit and non-audit businesses, to ensure maximum focus on audit quality.
4. A five-year review of progress by the regulator.

Interestingly, the report comments that the links between owners and managers of companies are distant, and ownership is diffuse, which makes it difficult for owners (i.e ultimately ordinary savers or pension-holders) to monitor and affect the performance of companies that they own. This is a very live and practical example of the issues of governance set out in the early chapters of this Handbook. The lack of choice between the four main big firms is a considerable factor on the ability to rotate audit firms as the choice of audit firm can be limited to as few as two or even on of these four, e.g. current auditor may be excluded due to the length of current service, another may be excluded due to the limit of the non-audit work that can be delivered.

The Independent Review by Sir Donald Brydon (April 2019) is looking to examine the existing purpose, scope and quality of statutory audit in the UK and on the extent of assurance that statutory audit in the UK currently provides to the users of financial statements, and how it might develop to meet better those users' needs to serve the interests of other stakeholders and the wider public interest. The review is will close in June 2019.

On 1 January 2015, the Statutory Audit Services for Large Companies Market Investigation (Mandatory Use of Competitive Tender Processes and Audit Committee Responsibilities) Order 2014 came into force for FTSE 350 companies. According to the Order, all such companies must put their statutory audit services engagement out to tender every ten years or earlier. This means that an auditor may not conduct more than ten consecutive statutory audits of a FTSE 350 company without a competitive tender process having taken place. In addition, it required that the terms of the statutory audit services agreement must have been negotiated and agreed between the audit committee and the auditor.

The principles of retendering are explored in *the FRC Audit Tenders: Notes on good practice* (February 2017), which adds that, apart from the regulatory requirement, feedback from companies that have changed auditors since the change in requirements indicates that there are benefits to be gained from fresh insight. Even if the incumbent firm is reappointed, experience suggests that the tender process itself can reinvigorate the audit approach.

The UK has not designated NHS organisations as public interest entities despite their significant public relevance, and so these regulations are not directly applicable to the NHS. Nevertheless, the recommendations for tenders demonstrate best practice. The FT guidance *Governance over Audit, Assurance and Accountability: Guidance for Foundation Trusts* (March 2015) also sets out good practice for maintaining independence of audit services. It recommends a three to five-year period of appointment and a market-testing exercise for the appointment of an auditor at least once every five years. The external audit should be subject to a tender process at least every ten years, and in most cases more frequently than this.

The *Local Procurement of External Auditors for NHS Trusts and CCGs* (March 2016) guidance states that the contract length can be anything from one to five years, with three to five years being 'normal' and considered an appropriate period for an auditor to develop a strong understanding of the organisation. Contracts can be awarded with an optional extension period, such as three years with an optional two-year extension. Whatever length of contract is chosen, it must be agreed at an early stage. It makes no stipulation as to retendering.

Audit partner rotation

An argument put forward by the major accountancy firms is that the requirement for rotation should apply, not to the firm of auditors, but to the individual partner of a firm in charge of the audit. For example, it might be acceptable for ABC Corporation to retain the services of Ernst & Young indefinitely, provided that the partner in charge of the audit is replaced every, say, five or seven years. Supporters of this argument claim that the independence of the audit is threatened by the personal relationship an audit partner builds up with the client organisation, not the length of association of the audit firm with the organisation.

A counter-argument, however, is that audit partner rotation would not have prevented the problem that arose between Andersen and its clients Enron and WorldCom. Although Andersen as a whole was not over-dependent on Enron, the company was a vital client for the firm's Houston office, which carried out the audit. Similarly, the Andersen office in Jackson, Mississippi was heavily dependent on the work that it did for WorldCom. To prevent loss of audit independence, audit partner rotation would almost certainly have been ineffective, whereas audit firm rotation might have been much more effective.

Currently, regulations in most countries favour audit partner rotation rather than audit firm rotation. In the UK, for example, the ICAEW's ethical standards require the rotation of various members of an audit team, including the rotation of the audit engagement partner at least every five years.

The audit committee

The UK Code requires that a board of directors should establish formal and transparent arrangements for considering how they should apply the corporate reporting and risk management and internal control principles, and maintaining an appropriate relationship with the organisation's auditors. These arrangements should be met by establishing an audit committee, which should be given certain responsibilities by the board. This does not detract from the unitary board principle and despite of the work of the audit committee, the board remains responsible for making the final decision.

The FRC Audit Guide has introduced the following requirements:

- The audit committee should consider key matters of its own initiative rather than relying solely on the work of the external auditor. It must satisfy itself that the sources of assurance and information it has used to carry out its roles to review, monitor and provide assurance or recommendations to the board are sufficient and objective.
- The board has ultimate responsibility for an organisation's risk management and internal control systems, but the board may delegate to the audit committee some functions to assist the board in meeting this responsibility.
- The need for an internal audit function should be regularly reviewed by the audit committee and where such a function is required then the audit committee should review and approve its role and mandate; approve the annual internal audit plan (which must be aligned to the risks of the organisation); and monitor and review the effectiveness of its work. The audit committee should review and approve annually the internal audit charter to ensure that it is appropriate to the current needs of the organisation.
- The audit committee should ensure that the internal auditor has a reporting line that enables it to be independent of the executive team and so be able to exercise independent judgement. The audit committee should ensure that the internal audit function has unrestricted scope and evaluates the effectiveness of the risk, compliance and finance functions as part of its internal audit plan. The audit committee may also wish to consider whether an independent, third party review of internal audit effectiveness and processes is appropriate.
- The audit committee should have primary responsibility for negotiating the fee and scope of the external audit, initiating a tender process, influencing the appointment of an engagement partner and making formal recommendations to the board on the appointment, reappointment and removal of the auditors (reflecting the CMA Order).
- More emphasis is placed on interactions with the external auditor around the areas of significant judgement and risks to audit quality.

- Set and apply a formal policy specifying the types of non-audit service for which use of the external auditor is pre-approved. The guidance reaffirms that such approval should only be in place for matters that are clearly trivial.
- The audit committee has a role in ensuring that shareholder interests are properly protected in relation to financial reporting and internal control. The committee should consider the clarity of its reporting and be prepared to meet investors.
- Remuneration should reflect the responsibility members bear and that a significant extra amount of time needs to be committed.

Reporting requirements for audit committees have also been updated to include:

- how the audit committee composition requirements have been addressed;
- how the performance evaluation of the audit committee has been conducted;
- the current external audit partner's name and for how long the partner has held the role;
- advance notice of any plans for retendering the external audit;
- the committee's policy for approval of non-audit services;
- the audit fees for the statutory audit of the company's consolidated financial statements and the fees paid to the auditor and its network firms for audit related services and other non-audit services, including the ratio of audit to non-audit work;
- for each significant engagement, or category of engagements, an explanation of the services provided and why the audit committee concluded that it was in the interests of the company to purchase them from the external auditor;
- explanations of how the committee has assessed the effectiveness of internal audit and satisfied itself that the quality, experience and expertise of the function is appropriate for the business;
- the nature and extent of interaction (if any) with the FRC's Corporate Reporting Review team; and
- that the FRC's Audit Quality Review team has reviewed a company's audit, disclosures about significant findings and the resulting actions they and the auditors plan to take. This disclosure should not include the audit quality category awarded.

Whilst these changes are not directly applicable within the NHS, they provide a benchmark of good practice and NHS audit committees must consider how the new requirements affect their own practice. There is a formal requirement, however, for every NHS board to establish an audit committee. The primary guidance for NHS Audit Committees is contained in the HFMA Handbook (2018) which is aligned to the UK Code and the FRC Audit Guide. The HFMA Handbook (2018) also includes considerations for the audit committee in relation to governance between organisations and in particular STPs, accountable care systems and accountable care organisations. The role of the audit committee in applying the principles of risk management and internal controls is described in Chapter 18; this chapter concentrates on the role of the audit committee is applying corporate reporting principles and maintaining an appropriate relationship with the external auditors.

Role and responsibilities of the audit committee

The UK Code describes the main roles and responsibilities of the audit committee as:

- monitoring the integrity of the financial statements of the company and any formal announcements relating to the company's financial performance;
- providing advice (where requested by the board) on whether the annual report and accounts, taken as a whole, is fair, balanced and understandable;
- reviewing the company's internal financial controls and internal control and risk management systems;
- monitoring and reviewing the effectiveness of the company's internal audit function or, where there is not one, considering annually whether there is a need for one and making a recommendation to the board;
- conducting the tender process and making recommendations to the board, about the appointment, reappointment, removal and remuneration of the external auditor;
- reviewing and monitoring the external auditor's independence and objectivity;
- reviewing the effectiveness of the external audit process;
- developing and implementing policy on the engagement of the external auditor to supply non-audit services; and
- reporting to the board on how it has discharged its responsibilities.

In the NHS, the two key areas that the audit committee should also provide assurance to the board on are the BAF and documents that are to be publicly disclosed (the AGS, registration evidence for the CQC, and the Quality Accounts).

In NHS organisations, there is usually an overlap between the work of the audit committee and the quality committee. Clarity on how these areas will be addressed by the two committees is vital to ensure that duplication of work is avoided and no gaps of assurance arise.

The board should decide just what the role of the audit committee should be, and the terms of reference should be tailored to the organisation's particular circumstances. A separate section of the annual report should describe the work of the committee. The audit committee should review its terms of reference and effectiveness annually and recommend any necessary changes to the board. The board should also review the effectiveness of the audit committee annually.

Composition of the audit committee

The specific requirements in respect of composition are set out in Chapter 7. However, the distinctive characteristic of the audit committee is that it comprises only NEDs.

The FRC Audit Guide suggests that appointments to the committee should be made by the board on the recommendation of the nomination committee, in consultation with the audit committee chair. Appointments should be made for a period of up to three years, extendable by no more than two additional three-year periods and so long as the director remains independent.

The UK Code states that a separate section of the company's annual report should describe the work of the audit committee. Similar recommendations are contained in the DHSC's model standing orders for NHS trusts and in the FT Code.

The organisation's management is under an obligation to make sure that the audit committee is kept properly informed and should take the initiative in providing the committee with information instead of waiting to be asked. The EDs should also have regard to their common law duty to provide all directors, including the audit committee members, with all the information they need to discharge their duties as directors of the organisation. This point is crucial: the audit committee can only do its work properly if it is kept properly informed by the EDs.

Remuneration, induction and training of committee members

Because audit committees carry out wide-ranging and time-consuming work, organisations must make the necessary resources available. This includes making suitable payments to the members of the audit committee in view of the responsibilities they have and the time they must commit to the work. The committee chair's responsibilities and time commitments will normally be greater than those of the other committee members, and this should be reflected in their remuneration.

The committee should have the support of the company secretary and should have access to the services of the organisation's secretariat. Audit committee members must also be given suitable induction and training. Ongoing training should include keeping the committee members up to date on developments in quality, performance and financial reporting and related NHS guidance or legislation.

Induction and training can take various forms, including attendance at formal courses and conferences, internal organisation talks and seminars and briefings by external advisers.

Audit committee meetings

The audit committee chair should decide the timing and frequency of committee meetings, in consultation with the company secretary. There should be as many meetings as the role and responsibilities of the committee require. The FRC Audit Guide suggests that there should be no fewer than three committee meetings each year, timed to coincide with key dates in the financial reporting and audit calendar. For example, meetings might be held when the audit plans are available for review and when interim statements, preliminary announcements and the full annual report are near completion. Most audit committee chairs will probably want to call meetings more frequently. In practice, most NHS audit committees meet quarterly, if not bi-monthly, to manage the significant workload carried by the committee. This is reflected in the HFMA Handbook.

Only the audit committee chair and members are entitled to attend meetings of the committee. It is for the committee to decide whether other individuals should be invited to attend for a particular meeting or a particular agenda item. It is expected that the external and internal audit lead partners and the organisation's finance director will be invited regularly to attend meetings.

The HFMA Handbook (2018) recommends that 'private discussion between audit committee members and each of the sets of the auditors and counter fraud specialists – without management present, is an important part of building a relationship of trust and supporting the independence of the audit functions These discussions should be formally scheduled and will generally take place before at one meeting per year.' Such meetings, which are not formally minuted unless a record is necessary, allow committee members and auditors freedom to discuss a wide range of issue without management influence and for the auditors to feedback to the committee on their own performance and the quality of the engagement of executive directors with the audit function. The Handbook recommends possible questions that this meeting might address.

The audit committee's role in quality, performance and financial reporting

It is the responsibility of management, not the audit committee, to prepare and complete accurate quality, performance and financial statements. It is the responsibility of the audit committee to review the significant reporting issues and judgements that are made in connection with these statements. Management should inform the committee about the methods they have used to account for significant or unusual transactions, particularly where the accounting treatment is open to different approaches. Taking the external auditors' views into consideration, the committee should consider whether the organisation has adopted appropriate accounting policies and made appropriate estimates and judgements.

The HFMA Handbook (2018) recommends that 'the role of the audit committee is to oversee, be aware of and ensure action plans relating to regulatory requirements are monitored and delivered.' The Handbook also lists the following areas that the audit committee would want to identify and consider appropriate assurances for as appropriate:

- STP dashboards (published annually)
- CCG IAF
- SOF
- CQC – use of resources assessment

If the committee is not satisfied with any aspect of the proposed reporting by the organisation, it should report its views to the board. The committee should also review related information presented with the quality, performance and financial statements, including the business review and the corporate governance statements relating to audit and risk management.

Appointment and removal of external auditors

Under the UK Code, the audit committee has the primary responsibility for making a recommendation to the board on the appointment, reappointment or removal of the external auditors. FRC Risk Guide recommends that the audit committee should 'oversee' the selection process if it recommends to the board that new external auditors should be selected. The committee's recommendation should be based on the qualification and expertise of the auditors, the resources of the auditors and the independence of the auditors.

Under the FRC Audit Guide, if the audit committee recommends that new external auditors should be selected, the committee should 'oversee' the selection process and its recommendation should be based on the qualification and expertise of the auditors, the resources of the auditors, the independence of the auditors and the effectiveness of the audit process. The assessment should cover all aspects of the audit service provided by the audit firm. In carrying out the assessment, the committee should obtain from the audit firm a report on its own internal quality control procedures. If the external auditors resign, the audit committee should investigate the issues that led to the resignation and consider whether any action is needed.

The audit committee should consider the terms of engagement of the external auditors and the remuneration to be paid to the auditors for their audit services. It should satisfy itself that the fee payable for the audit services is appropriate, and that an effective audit can be carried out for such a fee. The audit committee should then make a recommendation to the board of directors (or council of governors in the case of FTs). The committee is not required to negotiate terms and remuneration. The FRC Audit Guide also recommends that the committee should review and agree the engagement letter issued by the external auditors at the start of each audit, to make sure that it has been updated to reflect any changes in circumstances since the previous year. In addition, the committee should review the scope of the audit with the auditor. If it is not satisfied that the proposed scope is adequate, the committee should arrange for additional audit work to be undertaken.

For NHS trusts and CCGs, auditors have been appointed by the auditor panel under the Local Audit (Health Service Bodies Auditor Panel and Independence) Regulations 2015 and the selection/procurement process is set out in the *Local Procurement of External Auditors for NHS Trusts and CCGs* (March 2016) guidance.

Audit committee responsibilities and auditor independence

The Local Audit (Health Service Bodies Auditor Panel and Independence) Regulations 2015 and resulting NAO Code of Practice gives the audit committee the responsibility for monitoring and ensuring the independence of the external auditors. If the external auditors provide non-audit services to the organisation, the annual report should explain how auditor independence and objectivity are safeguarded. The audit committee should have procedures for ensuring the independence and objectivity of the external auditors annually.

The audit committee should also ensure that the provision of non-audit services by the organisation's audit firm will not impair the objectivity and independence of the auditors. It can do this by setting a formal policy specifying the types of non-audit work from which the external auditors are excluded and for which the external auditors can be engaged without referral to the audit committee. It should be established on a case-by-case basis and in these cases, it may be appropriate to give a general pre-approval for certain classes of work, subject to a fee limit decided by the audit committee and ratified by the board. If the external auditor subsequently provides any of these services, the engagement of the auditors should then be ratified at the next audit committee meeting. The policy may also set fee limits generally or for particular classes of non-audit work.

The FT Code states that, if the external auditors do provide non-financial services, the FT's annual report should explain to stakeholders how auditor independence and objectivity is safeguarded.

The audit committee and the annual audit cycle

The FRC Audit Guide goes into some detail on the annual audit cycle, and the relationship between the audit committee and the external auditors during this process. At the start of each annual audit, the audit committee should ensure that appropriate plans are in place for the audit. The committee should consider whether the auditors' overall work plan (including the planned levels of materiality and the proposed resources to carry out the audit) seems consistent with the scope of the audit engagement. This assessment should have regard to the seniority, expertise and experience of the audit team.

The audit committee should review, with the external auditors, the findings of their work. As a part of this review, the committee should:

- discuss with the auditors any major issues that arose during the audit (and whether these have been resolved);
- review key accounting or audit judgements; and
- review levels of errors identified during the audit and obtain explanations as to why certain errors might remain unadjusted.

Representation letters from the organisation's management are a part of the audit evidence collected and considered by the auditors. They contain information from management to the auditors. These deal with matters for which other audit evidence does not exist; therefore, the auditors are relying on what management tell them. Representations are required from the directors, acknowledging their collective responsibility for the financial statements and confirming that they have approved them. These should have regard to matters where knowledge of the facts is confined to management (e.g. management's intention to sell off a division of the business) or where there is a matter of judgement and opinion (for example, with regard to the trading position of a major customer and debtor, or the likely outcome of litigation in progress).

The audit committee should review these representations from management and assess whether (based on the knowledge of the committee members) the information provided seems complete and appropriate. At the end of the audit cycle, the audit committee should assess the effectiveness of the audit process.

Management reports to the audit committee

Management is accountable to the board (or the audit committee) for monitoring the system of internal control and for providing assurances that it has done so. To be effective, monitoring should be on a regular basis, and management should provide regular reports to the audit committee (or the board). These regular reports should each deal with a specific aspect of operations and provide an assessment of the significance of the risks and the effectiveness of the system of internal control for dealing with them. They should also report any significant control weaknesses or failings that have been identified, the impact these have had (or may have) on the organisation and the action that has been taken to deal with the problem.

The board or audit committee may also receive independent reports from the internal auditors. In addition to receiving regular reports from management on internal control, the board (or audit committee) should carry out an annual review of the effectiveness of the internal control system. The annual review should particularly consider:

- the changes that have occurred since the previous annual review – in what ways have the significant risks for the organisation changed, and how successful has the organisation been in responding to those changes;
- the scope and quality of monitoring of the control system by management; and
- the scope and quality of the investigations by the internal audit function, the weaknesses in the system identified by the internal auditors and the measures taken to implement recommendations of the internal auditors.

Raising concerns procedure

The UK Code states that the audit committee should 'review arrangements by which staff of the organisation may, in confidence, raise concerns about possible improprieties in matters of financial reporting or other matters'.

In other words, the audit committee should be responsible for the review of the provisions and procedures for raising concerns within the organisation. The UK Code specifies that the objective of the audit committee should be to ensure that there are satisfactory arrangements in place for the 'proportionate and independent investigation' of allegations, and appropriate follow-up action. The UK Code is referring to the adequacy of what the NHS has understood to be whistleblowing procedures within the organisation. This terminology has now changed and the NHS now refers to raising concerns in line with Code.

Health service governance and raising concerns

There is a strong connection between health service governance and raising concerns. An employee may honestly believe that there is (or has been, or could soon be) serious malpractice by someone within the organisation, but feel unable to report their concerns in the normal way. This could be because the individual to whom they normally report is involved in the suspected malpractice. Serious malpractice or a misdemeanour could be damaging to the organisation, such as:

- it might suffer financial loss if some employees are acting fraudulently;
- it might incur severe penalties as a consequence of employees breaking the law or regulations; or
- there could be damage to the organisation's reputation if the misdemeanour is made public.

The need for raising concerns arises when normal procedures and internal controls will not reveal the illicit activity because the individuals responsible for the activity are somehow able to ignore or 'get around' the normal controls.

However, although raising concerns procedures are an internal control, they are not an embedded control within the organisation's regular procedures. Their effectiveness relies on the willingness of staff to come forward with their allegations. The incidence of illicit or illegal behaviour should be uncommon; therefore, raising concerns should be an occasional event. Extensive inquiries into the baby heart unit at Bristol Royal Infirmary, the behaviour of the GP Dr Harold Shipman, and the concerns at Mid Staffs have raised questions about the protection provided to those, who raise concerns within the health service.

The *Freedom to Speak Up (FTSU): Raising Concerns (Whistleblowing) Policy for the NHS* (2016) creates a national guardian role that is intended to support local FTSU guardians and staff who have raised a concern with their NHS organisation and feel the concern has been poorly handled by their employer or other body. The priorities of the national guardian role includes establishing and supporting a strong network highlighting NHS providers that are successful in creating the right environment for staff to speak up safely and share this best practice across the NHS, and independently reviewing cases where NHS providers may have failed to follow good practice, working with statutory bodies to take action where needed. The policy also requires NHS organisations to have a named ED and NED with responsibility for whistleblowing and is clear that after raising a concern, feedback on the outcome should be provided in an open and transparent way.

The Guidance for boards on Freedom to Speak Up in NHS trusts and NHS foundation trusts (May 2018) set out the requirements in respect of raising concerns. The guidance recognises that having a healthy speaking up culture is an indicator of a well-led trust and is accompanied by a self-review tool. Alongside this guidance, the National Guardians Office has also produced a useful education and training guide to help develop skilled and expert guardians who can offer high calibre support.

Raising concerns: best practice

If an employee has a genuine, honest concern about something happening within the organisation that they believe to be unsafe or improper, there should be a way for the employee's concerns to be brought to the attention of management and dealt with in a constructive way. Having a system for listening to employees' concerns should be a part of an effective risk management system within the organisation, because diligent employees can act as an early warning system of problems.

There are several problems with raising concern procedures and policies. For example, experience in many organisations appears to show that an individual who reports concerns about illegal or unethical conduct is often victimised by colleagues and management. If the allegations are rejected, they might not receive the same salary increases as colleagues or could be overlooked for promotion. The attitude of colleagues and managers might also be hostile, making it difficult for the individual to continue in the job.

However, employees may deliberately make false claims about their colleagues or bosses, out of spite or a desire for revenge for some actual or perceived 'wrong'. It would be inappropriate to provide protection for individuals making malicious and intentionally false allegations. Organisations therefore need to establish a system that encourages employees to report illegal or unethical behaviour but discourages malicious and unfounded allegations.

An organisation might state its policy on raising concerns in the following terms.

- An employee is acting correctly if, in good faith, they seek advice about improper behaviour or reports improper behaviour, where it is not possible to resolve the individual's concerns through discussions with colleagues or line management. Raising concerns is appropriate if the employee does it in good faith and is not being malicious, and there is no other way to resolve the problem.
- The organisation will not tolerate any discrimination by employees or management in the organisation against an individual who has reported in good faith their concerns about illegal or unethical behaviour. This is a policy

statement that those who raise concerns will be protected if they have made their report in good faith.
- Disciplinary action will be taken against any employee who knowingly makes a false report of illegal or improper behaviour by someone else. Malicious reporting should not be tolerated.
- In practice, employees may feel obliged to take their concerns (possibly anonymously) to someone outside the organisation, risking the anger of the employer for breach of proper procedures if he is identified. An employee can be disciplined for making groundless complaints and allegations in bad faith about their employer. However, there is an 'official' raising concerns channel that provides a way of reporting concerns to someone outside the employer organisation provided by the government-funded whistleblowing helpline, which changed to a freephone service in January 2012.

Internal procedures for handling allegations

An organisation should have a fair system for dealing internally with accusations or allegations of concern so that an honest individual does not feel under threat. Employees ought to know what those procedures are. Since raising concerns is not a regular event, an organisation may simply try to deal with each case on its merits when it arises, without any formal procedures or channels of complaint being established. The employee will therefore not know whom to complain to, and will probably go to the most senior manager available – possibly the CEO.

A problem with dealing with raising concern incidents on an ad hoc basis is that the accusations may relate to senior members of staff or the EDs themselves. An employee who believes the CEO or finance director to be guilty of wrong-doing will have no option other than to resign or take the complaint to an external authority. It is, therefore, more appropriate to establish a formal internal channel for dealing with concerns that have been raised. This is the remit of the FTSU raising concerns policy, which should provide:

- documented internal procedures available to all employees who wish to raise a concern;
- the procedures by which an allegation will be investigated;
- a named person to whom employees should report their suspicions or concerns;
- an independent means of investigation;
- a statement that the employer takes malpractice or misconduct seriously, and is committed to a culture of openness in which employees can report legitimate concerns without fear of penalty or punishment;
- examples of the type of misconduct for which employees should use the procedure and set out the level of proof that there should be in an allegation (although positive proof might not be required, there should be good reasons for their concern);
- that false or malicious allegations will result in disciplinary action against the individual making them;

- that no employee will be victimised for raising a genuine concern. Victimisation for raising a qualified disclosure is a disciplinary offence;
- an external raising concern route, as well as an internal reporting procedure;
- that, as far as possible, anyone raising concerns will be informed about the outcome of their allegations and the action that has been taken; and
- that anyone raising concerns will be promised confidentiality, as far as this is possible.

Governance checklist

- Does the audit committee have the requisite skills, financial experience, resources, time commitment and robust independence to undertake its tasks?
- Does the audit committee review all financial statements, the Quality Accounts and any supporting audit assurance prior to their release?
- Does the audit committee control (or, in the case of FTs, support) the process of appointing and assessing the external auditors and is it satisfied as to their independence and effectiveness?
- Has account been taken of the ten-yearly audit tender requirements (five-yearly for FTs) and is the audit committee involved in the tender process?
- Is the external audit plan in place? Does the audit committee review and monitor the auditors' performance against that plan?
- Does the audit committee meet at least annual with the external and internal auditors without management being present?
- Is the internal audit team effectively and adequately resourced?
- Does the audit committee regularly challenge and review the effectiveness of the internal audit function?
- Is the internal audit function used effectively to provide objective assurance to the board on the key risks?
- Is the head of internal audit appointed by and accountable to the audit committee, and do they have unrestricted access to the audit committee and board chair? Is the management team responsive to their findings and recommendations?
- What action has the audit committee taken to review the raising concerns policy and procedures in the last 12 months?

Summary

Audit plays a key role in providing assurance to the board and wider NHS stakeholders. This critical role means that ensuring the independence of those functions is high on the agenda of the board and its audit committee. This, however, is only part of the role of the audit committee, which has a broad and extensive role that is not restricted to considering just the financial aspects of the organisation.

Glossary

Accountability – the requirement for a person in a position of responsibility to justify, explain or account for the exercise of his/her authority and his/her performance or actions. Accountability is to the person or persons from whom the authority is derived.

Accountable officer – the primary authority for providing financial management and accountability for NHS property and services.

Annual governance statement – the AGS is a mandatory disclosure for all central government entities that comply with the FReM. All public bodies (including NHS organisations) must provide assurance that they are appropriately managing and controlling the resources for which they are responsible. The AGS replaces the statement on internal control.

Apply or explain rule – similar to the comply or explain rule. Companies should apply the principles of a code or explain why they have not done so.

Audit committee – committee of the board, consisting entirely of independent non-executive directors, with responsibility (among other things) for monitoring the reliability of the financial statements, the quality of the external audit and the organisation's relationship with its external auditors.

Audit firm rotation – changing the firm of external auditors on a regular basis, say every seven years. Not common in practice.

Audit partner rotation – changing the lead partner (and possibly other partners) involved with an organisation's audit on a regular basis, typically every five or seven years.

Audit report – report for stakeholders produced by the external auditors on completion of the annual audit, and included in the organisation's published annual report and accounts. The report gives the opinion of the auditors on whether the financial statements present a true and fair view of the organisation's financial performance and position.

Balance of power – a situation in which power is shared out more or less evenly between a number of different individuals or groups, so that no single individual or group is in a position to dominate.

Board committee – a committee established by the board of directors, with delegated responsibility for a particular aspect of the board's affairs. For example, audit committee, remuneration/ compensation committee and nominations committee.

Board succession – the replacement of a senior director (typically the chair or CEO) when they retire or resign.

Box-ticking approach – an approach to compliance based on following all the specific rules or provisions in a code, and not considering the principles that should be applied and circumstances where the principles are best applied by not following the detailed provisions.

Bribery Act 2010 – UK Act of Parliament making it a criminal offence to give or receive bribes, to bribe a foreign public official for business benefit or to fail to prevent the payment of bribes by employees or agents.

Business ethics – standards of business behaviour, sometimes set out by companies in a code of corporate ethics.

Business risk – the risk from unexpected events or developments in a business or in the business environment, which are outside the control of management. In the NHS, business risks are to patient safety and financial security.

Business risk management – the management of business risks within a strategy based on risk appetite and risk tolerance. The board is responsible for business risk strategy and management is responsible for implementing the strategy within a business risk management system. The board is also responsible for monitoring the effectiveness of the business risk management system, at least annually according to the UK Corporate Governance Code.

Cadbury Code – a code of corporate governance, published by the Cadbury Committee in the UK in 1992 (and since superseded).

Care Quality Commission (CQC) – the safety and quality regulator for all health services, which is also responsible for the regulation of adult social care services.

Chair – leader of the board of directors. Often referred to as the 'company chair' in companies and 'chair' in public bodies and voluntary organisations.

Chief executive officer – the executive director who is head of the executive management team in an organisation.

Clinical commissioning groups (CCGs) – groups of GPs and other health professionals responsible under the Health and Social Care Act 2012 for commissioning most healthcare.

Combined Code – the UK code on corporate governance for listed companies from 1998 to 2010. It was revised in 2010 and re-named the UK Corporate Governance Code.

Comply or explain rule – requirement (e.g. in the UK, a requirement of the Listing Rules) for a company to comply with a voluntary code of corporate governance (in the UK, the UK Corporate Governance Code) or explain any non-compliance.

Connected person – a person with whom a director has an enduring and direct relationship, such as a family member, including a spouse, civil partner, children and step children (and equivalent relationships arising through civil partnerships) and companies in which the director has an interest of 20% or more.

Control totals – part of financial oversight regime that NHSI put in place for 2016/17 onwards which created annual financial targets that had to be achieved to unlock access to national funding and other financial benefits.

Corporate governance – the system by which a company is directed, so as to achieve its overall objectives. It is concerned with relationships, structures, processes, information flows, controls, decision making and accountability at the highest level in a company.

Council of governors – a council of governors is a several member group that oversees or manages the running of an institution. In the context of an NHS FT it is an elected body of members who hold the board of directors to account.

Davies Review – a government-sponsored report (published February 2011) recommending greater diversity on the boards of companies and in particular a greater proportion of women on the boards of FTSE350 companies.

Directors' report – the 'report' in the annual report and accounts of a company or organisation. A report by the board of directors to the stakeholders, contained in the annual report and accounts and containing a variety of reports and information disclosures, such as the business review and remuneration report.

Downside risk – a risk that actual events will turn out worse than expected. Downside risk can be measure in terms of the amount by which profits could be worse than expected. The expected outcome is the forecast or budget expectation.

Duty of skill and care – a duty owed by a director to the company or organisation. In the UK, this has been a common law duty, but became a statutory duty under the provisions of the Companies Act 2006. A question

GLOSSARY

can be raised, however, about what level of skill and care should be expected from a director.

Elective care – planned specialist medical care.

Emergency preparedness – emergency preparedness is a plan of what to do if a disaster that is unconnected with the organisation's business and outside the control of management occurs.

EU Directive – an instruction, devised by the European Commission and approved by the European Council and European Parliament. The contents of a Directive must be introduced into national law or regulations by all members states of the EU. Some Directives, such as the Shareholder Rights Directive, deal wholly or partly with corporate governance issues.

European Commission – the managing and administrative body of the EU.

Executive director – a director who also has executive responsibilities in the management structure. Usually a full-time employee with a contract of employment.

External audit – statutory annual audit of an organisation by independent external auditors.

Fairness – impartiality, a lack of bias. In a corporate governance context, the quality of fair ness refers to things that are done or decided in a reasonable manner, and with sense of justice, avoiding bias.

Fiduciary duty – a duty of a trustee. The directors of a company or organisation are given their powers in trust, and have fiduciary duties towards the company or organisation.

Financial risk – a risk of a failure or error, deliberate (fraud) or otherwise, in the systems or procedures for recording financial transactions and reporting financial performance and position, or the risk of a failure to safeguard financial assets such as cash and accounts receivable.

Fixed pay – the elements in a remuneration package that are a fixed amount each year, such as basic salary.

Going concern statement – a requirement of some corporate governance codes, such as the UK Corporate Governance Code. A statement by the board of directors that in their view the organisation will remain as a going concern for the next financial year.

Greenbury Report – report in the UK in 1995 by the Greenbury Committee, focusing mainly on corporate governance issues related to directors' remuneration.

Hampel Committee – committee set up in the UK to continue the review of corporate governance practices in the UK, following the Cadbury and Greenbury Committee Reports. The Hampel Committee suggested that the recommendations of all three committees should be integrated into a single code of corporate governance, which was published in 1998 as the Combined Code.

Health service governance – the system, practices and procedures by which power is shared and exercised by the board of directors (and the council of governors in foundation trusts) and how the holders of that power are held accountable for ensuring that the individual parts of the NHS achieve their objectives and are in line with public sector values such as value for money and providing universal and free healthcare benefits to all those in need.

Higgs Report – the 2003 UK Government commissioned review into the role and effective ness of non-executive directors.

Induction – process of introducing a newly appointed director into their role, by providing appropriate information, site visits, meetings with management and (where necessary) training.

Internal audit – investigations and checks carried out by internal auditors of an organisation. Internal audit is a function rather than a specific activity. However, the work programme of the internal audit team might reduce the amount of work the external auditors need to carry out in their annual audit, provided the internal and external auditors collaborate properly.

Internal control – a procedure or arrangement that is implemented to prevent an internal control risk, reduce the potential impact of such a risk, or detect a failure of internal control when it occurs (and initiate remedial action).

Internal control risk – a risk of failure in a system or procedure due to causes that are within the control of management. They can be categorised as financial risks, operational risk and compliance risks.

Internal control system – a system of internal controls within an organisation. The system should have a suitable control environment, and should provide for the identification and assessment of internal control risks, the design and implementation of internal controls, communication and information and monitoring. In the UK, the board of directors of a listed company has responsibility for the system of internal control.

International Corporate Governance Network (ICGN) – a voluntary association of institutional investors that has the objective of raising standards of corporate governance globally, to meet the requirements and expectations of global investors.

King Code – also called the King Report and King IV (because it is the fourth version of the Code/Report, issued in 2016). The corporate governance code for listed companies in South Africa.

Lead governor – the lead governor's role is to facilitate direct communication between Monitor and the NHS foundation trust's board of governors in a limited number of circumstances and in particular where it may not be appropriate to communicate through the normal channels.

Management board – a board of executive managers, chaired by the CEO, within a two-tier board structure. The chair of the management board reports to the chair of the supervisory board. The management board has responsibility for the operational performance of the business.

Modified audit report – audit report in which the auditors express some reservations about the financial statements of the organisation, because of insufficient information to reach an opinion or disagreement with the figures in the statements.

Money laundering – the process of transferring or using money obtained from criminal activity, so as to make it seem to have come from legitimate (non-criminal) sources. Companies are often used as a cover for money laundering.

Mutual society – a mutual, mutual organisation, or mutual society is an organisation (which is often, but not always, a company or business) based on the principle of mutuality. A mutual is therefore owned by, and run for the benefit of, its members – it has no external shareholders to pay in the form of dividends and, as such, does not usually seek to maximise and make large profits or capital gains.

Nomination committee – a committee of the board of directors (or council of governors in foundation trusts), with responsibility for identifying potential new members for the board of directors. Suitable candidates are recommended to the main board (or to the council of governors), which then makes a decision about their appointment.

Non-audit work – work done by a firm of auditors for a client organisation, other than work on the annual audit, such as consultancy services and tax advice. In the context of corporate governance, the independence of the auditors might be questionable when they earn high fees for non-audit work.

Non-executive director (NED) – a director who is not an employee of the company and who does not have any responsibilities for executive management in the company.

OECD Principles of Corporate Governance – general principles of corporate governance issued by the Organisation for European Cooperation and Development, which all countries are encouraged to adopt.

Policy governance theory – policy governance theory is an integrated set of concepts and principles that describes the job of any governing board. It outlines the manner in which boards can be successful in their servant-leadership role, as well as in their all-important relationship with management.

Primary care – the first point of healthcare such as GPs, dentists, pharmacists and optometrists.

Public benefit corporation – a public benefit corporation is usually a corporation created by the government that performs a specific function for the benefit of the public, such as a hospital or public library.

Quality Account – a Quality Account is a report about the quality of services provided by an NHS healthcare service. The report is published annually by each NHS healthcare provider, including the independent sector and made available to the public.

Quality governance – the combination of structures and processes at and below board level to lead on trust-wide quality performance including: ensuring required standards are achieved; investigating and taking action on sub-standard performance; planning and driving continuous improvement; identifying, sharing and ensuring delivery of best-practice; and identifying and managing risks to quality of care.

Remuneration committee – a committee of the board of directors (or council of governors in foundation trusts), with responsibility for deciding remuneration policy for top executives and the individual remuneration packages of certain senior executives, for example, all the executive directors (or non-executive directors in foundation trusts).

Reputation risk – risk to the reputation of a company or other organisation in the mind of the public (including customers and suppliers) when a particular matter becomes public knowledge.

Responsibility – having power and authority over something. A person in a position of responsibility should be held accountable for the exercise of that authority.

Risk appetite – the amount and type of business risk that the board of directors would like their organisation to have exposure to. Identifying risk appetite should be a part of strategic planning.

Risk assessment – an assessment of risks faced by an organisation, Typically risks are assessed according to how probably or how frequent an adverse outcome is likely to be in the planning period and the potential size of the losses if an adverse outcome occurs. The greatest risks are those with a high probability of an adverse outcome combined with the likelihood of a large loss if this were to happen.

Risk capacity – the maximum risk exposures that the organisation can accept without threatening its financial stability.

Risk committee – a committee of the board that an organisation may establish, with the responsibility of monitoring the risk management system within the organisation, instead of the audit committee. A risk committee may be established when the audit committee has too many other responsibilities to handle.

Risk management – a function of the administration of the NHS body directed toward identification, evaluation, and correction of potential risks that could lead to injury to patients, staff members, or visitors and result in loss or damage.

Risk tolerance – the amount of business risk that the board is willing to let their organisation be exposed to. Alternatively, the amount of risk that the organisation is able to accept without serious threat to its stability.

Sarbanes-Oxley Act – legislation, largely on corporate governance issues, introduced in the USA in 2002 following a series of corporate scandals such as Enron and WorldCom.

Secondary care – acute healthcare, either elective or emergency.

Secret profit – a profit that is not revealed. In the context of corporate governance, a director should not make a secret profit for his/her personal benefit and at the expense of the company or organisation.

Senior independent director – a non-executive director who is the nominal head of all the non-executive directors on the board. The SID may act as a channel of communication between the NEDs and the chair, or (in some situations) between major stakeholders and the board.

Severance payment – payment to a director (or other employee) on being required to resign (or otherwise leave the company).

Shareholder value approach – approach to corporate governance based on the view that the objective of its directors should be to maximise benefits for shareholders.

Smith Report – a report concerned with the independence of auditors in the wake of the collapse of Arthur Andersen and the Enron scandal in the US in

2002. It raised the important point that an auditor himself should look at whether a company's corporate governance structure provides safeguards to preserve his own independence.

Stakeholder – a stakeholder group is an identifiable group of individuals or organisations with a vested interest. Stakeholder groups in a company include the shareholders, the directors, senior executive management and other employees, customers, suppliers. In the NHS stakeholders will also include patients, employees, the regulators, the general public and the government.

Statutory duties – duties imposed by statute law.

Strategic risk – the risks of taking decisions on strategy that will result in exposures to excessive business risk and so could lead to losses or even business collapse.

Stress testing – testing the ability of a business to withstand the effects of extreme adverse events or developments in the business environment.

Succession planning – planning for the eventual replacement of a senior member of the board (chair, CEO and possibly finance director) by their successor.

Supervisory board – a board of non-executive directors, found in an organisation with a two-tier board structure. The supervisory board reserves some responsibilities to itself. These include oversight of the management board.

Sustainability – conducting business operations in a way that can be continued into the foreseeable future, without using natural resources at such a rate or creating such environmental damage that the continuation of the business will eventually become impossible.

Transparency – openness. Being clear about historical performance and future intentions, and not trying to hide information.

Turnbull Guidance – initially a report of the Turnbull Committee in the UK, giving listed companies guidance on how the directors should carry out their responsibility for the internal control system, as required by the UK corporate governance code. Now the responsibility of the FRC.

Two-tier board – board structure in which the responsibilities are divided between a supervisory board of non-executive directors led by the chair, and a management board of executives led by the CEO.

UK Corporate Governance Code – the code of corporate governance issued by the FRC in the UK, which is applied to UK listed companies. Formerly (until 2010) called the Combined Code.

GLOSSARY 453

UK Listing Rules – rules that apply to all listed companies in the UK. They include the 'comply or explain' rule on compliance with the UK Corporate Governance Code.

Ultra vires – in corporate law, ultra vires describes acts attempted by a corporation that are beyond the scope of powers granted by the corporation's objects clause, articles of incorporation or in a clause in its bylaws, in the laws authorising a corporation's formation, or similar founding documents.

Unitary board – board structure in which decisions are taken by a single group of executive and non-executive directors, led by the company chair.

Upside risk – a risk that actual events will turn out better than expected and will provide unexpected profits. Some risks, such as the risk of a change in foreign exchange rates, or a change in interest rates, or a change in consumer buying patterns could be 'two-way' with both upside and downside potential.

Variable pay – the elements in a remuneration package that vary each year according to the individual's performance, such as annual bonuses, and the grant of shares or share options.

Voluntary code of governance – a code of governance that is not enforced by law or regulation. However, as in the UK and South Africa, listed companies may be encouraged to adopt a voluntary code by means of a 'comply or explain' or 'apply or explain' regulation.

Walker Report – a report published in the UK in 2009 about corporate governance in banks and other financial services organisations, following the banking crisis of 2007–09.

Whistleblowing – the disclosure by a person, usually an employee in a government agency or private enterprise, to the public or to those in authority, of mismanagement, corruption, illegality, or some other wrongdoing.

Window dressing of accounts – applying accounting policies that are just within the limits of permissible accounting practice, but which have the effect of making the company's performance or financial position seem better than it would if more conservative accounting policies were used. For example, accounting policies might be used that recognise income at an early stage in a transaction process, or defer the recognition of expenses.

Women on Boards Report – a report highlighting the poor representation of women on boards, relative to their male counterparts, and raised questions about whether board recruitment is in practice based on skills, experience and performance. This report presents practical recommendations to address this imbalance.

Wrongful trading – wrongful trading occurs when a company continues to trade when the directors are aware that the company had gone into (or would soon go into) insolvent liquidation.

Index

2018 funding settlement 53–55
Accountability
   governance, and 7–8
Accountable/accounting officer
   role of 228–230
Accountable care organisations 346–347
Accountable Clinical Networks 349
Acute Care Collaborations 348
Agency theory 29–32
   earnings retention 30–31
   key elements 31–32
   level of effort 30
   moral hazard 30
   shareholder value approach 32
   time horizon 31
Alliance Agreement 354
Annual audit cycle
   audit committee, and 437–438
Annual governance statement 413–414
Annual report and accounts – CCGs 408–409
Annual report and accounts – FT 407
Apply or explain 114–116
Assurance 391–418
   meaning 391
Audit 419–443
   auditors' liability to third parties 426
   non-audit work for client by audit firm 428–429
   partner rotation 431
   rotation of firm 429–431
Audit Committee 144, 431–438
   annual audit cycle, and 437–438
   composition 434
   induction of members 434–435
   management reports to 438
   meetings 435
   remuneration of members 434–435
   reporting requirements 432–433
   requirements 431–432
   responsibilities 433–434
   role 433–434
   role in quality, performance and financial reporting 435–436
   training of members 434–435
Audit report 424

Board and culture 179–185
   attributes of healthy culture 179
   Boardroom Behaviours 182
   challenge function 181–187
   constructive challenge 181–187
   monitoring 1801–181
   NHS Leadership Model 184
   questions for consideration 180
   roles for effective healthcare boards 184
   sources of insights 180
Board assurance framework 414–417
Board effectiveness
   chair, role of 187–188
Board-level power, exercise of
   governance, and 11
Board committees 142–149
   protecting independence and effectiveness 148
   performance evaluation 201–206
   recommended standing committees 142
   UK Code's recommendations regarding membership 149
Board evaluation
   well-led, meaning 202–204
Board meetings 188–189
   agenda 188
   information 188–189
Board structures 134–138
   two-tier boards 135–138
   unitary boards 134–135
Board structure and committees 130–150
Boardroom Behaviours 182
   guidance 182–183

Boards 130–150
　appointments in corporate sector 193–194
　　Davies Report 194–195
　　nomination committee 195–197
　appointments to 139–192
　　assurance 190
　　diversity 190
　　fairness 191
　　fit and proper persons 191–192
　　integrity 190
　　merit 190
　　openness 190
　　procedures 190
　　selflessness 190
　balance of power 140
　CCGs 131
　characteristics 130
　composition 140–142
　delegation, approach to 139
　effective 178–207 *see also* Maintaining an effective board
　foundation trusts 131
　governance checklist 149
　grounds for termination of appointment 192–193
　matters reserved for 138–139
　performance evaluation 201–206
　refreshing membership 197–199
　responsibilities according to voluntary codes 132–134
　risk management, and 374–375
　role of 132–134
　size 139–140
　succession planning 197–199
　suspension or removal from office 192–193
　techniques and practices supporting and hindering 183–184
Bribery Act 2010 106–107
　guiding principle 106–107
Buddying 347

Cabinet office
　Consultation Principles 99
Cadbury Code 13–14
Care Act 2014 90–92
　implications 91
　statutory duty of candour 91–92
Care Quality Commission 81–83
Carter Review 55
CCGs 67, 315–343
　accountable officer 333–334
　audit committee 330
　being membership organisation 341
　board 131
　chair of governing body 332–333
　clinical engagement, and 317–318
　codes of governance 319–320
　committees 328–331
　company secretary 334
　complementary duties 92
　conflicts of interest, and 169
　duties 315–316, 331
　financial duty 316
　Good Governance Institute 335–336
　Good Governance Standard 320
　governance challenge 336–341
　governing body 324–327
　　appointments 325–326
　　composition 324–325
　　disqualification 326–327
　　elections 325–326
　　ICSA specimen code of conduct 327
　　tenure 326
　history 316–317
　ICSA Code of Governance 320–321, 322
　internal audit 330–331
　key actions 93
　legal and regulatory framework 318–321
　legal duty to involve 95–101
　maintaining effective governing body 331–336
　managing conflicts of interest 337–340
　Members' Council 323–324
　Members' Forum 323–324
　membership 321–324
　　liability 324
　model core constitution 318–319
　NHS Clinical Commissioners 334–335
　non-executive members and independence 336–337
　pay ranges 236
　powers 331
　procurement 341
　remuneration committee 328–330
　rights 331
　services commissioned 315
　structure 3
CEO 227–230
　chair of the board, and 216–218
　pay ranges for 235
　role of 227–230
Chair of the board 208–223
　annual meeting 222

annual report 221–222
appointment 215
CEO, and 216–218
commitments 212
company secretary, and 218–219
effective, behaviour of 212–215
  be a representative with shareholders, not a player 214
  be the guide on the side 212–213
  don't be the boss 214
  measure the inputs, not the outputs 214
  own the prep work 213
  practice training 213
  remain impartial 213–214
  take committees seriously 213
evaluation 215
independence 211–212
responsibilities 210–211
role 208–210
senior independent director, and 219–221
stakeholder, and 221–222
Charity Governance Code 24–26
Chief finance officer
  role of 230–231
Clinical commissioning groups *see* CCGs
Clinical private practice
  declaration 175
Clinical senates 81
Codes for health service governance 116–126
Combined Code 14–15
Commissioning care 66–71
Commissioning support units (CSUs) 69–70
Committees in common 351
  advisory committee 351
  decision-making committee 351
Companies Act 2006 109
Company secretary 267–287
  additional duties 275
  administrative function 279
  chair of the board, and 218–219
  challenges 268
  compliance 279
  conscience of company 275–276
  conscience of organisation 279
  core duties 281–285
  development in NHS 278–285
  fit for the future 285–286
  governance 279
  governors, and 279
  in-house lawyer, and 277–278

increased profile 267
independence 276–277, 280–281
officer of company, as 269–271
required skills and knowledge 268–269
responsibilities 271–275
  FRC Board Guide 274
  ICSA Guidance 271
  statutory and regulatory compliance 274–275
  UK Code 272–274
Company purpose 130–134
Company regulation
  voluntary best practice, and 112–116
Comply or explain 114–116
Conflicts of interest 168–176
  CCGs 169
  clinical private practice 175
  decision-making staff, and 172
  declaration of interests 172–173
  effectiveness of board, and 189
  financial interests 171
  indirect interests 171
  management of 169
  managing 175–176
  meaning 170–172
  NHS guidance 168
  non-financial personal interests 171
  non-financial professional interests 171
  outside employment 174–175
  ownership interests 175
  shareholdings 175
Constructive challenge 185–187
  effective decision-making, and 185
  extra steps 186
  questions for boards to consider 185–186
  risk factors for poor decision-making 185
Contractual joint ventures 353–354
Corporate companions 4–5
Corporate culture
  long-term business success, and 178
Corporate governance statement 412–413
Corporate joint ventures 349–351
Corporate Manslaughter and Corporate Homicide Act 2007 105
CQC inspections 395–397
  fundamental standards 82–83
    complaints 83
    consent 83
    dignity and respect 82
    display of ratings 83
    duty of candour 83
    fit and proper staff 83

food and drink 83
good governance 83
person-centred care 82
premises and equipment 83
safeguarding from abuse 83
safety 83
staffing 83
principal function 82
Corporate social responsibility 12–13
CSUs
specialist support services 69

Dalton Review 53–55
Darzi Report 402
Davies Report 16, 194–195
Declaration of interests 172–173
Deprivation of Liberties Safeguards (DoLS) 105
DHSC
purpose 62
stewardship role 62–63
Directions to NHS bodies on Counter Fraud Measures 2004 89
Director of Finance
role of 230–231
Directors 151–177
agents, as 151
borrowing powers 163
civil liability to third parties 165
claims by NHS organisation, and 165–166
common law duties 155–157
criminal liability 164–165
duties 151–177
duties to organisations 154–155
duty not to accept benefits from third parties 161–162
duty of skill and care 156–157
duty to act within powers 158
duty to avoid conflicts of interest 160–161
duty to break even 163–164
duty to declare interests in proposed transactions with organisation 162
duty to exercise independent judgment 159
duty to exercise reasonable care, skill and diligence 159
duty to improve quality 164
duty to promote success of organisation 158
fiduciary duty 155–156
indemnity 166
induction 199–200
liabilities 151–177
liability 164–166
NHS
fit and proper persons test 152–154
performance evaluation 201–206
powers 154
professional development 200
related party transactions 162–163
responsibilities to third parties 162
statutory duties 157–162
training 200
UK Disclosure and Transparency Rules 162–163
who can be 151–152
Directors' remuneration report 247–248

Effective decision-making
stakeholder engagement, and 187
Employment Rights Act 1996 101
Enhanced health in care homes 348
Equality Act 2010 105–106
protected characteristics 106
EU company law directives 109
EU Directives 108
Executive directors 224–249
appointment 225–227
appraisal 243
evaluation 243
induction of executive manager as 226–227
lead clinician 231–232
remuneration 232–243
component elements 242
consultants 243–244
corporate sector 232–234
governance issue 238–239
Hutton Review 240–241
NHS 234–235
people 235
performance 235
principles 239–242
public attitudes 237
rewards for failure 237–238
vision 235
role of 224–225
External audit 422–431
appointment of auditors 436–437
function 423
independence 426–427
reliance of work on internal audit 423
removal of auditors 436–437

responsibilities
  auditor independence, and 437
  responsibility for detecting errors and fraud 425–426
  role 422–431
  scope 423

Failure regimes 397–402
  new models of care, and 401–402
Fair consultation process
  overview of what constitutes 98–99
Fairness
  governance, and 6–7
Federations 347–348
Financial reporting 406–412
  responsibilities of directors 409–410
  UK Code 406
Financial special measures 400–401
Five Year Forward View 53–55, 345–346
  closing funding and efficiency gap 55
  delivering 56–57
  key principles 345
  new organisational models 54
  principles for change 53
Formal agreement 355
Foundation groups 348
Foundation trusts 66 *see also* NHS foundation trusts
  board 131
FRC Guidance 18, 127
FRC Guidance on Audit Committees 15–16
Freedom of Information Act 2000 102–104
  exemptions 104
  model publication scheme 103
  public interest test 104
  refusal of requests 103–104
FT Code 121–123
  accountability 123
  effectiveness 123
  leadership 123
  relations with stakeholders 123
  remuneration 123
  G20/OECD Corporate Governance Principles 127–128
  GDPR 2016 108–109
    processing personal data 108–109

Generative governance theory 42–43
  governance as leadership approach 42–43
Glossary 444–454
Going concern statement 410–412

Good Governance Standard for Public Services 22–24
Governance
  accountability 7–8
  balance of power 2–3
  board-level power, exercise of 11
  corporate companion 4–5
  defining 1–2
  fairness 6–7
  good, principles of 6–9
  importance of 5
  key issues 9–13
  management, and 5–6
  membership 2–3
  public sector 19–20
  responsibility, and 8
  risk management 11–12
  stakeholder engagement 12
  stakeholders, interests of 3–4
  transparency, and 8–9
  transparent reporting and auditing 10–11
  UK law, and 18–19
  voluntary sector 19–20
Governance and the law 86–109
Government regimes
  arguments for and against 26–27
Greenbury Report 14
Guidance on Board Effectiveness 15

Health Act 1999 88
Health Act 2009 89–90
Health and safety regulations 107–108
Health and Social Care Act 2001 88
Health and Social Care Act 2008 89
Health and Social Care Act 2012 90
Health and Social Care (Community Health and Standards) Act 2002 88–89
Health and wellbeing boards (HWBs) 74–75
  powers 74
  The Power of Place 75
Health Authorities Act 1995 88
Health Education England (HEE) 80–81
Health Overview and Scrutiny Committee (HOSC) 73–74
Health service governance
  defining 45–46
  importance of 46–49
  poor governance, common themes 49
Health Services Act 1980 87
Healthcare law 87–101
Healthwatch England 76–77

Healthy NHS Board: principles for good governance 120–121
Higgs Report 15
  non-executive directors 259
Hospitality & gifts policy 173
  declaration 174
Human Fertilisation and Embryology Authority 80
Human Rights Act 1998 102
Human Tissue Authority 84
Hutton Review 240–241

ICGN
  Global Corporate Governance Principles 220–221
Improving public health 71–73
In-house lawyer
  company secretary, and 277–278
Insolvency 109–110
Integrated care 346–347
Integrated care partnerships 346
Integrated care systems 346
Integration Agreement 354
Intelligent Board 116–117
Integrated governance
  definition 117–118
  development programme 119
Integrated Governance Handbook 117–119
  key themes 118
  standing committees 118–119
Internal audit 419–422
  function 420–421
  independence of auditors 421–422
  investigation of internal financial controls 421
  objectivity of auditors 421–422
  review of effectiveness of function 422
  role 419–420
  scope 420–421
Internal control risks 372–375
  compliance risks 374
  financial risks 373
  operational risks 373

Judicial review 99–100
  remedies 100

King IV Code 129
  integrated approach 36

Laws on patient and public involvement 92–101

Learning and clinical networks 348
Local authorities 70–71
  duties 70–71
  functions 70–71
  responsibilities 70–71
Local Authority (Public Health, Health and Wellbeing Boards and Health Scrutiny) Regulations 2013 100
Local Government and Public Involvement in Health Act 2007 89
Local Healthwatch 76–77

Maintaining an effective board 178–207
Management
  governance, and 5–6
MCP/PACS Contract 354–355
Medicines and Healthcare Products Regulatory Agency 80
Mental Capacity Act 2005 104–105
Mergers and acquisitions 353
Mid Staffordshire NHS Foundation Trust 47–49
Models of care 347–349
Money-laundering 110
Multi-speciality Community Providers 348

National Health Service Act 1948 87
National Health Service Act 1977 87
National Health Service Act 2006 89
National Health Service and Community Care Act 1990 87
National Health Service Report and Health Care Professions Act 2002 88
National Institute for Health and Care Excellence (NICE) 79–80
New models of care 344–364
  accountability 357
  audit and assurance 358
  balancing tension between making decisions quickly, openly and transparently 358
  clinical voice 358
  complexity 358–359
  governance implications 356
  independent scrutiny 358
  legal structures 344
  legislative change 359
  local government 357
  patient and public engagement 357
  practical change 360–361
  regulation 355–356

regulatory change 359–360
scale 358–359
tackling governance challenges 361–362
guiding principles 61
how the money flows 72
providing care *see* Providing care
Statement of Accountability 61–64
structure 60–85
NHS board composition 141–142
NHS Blood and Transplant Authority 79
NHS Code of Conduct and Accountability 167–168
NHS Constitution 49–53
 key responsibilities 51–52
 principles of the NHS 51
 rights, responsibilities and pledges 51–52
 staff rights, pledges and expectations 52–53
 values 50–51
NHS England 67–69
 board 68
 complementary duties 92
 key actions 93–95
 key responsibilities 67–68
 legal duty to involve 95–101
 operational independence 68
 regional teams 68
 special measures 397–398
 ten principles of participation 96–97
 vision for the future 68
NHS foundation trusts 288–314
 accountabilities 290
 appointed governors 297
 appointment of auditors 299
 approval of appointment of CEO 300
 balancing tension in board's general duty 311
 board committees 308
 board composition 306–308
 board structure 305–309
 capacity and capability of governors 312–313
 chair 296
 chair of board 309–310
 codes of conduct for governors 305
 committees 295–300, 305–309
 company secretary 310–311
 council 309–310
 council of governors 295–300
  duties 300–305
  initiatives 300
  powers 300–305
  rights 300–305
 elections 294–295
 FT Code 292–293
 governance arrangements 307
 governance challenge 311–313
 history 289
 lead governor 296–297
 legal and regulatory framework 290–293
 local accountability 289–290
 maintaining effective board 309–311
 membership 293–295
 model core constitution 291–292
 nomination committee 297–298
 planning guidance 288
 provider licence 290–291
 public governors 297
 remuneration committee 298–299
 reporting requirements 290–291
 significant transactions 302–305
 staff governors 297
 statutory duties of director 308–309
 training and support for governors 313
 who owns 312
NHS funding 2019/20 to 2023/24 57
NHS Improvement 78
 special measures 398
NHSI's Improvement and Assessment Framework 394–395
NHSI's Single Oversight Framework 392–394
NHS Long Term Plan 57–58
NHS Reorganisation Act 1973 87
NHS Resolution 78–79
NHS structure 65
 education and training 80–81
 empowering people and local communities 73–77
 national bodies 79–80
 supporting health and care system 77–80
NHS trust boards
 functions 132
NHS trusts 66
NHS Trusts (Membership and Procedures) Regulations 1990 88
Nolan's Principles of Public Life 20–21
Nomination committee 145, 195–197
 criteria for appointment to board 197
 main duties 196–197
 recommendations 196
Non-executive directors (NEDs) 250–266
 accepting offer of appointment 252–253
 appointment 251–255

barriers to effectiveness 261–263
  delays in decision-making 262
  inherent tension 263
  insufficient knowledge 261
  insufficient time 262
  overriding influence of executive directors 262
effectiveness 259–261
evaluation 251–255
FRC Board Guide 260
Higgs Report 259
independence 256–258
  criteria for judging 257–258
  serving directors 258
induction 251–255
key elements of role 263
key board level competencies 255
key questions 255
key questions for evaluation 255
remuneration 263–265
resignation 265
role 250–251
terms of engagement 253–254
time commitment 251–252
UK Code 260
Walker Review 260–261
NYSE 19

OECD 19, 34
Overview and scrutiny committees (OSCs) 73–74

Parliamentary and Health Service Ombudsman (PHSO) 75–76
Performance evaluation 201–206
  annual, requirement for 201–202
  using results 205
Primary and Acute Care Systems 348
Principles of the NHS 51
Primary care 64
Providing care 64–66
  primary care 64
  secondary care 64–66
Professional regulators 84
Protected disclosure 101
Public Health England (PHE) 71–73
Public Interest Disclosure Act 1998 102
Public participation
  commissioning cycle, and 94

Quality accounts 404–405
Quality governance 402–406

5YFV framework 403
Darzi Report 402
special measures 398–400
Quality report 405–406

Raising concerns procedure 439–442
  best practice 440–441
  health service governance, and 439–440
  internal procedures 441–442
Regulatory reporting 392–397
  information requirements for monitoring 393
  new models of care 395
Remuneration committee 146–148, 242–243
  annual report, and 147
  composition 146
  practice 244
  principal duties 147–148
  process 244
  requirement for 243
  review by 146–147
  severance payments 244–247
Responsibility
  governance, and 8
Risk appetite 369–370
Risk committees 375–376
Risk management 365–390
  board 374–375
  business continuity 383–385
  business continuity incident 385
  critical incident 385
  emergency preparedness 383–385
  FRC Guidance 365–366, 367–368
  governance, and 11–12
  high reliability organisations 386–388
  internal control systems and procedures 379–383
    compliance controls 383
    operational controls 382–383
    segregation of duties 381
    SPAMSOAP 381–382
  major incident 385–386
  regulatory framework 366–368
  reviewing effectiveness 383
  risk assessment process 377–379
  risk, nature of 368–369
  risk, relevance of 370
  systems and procedures 376–379
  Turnbull Guidance 366–367

types of risks 371–374 *see also* Risks, types of
UK Code 368
Risk registers 376–377
Risk tolerance 369–370
Risks, types of 371–374
  behavioural risk 371
  categories of business risk 371–372
  external risk 372
  financial risk 371
  internal control risks 372–375
  operational risk 371
  reputational risk 371
  third-party or competition risk 371

Safeguarding patients' interests 81–84
Secretary of State for Health and Social Care 62
Section 75 agreements 355
Senior independent director (SID) 219–221
  chair of the board, and 219–221
  intervention by 220
  role of 219–220
Severance payments 244–247
  NHSI guidance 245
  proposal for 246
Six principles for engaging people and communities 97–98
Smith Report 15–16
South Africa
  King Committee 19
SPAMSOAP 381–382
Special health authorities 77–79
Special measures 397–402
  financial 400–401
  NHSE 397–398
  NHSI 398
  quality of care 398–400
Speciality franchises 349
Staff rights, pledges and expectations 52–53
Stakeholder engagement
  effective decision-making, and 187
  governance, and 12
Stakeholder theory 33–36
  enlightened shareholder approach 35–36
  focus of 33
  King Code: integrated approach 36
  OECD Principles of Corporate Governance 34
  pluralist approach 34–35
  stakeholder approach 34–35

Stakeholders
  chair of the board, and 221–222
  interests of 3–4
Standards for NHS board members 22
Statement of Accountability 61–64
Stewardship theory 37–39
  policy governance approach 37–39
Stress testing 377
Structure of the NHS 60–85

Taking it on trust 119–120
  recommendations 120
The Power of Place 75
Transaction cost theory 39–42
  bounded rationality 40–41
  opportunities 41–42
Transparency
  governance, and 8–9
Transparent reporting and auditing
  governance, and 10–11
Turnbull Guidance 15, 366–367
Two-tier boards 135–138
  criticisms 137–138
  main concerns 137
  management board 136
  supervisory board 136

UK Corporate Governance Code 17–18, 126–127
  areas of guidance 128
UK Stewardship Code 16–17
Unitary boards 134–135
  dangers of not using 134
  key strength 135
  purpose 134
Urgent and Emergency Care Networks 348

Values of the NHS 50–51
Voluntary best practice
  compulsory registration, and 112–116
Voluntary codes of best practice 112–129
Voluntary governance frameworks 113
  'apply or explain' 114–116
  'comply or explain' 114–116

Walker Report 16
Well-Led Framework 123–126
  developmental reviews 124
  external facilitator 125
  eight KLOEs 124
Whistleblowing 101
Wrongful trading 157

www.ingramcontent.com/pod-product-compliance
Ingram Content Group UK Ltd.
Pitfield, Milton Keynes, MK11 3LW, UK
UKHW020857160426
5217IPUK00036B/1630